2009

Accreditation Process Guide for Long Term Care

Includes the Compliance Assessment Checklist!

The Joint Commission

Joint Commission Resources

http://www.jcrinc.com

Joint Commission Resources Mission

The mission of Joint Commission Resources is to continuously improve the safety and quality of care in the United States and in the international community through the provision of education and consultation services and international accreditation.

Joint Commission Mission

The mission of the Joint Commission on Accreditation of Healthcare Organizations is to continuously improve the safety and quality of care provided to the public through the provision of health care accreditation and related services that support performance improvement in health care organizations.

Joint Commission Resources educational programs and publications support, but are separate from, the accreditation activities of the Joint Commission. Attendees at Joint Commission Resources educational programs and purchasers of Joint Commission Resources publications receive no special consideration or treatment in, or confidential information about, the accreditation process.

Joint Commission Resources, Inc. (JCR), a not-for-profit affiliate of the Joint Commission on Accreditation of Healthcare Organizations (Joint Commission), has been designated by the Joint Commission to publish publications and multimedia products. JCR reproduces and distributes these materials under license from the Joint Commission.

Printed in the U.S.A. 5 4 3 2 1

ISBN-10: 1-59940-268-0
ISSN: 1546-1106

For more information about Joint Commission Resources, please visit http://www.jcrinc.com. For more information about the Joint Commission on Accreditation of Healthcare Organizations, please visit http://www.jointcommission.org.

Contents

☑ Introduction

Welcome to The Joint Commission accreditation process. Our accreditation model is data driven and emphasizes continuous improvement and ongoing standards compliance. You will notice this emphasis on continuous compliance and improvement throughout the descriptions of activities and processes in this book. By focusing on continuous compliance, you can use the accreditation process as a systems improvement management tool, wherein accreditation becomes a byproduct of quality improvement.

If you are seeking accreditation for the first time, you may be unfamiliar with some of the highlights of the new process, which include the following:

- Annual submission of an assessment of standards compliance—Periodic Performance Review* (PPR)—to promote ongoing standards compliance
- A Priority Focus Process (PFP) that integrates organization-specific data to help surveyors focus on areas relevant to your organization's unique characteristics
- An *unannounced*† on-site survey process that evaluates organization performance in terms of both standards compliance and the resident's experience of care
- A strong educational role for surveyors
- Revised accreditation reports

The on-site survey is only one element of the accreditation process, and it is important to understand all the elements and how they fit together cohesively. *The Accreditation Process Guide for Long Term Care* helps you do that.

Part 1

Part 1 of this book focuses on the PPR component of The Joint Commission's accreditation process. The following elements are included in Part 1:

- Explanation of the PPR process, including full PPR, Option 1, Option 2, and Option 3
- Time lines noting significant events for full PPR, Option 1, Option 2, and Option 3
- Tips on writing Plans of Action and Measures of Success (MOS), including structure, phrasing, and examples
- Explanation of how to conduct the PPR using the electronic PPR tool, including how to use time effectively and which staff members to involve
- Strategies on how to assess compliance across multiple sites and services in an organization, how to involve staff members from those sites, and how to note observations in the electronic PPR tool and in this book
- Explanation of how to determine compliance with a standard (scoring information)

Part 2

Part 2 of this book will help organizations assess their compliance with the 2009 accreditation standards and elements of performance (EPs). It contains questions that address the standards and EPs from the *Comprehensive Accreditation Manual for Long Term Care* (*CAMLTC*). This means that questions have been updated to reflect the new Leadership, Life Safety, National Patient Safety Goals, and Accreditation Participation Requirements chapters, as well as the new six-digit standard numbering for these chapters. All checklist questions also include the new scoring information. An update to the 2008 edition, this easy-to-use workbook format lets you note actions needed, identify who is responsible for implementing improvements, and track progress toward compliance. The checklist also identifies EPs in which MOS are needed. Part 2 of this book can be used as a planning tool for the PPR process in the following ways:

- For full PPR: Organizations can use Part 2 to guide their self-assessment so they are ready to effectively complete the PPR extranet tool in the allotted three-month time frame.
- For Option 1: Because organizations will not be able to use the assessment portion of the PPR extranet tool, they can use Part 2 to document their actual PPR, noting where Plans of Action and MOS must be written so they can attest to the completion of a PPR and have their MOS ready for the surveyor at the time of their on-site survey.
- For Options 2 and 3: Organizations can use Part 2 as a self-assessment to identify standards compliance before the on-site survey.

Organizations can use Part 2 to promote continuous compliance and improved safety and quality of care while continually assessing themselves against the standards and

*Annual submission of the PPR is not applicable to the Medicare/Medicaid certification–based long term care accreditation option.

† For more information about the exceptions to unannounced surveys, *see* page 290.

EPs. This book will help organizations be ready to efficiently and effectively complete an annual PPR.

Part 3

Part 3 leads you through the steps in the unannounced, on-site survey portion of the accreditation process—from your application for accreditation to your on-site survey to post-survey reports and your accreditation decision. This edition of the *Accreditation Process Guide* also provides extensive information on the postsurvey process should your organization meet a decision rule for Conditional Accreditation or Preliminary Denial of Accreditation. Part 3 tells you what to expect during each phase of the accreditation process and includes descriptions of the activities that will take place during your unannounced, on-site survey. The goal of this section is to demystify the survey portion of accreditation and give you the information you need to make your transition (or introduction) to unannounced surveys and the tracer methodology as easy as possible.

In addition, Part 3 includes program-specific examples of tracers and a tracer narrative from the surveyor's perspective with pullout questions to show you how the tracer was conducted. You also will find example questions that can be asked during a tracer and which should be used as an educational tool to help you become more familiar with tracer methodology.

Whether your organization is already accredited or is seeking accreditation for the first time, the book's easy-to-use format helps you find what you are looking for at each stage of the process. For each on-site activity, you will find a brief explanation of its purpose, a list of staff members who will need to be available, an estimated time for completion of the activity, and a summary of what will actually occur. There is no formal document review session, but you may be asked for required policies and procedures at any time. For those activities that do include some document review, a list of what you need to have on hand is provided.

Finally, Part 3 contains sample agendas that will give you an idea of how the most common types of long term care surveys may be organized. Please remember that your survey agenda will depend on the size of your organization.

Appendices

For your convenience, Appendix 1 lists all the EPs that have MOS attached to them. To help organizations logistically prepare for the unannounced survey, worksheets pertaining to several different survey activities (such as the Opening Conference and Orientation to the Organization, the competency assessment process, and the individual-based system tracers) have been provided in Appendix 2: "Worksheets to Facilitate Survey Logistics Planning."

All elements of the accreditation process are under ongoing review by The Joint Commission, and improvements will be made as new information becomes available. Be sure to monitor *The Joint Commission Perspectives®* for changes and revisions.

Important Phone Numbers

If you have questions at any stage of the accreditation process described in this guide, the list below provides phone numbers for Joint Commission departments and the topics for which they can provide information and clarification.

Main Joint Commission Number	630/792-5000
Business Development	630/792-5286
Customer Service ■ General information ■ Ernest A. Codman Award program/applications ■ Current accreditation decision for organizations ■ Help with *The Joint Commission Connect™* extranet or the Joint Commission Web site (http://www.jointcommission.org)	630/792-5800
Department of Communications ■ Publicizing accreditation	630/792-5633
Disease-Specific Care Certification Program	630/792-5291
Division of Standards and Survey Methods ■ Field review for new standards	630/792-5912

Federal Relations (Washington, DC, office) ■ Business associate agreement ■ Regulations/legislation	202/783-6655
Accreditation Operations ■ Applications for accreditation, scheduling, agendas, and process; accreditation report content/status ■ Presurvey materials	630/792-3007 630/792-5798
Management Support Unit ■ Priority Focus Process (PFP) inquiries ■ Orders for certificates	630/792-5649
Media Relations	630/792-5175
Office of Quality Monitoring (complaint hotline)	800/994-6610
ORYX® initiative ■ Requirements ■ Performance measurement systems ■ Data submission	630/792-5085
Pricing Unit ■ Survey fees ■ Invoices and billing information	630/792-5115
Sentinel Event Hotline ■ Self-reporting ■ Sentinel event policy	630/792-3700
Speakers' Bureau	630/792-5633
Standards Interpretation Group ■ Standards and elements of performance compliance ■ Credentialing ■ Periodic Performance Review (PPR) ■ Electronic Statement of Conditions™ (e-SOC)	630/792-5900
State Relations ■ Regulations/legislation	630/792-5261
Other Joint Commission accreditation programs ■ Ambulatory care ■ Behavioral health care ■ Critical access hospitals ■ Hospitals ■ Home care ■ Laboratories ■ Office-based surgery	630/792-3007 Corporate customers: Call your account representative directly. If you do not know who your account representative is, call 630/792-5778.

Part 1
Guide to the Periodic Performance Review

- ☑ **Overview of the PPR**
  - APR.03.01.01
  - Full PPR
  - Option 1
  - Options 2 or 3
- ☑ **Planning for the PPR**
- ☑ **Conducting the PPR**
- ☑ **Developing Plans of Action**
- ☑ **Submitting the PPR and Following Up**

☑ Overview of the PPR

Within The Joint Commission's accreditation process, The Joint Commission assesses an organization's continuous compliance with all applicable standards using elements of performance (EPs), Accreditation Participation Requirements (APRs), and National Patient Safety Goals. The Joint Commission's focus on continuous compliance represents a paradigm shift from the previous accreditation process in which most organizations "ramped up" operations a few months before their survey.

Not only was the ramping up process expensive, it also put resident safety and quality of care in jeopardy. Organizations that focused on the standards only around the time of survey could miss issues that arose at other times. By encouraging organizations to maintain continuous compliance, The Joint Commission hopes to help reduce costs associated with the ramp up for survey and, more importantly, help organizations improve resident safety and quality.

The Periodic Performance Review (PPR) is designed to promote continuous standards compliance. This tool, available to organizations seeking accreditation for the first time after they submit their e-App and deposit, allows the organization to assess its compliance with standards and APRs. The PPR process encourages the organization to carefully review the standards, assess its compliance, develop Plans of Action, and put them into motion. By participating in thorough reviews of standards and systems throughout their accreditation cycle, organizations are more likely to incorporate the standards into routine operations, which ultimately can improve the safety and quality of care.

If you choose the Medicare/Medicaid certification–based accreditation option, conducting or submitting the PPR is not required. However, this publication allows organizations to conduct a self-directed assessment of standards compliance that will prove to be beneficial in identifying areas for ongoing improvement. The standards that apply to organizations seeking The Joint Commission's Medicare/Medicaid certification–based long term care accreditation are identified with a "☆," in the checklist section of this book (Part 2).

The PPR process is not designed to add more work to your organization's already full schedule. In fact, most organizations currently have some internal process in place to assess and attest to their compliance with Joint Commission standards. The PPR just formalizes the assessment process and encourages continuous systems improvement. Numerous accredited organizations have recognized the value of performing on-site evaluations to help close the gap between potential and actual organization performance, thus expanded survey options (under PPR Options 2 and 3) are now available.

APR.03.01.01

In the *Comprehensive Accreditation Manual for Long Term Care (CAMLTC)*, APR.03.01.01 requires organizations accredited under the traditional long term care accreditation route to complete a PPR* and develop appropriate Plans of Action and necessary Measures of Success (MOS) for any standards out of compliance. According to this APR, completing the PPR is required annually during an organization's accreditation cycle. Note that the due date of your PPR submission is subject to change based on the anniversary date of your last full survey.†

Within this APR, The Joint Commission's Accreditation Committee included language clarifying the attestation requirement that organizations choosing PPR Options 1, 2, or 3 must attest that, after careful consideration with legal counsel,‡ they have decided not to participate in the full PPR. It is up to each organization to determine the appropriate PPR option for the organization and determine the level of involvement that is appropriate for staff. *See* APR.03.01.01 in Sidebar 1 on page 4.

* The PPR is not required for submission for the Medicare/Medicaid certification–based long term care accreditation option.

† In certain circumstances, your organization may not have to submit a PPR in 2009. For example, if your organization's PPR due date is May 15, 2009 but your full survey takes place April 13–14, 2009; the survey event would cause the PPR schedule to reset, and the next PPR would be due on April 14, 2010.

‡ When an organization selects a full-length PPR Option 2 or 3 survey, it may independently select one of these options without advice of legal counsel.

Sidebar 1. APR.03.01.01*

The organization fulfills requirements for Periodic Performance Review.

Rationale for APR.03.01.01
The Periodic Performance Review (PPR) helps organizations incorporate The Joint Commission standards into routine daily operations. When organizations use the PPR tool to self-assess, monitor and improve services, their residents are more likely to receive safe, high-quality care on a constant basis.

Elements of Performance for APR.03.01.01

1. The organization annually updates and transmits to The Joint Commission the full Periodic Performance Review (PPR) and its Plan of Action on any recommendations cited. (Refer also to "PPR Options" in "The Accreditation Process" (ACC) chapter of your accreditation manual.)

   Note: *For organizations that select Options 1, 2, or 3, the requirement to transmit the PPR and its Plan of Action to The Joint Commission may not apply in part or in whole.*

3. The organization exercising Option 1, 2, or 3 for the Periodic Performance Review (PPR) annually attests that, after careful consideration with legal counsel, the organization has decided not to participate in the full PPR and instead intends to undergo a limited survey.

4. The organization exercising Option 1 for the Periodic Performance Review (PPR) completes a PPR and Plan of Action.

   Note: *The organization does not submit this information to The Joint Commission.*

6. The organization exercising Option 2 for the Periodic Performance Review agrees to undergo a limited survey and submits a Plan of Action for recommendations cited as a result of the survey.

7. The organization exercising Option 3 for the Periodic Performance Review agrees to undergo a limited survey.

   Note: *The organization does not receive a written report after the survey.*

* Note, the PPR is not required for long term care organizations seeking accreditation by the Medicare/Medicaid certification-based long term care accreditation option. Please check future issues of *The Joint Commission Perspectives®* for additional revisions beyond this book's publication.

PPR Options

Organizations can fulfill the PPR requirement* in the following ways with new options for either a limited PPR survey or a full-length PPR survey under PPR Options 2 and 3:

- The full PPR, in which organizations assess themselves against the standards and EPs applicable to them and submit their assessment electronically to The Joint Commission using the PPR extranet tool. Because The Joint Commission may request a conference call even if an organization does not request one, organizations need to specify their conference call "avoid dates."
- Option 1, in which organizations assess themselves against the standards and EPs applicable to them and attest to their assessment without submitting their data to The Joint Commission
- Option 2, in which organizations can request and undergo either a limited on-site visit from The Joint Commission or a full-length announced or unannounced PPR survey and then participate in an optional follow-up call with Joint Commission staff. If your organization chooses this option, you must submit a Plan of Action with applicable MOS for not compliant standards identified at the on-site visit. When an organization selects a full-length PPR Option 2 survey, it may

* The PPR is not required prior to an initial survey. However, the following information will help those organizations undergoing an initial survey (under the Early Survey Policy) understand what will be expected of them after the initial survey. In addition, those organizations undergoing an initial survey will have access to the PPR and can use the PPR to help prepare for the initial survey. Note, the PPR is not required for long term care organizations seeking accreditation by the Medicare/Medicaid certification–based long term care accreditation option.

independently select this option without advice of legal counsel. Organizations that choose an Option 2 survey will be charged a fee. All PPR surveys incur a fee.

- Option 3, in which organizations can request and undergo either a limited on-site visit from The Joint Commission or a full-length announced or unannounced PPR survey and then participate in an optional follow-up call with Joint Commission staff. All findings from the on-site visit are communicated verbally and no written report is provided to the organization or transmitted to The Joint Commission. When an organization selects a full-length PPR Option 3 survey, it may independently select this option without advice of legal counsel. Organizations that choose an Option 3 survey will be charged a fee.

The PPR was created to help organizations shift from a mentality of survey preparation to one of continuous improvement. The Joint Commission hopes to transfer the focus from getting a "score" on an "exam" to using standards to achieve and maintain excellent performance. Regardless of the method you choose to fulfill the PPR requirement, it is a good idea to implement a self-assessment component to your process in which your organization systematically reviews each EP for each standard, APR, and National Patient Safety Goal. This review can help identify and correct problems well in advance of the survey.

Some standards and EPs do not apply to a particular type of organization. In this book, standards and EPs that do not apply to long term care organizations are simply skipped. Your organization is not expected to comply with these standards and EPs. In addition, some standards and EPs that do apply to long term care organizations may not apply to the specific care, treatment, and services that your individual organization provides. Although these standards and EPs are included in the *CAMLTC* and in this book, you are not expected to comply with them. If you are unsure about the standards or EPs that apply to your organization, please contact The Joint Commission's Standards Interpretation Group (SIG) at 630/792-5900.

Annual Periodic Performance Review Due Dates

For complex organizations, the PPR tool contains all accreditation programs applicable to the organization that are required for PPR submission. The PPR tool is due for submission annually at the time of the primary program's due date. The selection of which PPR option the organization elects to submit applies to all programs included in the tool; different PPR options may not be selected for different programs.

Annual PPR due dates are derived from the end date of the last full survey for the organization's primary program. If an organization's unannounced full survey* (primary program) precedes the annual PPR due date, then the PPR due date will automatically be reset to one year from the end date of the primary program's new cycle survey. If the "Begin Submission" link had been visible in the left navigation bar of the PPR tool prior to the full survey event, the link will be removed when the PPR due date is reset (this will occur automatically on the second day of the full survey). The organization will continue to have access to its open PPR tool.

Contracted Services

Although an organization's accredited services are typically provided directly by the organization, certain services can be provided on behalf of the organization, through contractual or other arrangements (for example, laboratory and diagnostic services, home care services, dialysis services, or other services). The contracted services can be provided on site at the contracting organization or at an off-site location. The contracted organization is responsible for meeting Joint Commission Standard **LD.04.03.09**, which requires that care, treatment, and services provided through contractual agreement are provided safely and efficiently.

Organizations accredited for services that are provided under contractual or other arrangement must include those services in their assessment of compliance when submitting their PPR. Organizations must assess and score each standard and EP that is applicable to the contractual services and enter a score and any findings, Plans of Action, and required MOS for all EPs of a standard determined to be not compliant. It is not acceptable for the organization to score the EP and standards as not applicable for those contracted services, even when the service is provided by a Joint Commission–accredited organization. Organizations that use contracted services are responsible for ensuring that these services meet the requirements of Joint Commission accreditation and thus must submit a PPR that evaluates the services provided to residents by contractors.

Full PPR

The PPR consists of much more than just a self-assessment. Within the full PPR, your organization must perform the following actions:

- Assess its own compliance with all applicable standards, APRs, and the National Patient Safety Goals using the automated PPR tool
- Create Plans of Action to bring not compliant standards into compliance

* For more information about the exceptions to unannounced surveys, *see* page 290.

Sidebar 2. Continuous Periodic Performance Review Access

Your organization has continuous access to the PPR tool via *The Joint Commission Connect*™ extranet site, a secure section of The Joint Commission's Web site. This continuous access can help your organization gain familiarity with the tool and begin work on assessing compliance with all relevant standards and APRs earlier in the process. Although your organization cannot actually submit the PPR to The Joint Commission until provided with access to a "Submit" button at the 90-day point before your organization's due date, you can use the PPR for standards compliance assessment at any time.

The tool houses a list of all standards and EPs with which organizations must comply. This list is the same one used by surveyors in the on-site survey. The Joint Commission has designed the tool to be Windows® based and user friendly. It offers point-and-click data entry and a user manual to provide easy instruction. The extranet site that hosts the tool is password protected to maintain confidentiality. The PPR on the extranet is never accessible to The Joint Commission, so if you use the tool to assess standards compliance, The Joint Commission cannot see the content.

Note: *Organizations undergoing initial accreditation will get access to the PPR tool after The Joint Commission receives the e-App and deposit and after the account representative reviews the e-App.*

- Identify ways to measure the success of those plans
- Implement the plans to bring all standards and APRs into compliance
- Demonstrate a track record for all MOS from the date of the approved Plan-of-Action start date to the time of survey
- Demonstrate that physicians were appropriately involved in the completion of the PPR and in development of Plans of Action
- Engage in a phone call with Joint Commission staff to review and receive approval for Plans of Action and applicable MOS. (**Note:** *This step is optional.*) If a conference call is not requested, the data will be reviewed by Joint Commission staff members. However, should they determine a conference call is needed, your organization will be contacted to schedule the call. Therefore, it is important that your organization identify conference call avoid dates in the PPR tool.

The Joint Commission sends your organization an e-mail to the extranet site indicating the due date of the PPR three months before the due date. Three months before the PPR due date, your organization can begin the formal PPR submission process, although you have the ability to access the tool continuously through your extranet (*see* a description of this access in Sidebar 2, above, and Figure 1 on page 7). Your organization has three months to submit the PPR, including assessing all applicable standards and developing any necessary Plans of Action.

For each standard found not compliant in the full PPR, your organization must develop and submit a Plan of Action that addresses each EP found not compliant or partially compliant. Each Plan of Action should succinctly describe why an EP was found not or partially compliant, how your organization plans to address the issue(s) identified, and in what time frame you will achieve compliance. Some EPs require specific MOS that outline how your organization will measure any improvements implemented through the Plans of Action. For more information on how to create and submit Plans of Action, *see* pages 24–25.

After the self-assessment data and Plans of Action are submitted, a representative from The Joint Commission reviews your PPR to ensure that it is complete and comprehensive. Within approximately one month, your organization could participate in a scheduled phone conference with Joint Commission's SIG. This call is optional, however, and may take place if any standards are out of compliance or another problem is identified. The SIG staff member reviews the assessment with you and offers comments and suggestions on any Plans of Action. He or she indicates whether the Plans of Action, MOS, and time frames are acceptable. More information on the conference call with SIG appears on page 27.

During your organization's on-site survey, surveyors will review any MOS for not compliant standards identified through the PPR. At the time of survey, your organization must illustrate a track record of compliance with all stan-

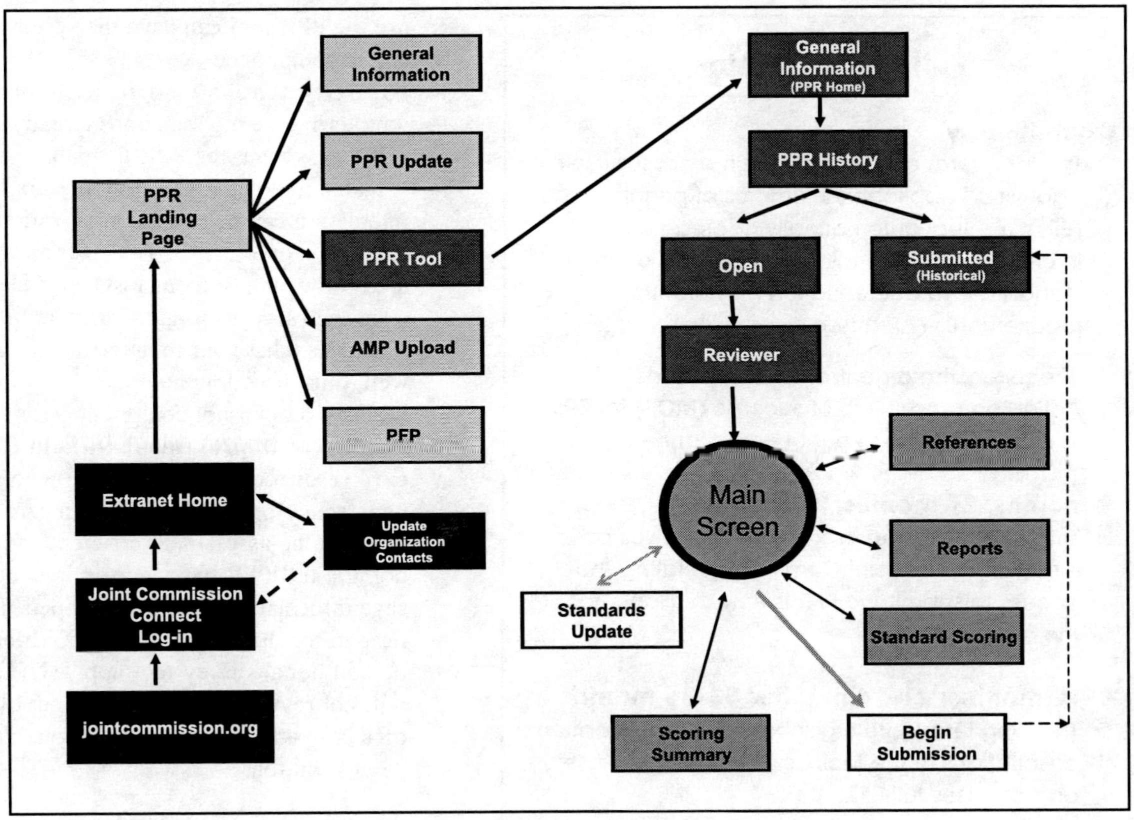

Figure 1. *Screen flow overview of the Periodic Performance Review tool.*

dards from your approved Plan of Action compliant by date. Standards found not compliant at the time of survey are scored appropriately.

The full PPR is one component of the entire accreditation process. It is an annual step in the accreditation cycle. Figure 2 on page 8 illustrates the important deadlines associated with the different components of the full PPR as well as where the process fits into the accreditation cycle.

The Benefits of the Full PPR

The PPR process is designed to enhance the relevance of standards and the accreditation process, to encourage continuous compliance with the standards, and to reduce health care organization costs. These benefits are realized when a long term care organization takes the time to conduct a thorough, well-thought-out review. Performing the full PPR provides the following benefits:

- **Maximized educational benefit for staff and leaders.** Data continue to show that the majority of health care organizations chooses to complete the full PPR. If your long term care organization submits your plan for Joint Commission review, the staff can tap into The Joint Commission's resources to create the most achievable and efficient Plans of Action. In addition, the full PPR process helps individuals identify strengths and weaknesses in their performance and encourages participation and ownership in the process. The full PPR process provides valuable insight into the link between Joint Commission standards and daily operations. One organization staff person who went through the full PPR said, "The participants certainly became more invested in both the quality improvement process and the outcome as compared with having an outside surveyor coming in to conduct the evaluation. There's a big difference between watching somebody else do this and having the responsibility for doing it yourself and learning it well enough to be able to actually complete the task."*
- **Time efficiency.** By obtaining Joint Commission feedback, your long term care organization does not waste time implementing inappropriate Plans of Action. Staff time is well spent, and the standards are met. This efficiency can help control or lower health care organization costs.

* **Source:** Carol Wilinski, M.P.A., senior director of Education and Performance Improvement for the Palliative Care Center and Organization of the North Shore, Evanston, IL.

Full PPR Time Line

Continuously

- ❑ The long term care organization assesses itself against all applicable elements of performance (EPs). The tool automatically aggregates information to determine compliance at the standard and accreditation participation requirements (APR) levels.
- ❑ If required, the organization writes Plans of Action and measures of success (MOS) for EPs in standards scored out of compliance.

9 months; 21 months; 33 months

- ❑ The long term care organization receives an e-mail from The Joint Commission stating that access to submit the PPR is now available to the organization.

9–12 months; 21–24 months; 33–36 months

- ❑ The long term care organization explores option descriptions in the tool, as well as the tool itself, and chooses full PPR.

12 months; 24 months; 36 months

- ❑ The long term care organization submits all data to The Joint Commission through the extranet PPR tool.

13 months; 25 months; 37 months

- ❑ If the long term care organization submitted Plans of Action and MOS, the organization may participate in a scheduled conference call with The Joint Commission to discuss and approve Plans of Action and MOS. (This step may also occur if The Joint Commission's Standards Interpretation Group [SIG] determines it necessary.)

36 months

- ❑ During the full, on-site survey, the surveyor(s) reviews the MOS to ensure that the Plans of Action were implemented and that performance has been sustained.

Figure 2. *Full PPR time line.*

- **Technological efficiency.** By using the PPR tool to its full extent, the long term care organization can capitalize on the electronic format and efficiencies of the extranet. For example, rather than determine compliance manually, long term care organizations that fully use the PPR tool can have the system automatically calculate compliance.
- **Focused attention on priority issues.** Although most long term care organizations already have some form of self-assessment, the PPR formalizes the task and adds a valuable interactive discussion with SIG staff. This interaction can help your organization focus efforts more effectively. If the PPR is thorough, it identifies areas on which to focus instead of having you guess what the surveyor might find. The full PPR process also identifies what your long term care organization does well, thus providing an opportunity to transfer lessons learned to other not compliant areas.
- **Facilitated improvement without draining long term care resources.** Because the PPR tool capitalizes on new technology, your long term care organization can perform the assessment efficiently. The organization doing a full PPR can work on it as time allows and save information as it is developed. The only tool needed for the full PPR is the Web-based program and no additional survey fees apply. The Joint Commission will not review any information until the organization officially attests to its completion and clicks the "Send" button.

Option 1

Although the full PPR process should result in the most benefit to your long term care organization, The Joint Commission does offer three options other than the full PPR approach. Option 1 requires the long term care organization to attest to completing a self-assessment of all applicable standards and to create Plans of Action and MOS as needed. The long term care organization, however, will not submit the data findings to The Joint Commission via the extranet PPR tool or automatically engage in a dialogue with Joint Commission staff regarding any of its own specific standards compliance issues. Long term care organizations may submit standards-related issues for discussion with Joint Commission staff members without indicating their own levels of standards compliance.

Option 1 was created so organizations can still benefit from the process of conducting a self-assessment, but can retain their data in house. This was developed in response to concerns about whether sharing information with The Joint Commission can waive state law protection from discovery. Figure 3 on page 9 shows the deadlines associated with the different components of Option 1.

As previously mentioned, this option deviates from the full PPR process in the submission aspect. Following are the requirements specific to this option:

- The long term care organization must attest that it assessed its compliance with all relevant standards and

Option 1 Time Line

Continuously

- ❑ The long term care organization assesses itself against all applicable elements of performance (EPs) but does not enter findings in the tool.
- ❑ The long term care organization writes Plans of Action and any required measure of success (MOS) for standards scored out of compliance.

9 months; 21 months; 33 months

- ❑ The long term care organization receives an e-mail from The Joint Commission communicating that access to submit the PPR is now available to the organization.

9–12 months; 21–24 months; 33–36 months

- ❑ The long term care organization explores option descriptions in the tool, as well as the tool itself, and selects Option 1.

12 months; 24 months; 36 months

- ❑ The long term care organization submits attestation of completion of the PPR and that it, after careful consideration with legal counsel, has decided not to participate in the full PPR.
- ❑ The long term care organization may submit standards-related issues for discussion with Joint Commission staff, if it chooses.

13 months; 25 months; 37 months

- ❑ If it submitted standards-related issues for discussion, the long term care organization participates in a conference call with The Joint Commission. This call is about standards-related issues without indicating the organization's own levels of standard compliance.

36 months

- ❑ During the full, on-site survey, the surveyor(s) will review the MOS.

Figure 3. *Option 1 time line.*

APRs, has developed Plans of Action for standards found not in compliance, and has developed MOS for any required areas. It submits this attestation to The Joint Commission via the PPR tool.

- Although the long term care organization has access to the continuous PPR extranet tool, the long term care organization must select a PPR option annually. Option 1 requires long term care organizations to attest that they, after careful consideration with legal counsel, have decided not to participate in the full PPR.
- If a long term care organization has compliance questions, it can submit any questions about process designs to The Joint Commission for discussion without indicating its own level of standards compliance. The Joint Commission staff does not identify any of the standards discussed to surveyors assigned to the organization's on-site survey. If the long term care organization does not submit any issues, no follow-up phone call is scheduled with Joint Commission staff. If the long term care organization has opted to have a phone call with The Joint Commission, it can and should submit any standards-related questions or issues for discussion. This enables The Joint Commission to ensure that the appropriate staff members are available for the conference call.
- During the on-site survey, surveyors still request and review MOS data collected by the long term care organization related to standards found not compliant during PPR.

Options 2 or 3

PPR Options 2 and 3 provide for an organization to choose either a limited on-site announced survey or a full-length announced or unannounced survey in place of a self-assessment activity. Some long term care organizations feel that the completion of the PPR in and of itself, whether or not shared with The Joint Commission, would put them at risk for disclosure of information. In response to this concern, The Joint Commission created these options so that these long term care organizations could still benefit from an annual evaluation, and thus more continuous compliance with standards, without engaging in any activity that the long term care organization feels would put it at risk. Options 2 and 3 share the characteristics listed below, followed by some specific to each:

- If the long term care organization chooses this option in the PPR tool, the decision triggers The Joint Commission to schedule a survey. Organizations may switch options annually.
- Although the long term care organization has access to the continuous PPR extranet tool, the long term care organization must select a PPR option annually. Option 2 requires the long term care organization to attest that, after careful consideration with legal counsel, it will not complete the full PPR.
- The limited-survey length is approximately one-third the usual length of the long term care organization's full survey and is usually conducted by one surveyor. Alternatively, organizations may select a full-length survey.

- The limited survey is conducted primarily through tracer methodology, as guided by the long term care organization's Priority Focus Process (PFP) output.
- When an organization selects a full-length PPR Option 2 or 3 survey, it may independently select one of these options without advice of legal counsel.

Option 2 Only

- The surveyor leaves a written report of findings.
- The long term care organization must submit the tool again within 30 days of the survey. This submission addresses not compliant standards, choice of conference call, and any other topics for discussion with The Joint Commission staff.
- Long term care organizations are required to submit to The Joint Commission a Plan of Action (with an MOS, if required) within 30 days of the survey for any standards found not compliant.
- Long term care organizations may elect to participate in a conference call with The Joint Commission staff to discuss the Plan(s) of Action and MOS. If a conference call is not requested, Joint Commission staff members will review the data. Should they determine a conference call is needed, your organization will be contacted to schedule the call. Therefore, it is important that your organization identify conference call avoid dates in the PPR tool.
- If the surveyor does not identify any not compliant standards, the long term care organization may submit a request for a conference call to review general topics for discussion.
- The organization is charged a fee to cover the costs of conducting this survey.

Figure 4 at right shows the time line for Option 2.

Option 3 Only

- The long term care organization must submit the PPR tool again within 30 days of the survey. This submission addresses the choice of a conference call and any topics for discussion with The Joint Commission staff. Conference call avoid dates should be included in the PPR tool.
- Following the survey, the long term care organization may elect to participate in a conference call with The Joint Commission staff to discuss standards issues and process designs. All findings from the on-site visit are communicated verbally to the long term care organization and no written report is provided to the long term care organization or transmitted to The Joint Commission.
- At the time of the long term care organization's full survey, the surveyor(s) receives no information relating to the long term care organization's Option 3 survey findings.

Note: *All conference calls are optional.*

Option 2 Time Line

Continuously

- ❑ The long term care organization can access the PPR extranet tool.

9 months; 21 months; 33 months

- ❑ The long term care organization receives an e-mail from The Joint Commission communicating that the choice to submit the PPR is now available to the organization.

9-12 months; 21-24 months; 33-36 months

- ❑ The long term care organization explores the option descriptions.
- ❑ The long term care organization chooses Option 2, which triggers the scheduling of an on-site visit.

12 months; 24 months; 36 months

- ❑ The on-site visit is held.
- ❑ The surveyor assesses the long term care organization against all elements of performance (EPs) applicable to the organization using the PPR extranet tool. The tool automatically aggregates information to determine compliance at the standard and Accreditation Participation Requirements (APR) level.
- ❑ The long term care organization writes Plans of Action and measure(s) of success (MOS)—if required—for standards out of compliance. The long term care organization submits this information to The Joint Commission.
- ❑ If the long term care organization must write Plans of Action, it has the option of participating in a conference call with The Joint Commission to discuss and approve Plans of Action and MOS. (The organization must submit the PPR tool again within 30 days of survey to address not compliant standards, choice of conference call, and any other topics for discussion with Joint Commission staff.)

36 months

- ❑ During the full, on-site survey, the surveyor(s) reviews the MOS to ensure that Plans of Action were implemented and that performance has been sustained.

Figure 4. *Option 2 time line.*

TIP *The Joint Commission allows organizations to videotape or audiotape the exit briefing for PPR Option 3 because the surveyor does not provide a written report.*

As with PPR Option 2, PPR Option 3 provides for an on-site survey in place of a self-assessment activity. Figure 5 at right shows the time line for Option 3. Option 3 has the following characteristics:

- If the long term care organization chooses this option in the PPR tool, this decision will trigger The Joint Commission to schedule an annual survey.
- While the long term care organization will have access to the continuous PPR extranet tool, the long term care organization will be required to select a PPR option annually. Option 3 requires the long term care organization to attest that, for substantive legal reasons, it was advised not to complete the full PPR.
- The limited survey length is approximately one-third the usual length of the long term care organization's full survey and is usually conducted by one surveyor. Alternatively, organizations may select a full-length survey.
- The limited survey is conducted primarily through tracer methodology, as guided by the long term care organization's PFP output.
- Following the survey, the long term care organization may elect to participate in a conference call with The Joint Commission staff to discuss standards issues and process designs. (Organizations must submit the PPR tool 30 days after survey to address the choice of a conference call and any topics for discussion with Joint Commission staff.) All findings from the on-site visit are communicated verbally to the organization and no written report is provided to the organization or transmitted to The Joint Commission.
- At the time of the long term care organization's full survey, no review of the PPR survey findings occurs.
- The long term care organization is charged a fee to cover the costs of conducting this survey.

The main elements of the PPR are consistent across the full PPR, Option 1, Option 2, or Option 3. To efficiently address these elements and to reap the most benefits from the process, certain specific steps your long term care organization may wish to take include the following:

- Planning for the PPR
- Conducting the assessment
- Reporting the results
- Correcting any identified problems

There is a variety of ways to accomplish these four steps. The following sections will provide tips for successful implementation.

Option 3 Time Line

Continuously

- ❑ The long term care organization can access the PPR extranet tool.

9 months; 21 months; 33 months

- ❑ The long term care organization receives an e-mail from The Joint Commission communicating that access to submit the PPR is now available to the organization.

9–12 months; 21–24 months; 33–36 months

- ❑ The long term care organization explores the option descriptions in the tool, as well as the tool itself.
- ❑ The long term care organization chooses Option 3, which triggers the scheduling of an on-site visit.

12 months; 24 months; 36 months

- ❑ The on-site visit is held.
- ❑ The surveyor assesses the long term care organization against all elements of performance (EPs) applicable to the long term care organization using the PPR extranet tool. The tool automatically aggregates information to determine compliance at the standard and APR level. The surveyor delivers verbal results to the organization.
- ❑ The long term care organization may choose to participate in a conference call with The Joint Commission to discuss standards-related issues.

36 months

- ❑ During the full, on-site survey, the surveyor(s) does not review the measures of success (MOS).

Figure 5. *Option 3 time line.*

Table 1 on pages 12–13 compares features of the full PPR, Option 1, Option 2, and Option 3. *See* Sidebar 3, page 14, for a description of what features the PPR options share.

Table 1. Comparison of the Full Periodic Performance Review, Option 1, Option 2, and Option 3

The following table compares features of the full PPR, Option 1, Option 2, and Option 3.

NO.	FEATURE	FULL	OPTION 1	OPTION 2	OPTION 3
1	At the 9th, 21st, and 33rd months in an organization's accreditation cycle, The Joint Commission notifies a long term care organization via e-mail that it must advise The Joint Commission no later than the 12th, 24th, and 36th months in its cycle whether it intends to participate in the full PPR,* Option 1, Option 2, or Option 3.	Yes	Yes	Yes	Yes
2	By the 12th, 24th, and 36th months in its accreditation cycle, the long term care organization either submits a completed PPR or notifies The Joint Commission that it chooses Option 1, Option 2, or Option 3.	Yes	Yes	Yes	Yes
3	The long term care organization must affirm that, after careful consideration with legal counsel, the organization has decided not to participate in the full PPR.	NA*	Yes	Yes†	Yes†
4	A long term care organization is required to conduct a self-assessment of compliance with Joint Commission standards annually.	Yes	Yes	No	No
5	The long term care organization is required to use The Joint Commission's automated tool to score standards and EPs* and to document Plans of Action and MOS.*	Yes	No	Yes, for completion of the Plan of Action, MOS	NA
6	The Joint Commission schedules an on-site survey.	NA	NA	Yes	Yes
7	The long term care organization undergoes an on-site survey conducted by Joint Commission surveyor(s) in lieu of conducting any self-assessment activities. The survey (1) is either approximately one-third the usual length of survey for the organization or an announced or unannounced full-length survey, and (2) uses the tracer methodology guided by the organization's PFP.* The organization is charged a fee to cover the costs of conducting the survey.	NA	NA	Yes	Yes
8	The surveyor(s) identifies EPs found not in compliance in the PPR tool.	NA	NA	Yes	Yes
9	The surveyor(s) provides a report.	NA	NA	Yes	No

* PPR, Periodic Performance Review; NA, not applicable; EPs, elements of performance; MOS, Measure of Success; PFP, Priority Focus Process; SIG, Standards Interpretation Group.

† When an organization selects a *full-length* PPR Option 2 or 3 survey, it may independently select one of these options *without* advice of legal counsel.

Table 1. continued

NO.	FEATURE	FULL	OPTION 1	OPTION 2	OPTION 3
10	The surveyor(s) only verbally communicates the survey findings to the organization and no written report is provided to the organization.	NA	NA	No	Yes
11	For any standards found through the full PPR or the Option 2 survey to be not compliant, the long term care organization is required to formulate and submit a Plan of Action addressing each EP scored in partial or insufficient compliance. This plan should state how the matter will be corrected and how the success of the Plan of Action will be evaluated, if an MOS is required.	Yes	NA	Yes	NA
12	The long term care organization affirms that it has self-assessed compliance with all relevant standards, developed appropriate Plan(s) of Action for identified areas of noncompliance, and identified MOS for all such standards as required.	NA	Yes	NA	NA
13	The organization may elect to participate in a conference call with The Joint Commission's SIG* staff to discuss the standards not in compliance and reach approval on the Plan of Action.	Yes	No	Yes	No
14	The organization may elect to participate in a conference call with The Joint Commission's SIG to discuss the standards-related issues.	Yes	Yes	Yes	Yes
15	All standards found not in compliance, whether through an organization's self-assessment or an Option 2 or Option 3 survey, do not affect an organization's accreditation decision. If an immediate threat to health or safety is identified, The Joint Commission initiates a special survey. (*See* Sidebar 4, page 14)	Yes	Yes	Yes	Yes
16	At the time of the organization's annual survey, the organization's MOS is validated throughout the survey.	Yes	Yes	Yes	No
17	Results of the annual review (PPR) feed into the PFP.	No	No	No	No

* PPR, Periodic Performance Review; NA, not applicable; EPs, elements of performance; MOS, Measure of Success; PFP, Priority Focus Process; SIG, Standards Interpretation Group.

Sidebar 3. Key Characteristics of the Full Periodic Performance Review and Options 1, 2, and 3

Several things that the full PPR and its options have in common include the following:

- All long term care organizations develop Plans of Action and Measures of Success (MOS), as required annually.
- All long term care organizations share completed MOS results with surveyors at the time of the full survey except for those organizations choosing to complete Option 3.
- All long term care organizations demonstrate at the time of the full survey a track record of standards compliance from their approved Plan of Action compliant by date.
- Any area of noncompliance discovered at the time of full survey is documented.

Sidebar 4. An Immediate Threat to Health or Safety

No matter what PPR option you choose, if The Joint Commission or your organization during the course of the PPR process identifies a continuing situation that represents a potential threat to health or safety, a special survey is initiated to facilitate resolution of the situation.

☑ Planning for the PPR

A well-planned PPR, regardless of the option you choose, is easier to implement than a haphazardly structured one. Understanding the process, having all the staff on board, and outlining the steps involved helps your long term care organization complete the process most efficiently.

Depending on the long term care organization, the PPR planning process may be formal or informal, complex or simple. Because of their size and variety of care services, large long term care organizations may need to plan differently from smaller ones. More people might be involved in the PPR process in a large long term care organization. With more people comes a greater possibility for efficiency as well as greater possibilities for confusion. Similarly, a long term care organization with multiple sites may have unique challenges to address in the planning process. *See* Sidebar 5, on page 16, for strategies on how to tackle a PPR involving multiple sites and services. Although The Joint Commission leaves it to the long term care organization to choose how to approach the PPR process, it is important to consider the approach before jumping in.

TIP *Reviewing the automated PPR tool to become familiar with its features and requirements can be helpful in determining what option to select, what approach to use, who will be involved, what data will be needed for the review, and what types of reports will be helpful. Careful planning prevents feeling rushed and makes the PPR process more meaningful to your long term care organization. Because you have access to the PPR tool continuously, you can better plan a strategy for submitting and completing, and can easily train new staff on the PPR process. In addition, because you can enter data into the tool at any time, your organization can continuously monitor standards compliance and identify areas for improvement. You can review your PPR history by accessing any previously submitted PPRs. This feature allows your organization to compare performance over time. It is important to note that The Joint Commission can never access the information you enter into the PPR tool unless you submit it to The Joint Commission.*

Several steps are involved in planning a PPR. Your long term care organization needs to decide on an approach (including the who, when, and how), develop a data collection strategy, and schedule assessment activities. Your long term care organization should also consider a high-level strategy to implement any Plans of Action generated. The following sections discuss the steps of the planning process in more detail.

All of these planning steps can be relevant for the full PPR, Option 1, Option 2, or Option 3. In each case, your long term care organization's goal should be to promote continuous standards compliance by continually assessing yourself. Therefore, even if you choose Option 2 or 3, for example, you can follow the tips outlined here so that you are able to review your performance on a more consistent basis. That way you will know where you stand, and you can support your goal of being in compliance with the standards 100% of the time.

Determining the Staff Involved

The full PPR and Option 1 are designed to be conducted by internal staff. This internal process makes sense both financially and logically and provides many benefits including the following:

- Flexibility in how the process is approached. The PPR is a dynamic process, and using internal staff allows the long term care organization to change the way of implementing the PPR as necessary.
- Enhanced individual learning by those involved in the process. By reviewing and assessing all standards and APRs, the staff becomes more familiar with them and what determines compliance.
- An opportunity for greater focus on areas of concern. Your staff members, more than anyone, are aware of problems and issues within a facility. This process gives your long term care organization an opportunity to capitalize on staff knowledge in a positive, proactive way.
- An environment of open and honest discussion of concerns and problems. This can help reinforce a blame-free culture that is crucial in today's health care environment.
- Greater buy-in to improvement activities by the staff involved in the PPR. By assessing yourself against all standards and EPs, staff understands the need for improvement activities more fully.

Determining that internal staff will conduct the PPR process is not enough. Your long term care organization should also determine the approach to the project. The

Sidebar 5. Strategies for Long Term Care Organizations Under More Than One Accreditation Manual

The PPR is an organization-level self-assessment tool. If an accredited organization has a requirement for PPR submission, it is contained within the single PPR extranet tool. All accredited components are therefore included in the annual PPR submission. For example, if your organization is accredited under both the long term care and hospital programs, it would find a drop-down menu within its PPR tool on its secure extranet site that allows it to select either long term care or hospital standards.

The following strategies may also help long term care organizations with multiple sites or services complete the PPR accurately and efficiently:

- Designate one or two key people to oversee the PPR process across the site.
- Designate one or two key people to monitor data entry into the tool.
- Create phone/e-mail lists of key staff members involved in the PPR process.
- Plan biweekly meetings involving key staff members. These meetings can be by conference call, if necessary.
- Distribute minutes from these meetings to all staff members involved in the PPR.
- Start the planning process as far ahead of your required submission as possible. Planning will take more time when multiple sites/services are involved.

approach you choose will depend on a variety of characteristics of your long term care organization including the following:

- Size
- Complexity
- Programs and services
- Organization culture
- Resources
- Leadership
- Expertise and knowledge

In determining the appropriate approach, your long term care organization must decide whether you are going to have an individual or multiple staff spearhead the project. Each of these approaches has advantages and disadvantages. For example, your long term care organization may choose to have one individual designated as the project leader on the PPR process. This individual will probably have in-depth knowledge of the standards and their interrelationships. He or she will be ultimately responsible and accountable for the proper assessment of the standards and APRs. This might be appropriate for a small long term care organization where staff is limited in size and the services provided are small in scope. The disadvantage to this approach is the time commitment required of this individual and the potentially one-dimensional perspective of the review. In a large long term care organization, the PPR is likely to require that several individuals or groups within the organization be involved.

Instead of an individual approach, your long term care organization may want to use a team approach to the PPR. In this approach, an individual or group is assigned the portion of the PPR with which it has knowledge and expertise. It is responsible for spearheading the PPR process as it relates to the assigned area. For example, health information management staff could be put in charge of assessing and completing the assessment and scoring of the Management of Information standards. One advantage of this approach is that each department/unit lends its expertise and familiarity with standards to the assessment process. The team approach provides varied input and more focus on each individual standard and APR. However, this approach may also yield some inconsistency in how the standards are reviewed and assessed. One department/unit may "set the bar higher" for compliance than another. Issues of redundancy may also arise in this scenario because multiple departments/units may address the same standards. In cases where standards cross functions, opportunities for collaboration may be missed.

Still another approach to the PPR also involves an interdisciplinary team. In this approach, a group composed of members of different areas of the long term care organization such as nursing, physical therapy, nutrition, and building services reviews all standards and APRs, identifies compliance issues, and develops Plans of Action where appropriate. Although this method offers a structured approach, multiple viewpoints, and shared responsibility, it

Sidebar 6. Securing the Medical Director's Participation

- **Educate.** To secure the medical director's participation, your organization must show physicians how the PPR will ultimately affect and improve resident care. This can be accomplished through education. An interactive approach might be helpful, allowing for questions, explanations, and discussions.
- **Engage.** By making an open-ended invitation to participate in the PPR process, your organization may not gain the medical director support you seek. Organizations that supply the reasons why participation is beneficial, identify the medical director's role in the process, and describe the expected time commitment will gain more support. Your organization may wish to use the medical director as a champion to stimulate interest.
- **Empower.** As with other health care providers, the time that a medical director has for performance improvement is limited. Organizations that involve the medical directors where their input can make the biggest impact on clinical care will reap the benefit of their participation. The medical director may be more interested in participating in the PPR process if he or she thinks he or she can make a difference in the health and safety of residents.

also requires a time commitment from each team member and increased long term care organization resources. The interdisciplinary team method might work well for large long term care organizations; however, this approach might not be practical for smaller ones, simply because there are not as many staff members from different disciplines.

Regardless of the approach selected, leaders should play a prominent role in the PPR process. Leaders may include the long term care organization chief executive officer, governing body leader, senior managers, and any administrative or nursing leaders. Many of the issues that are uncovered in the PPR may require attention from these individuals. In addition, Plans of Action may require ongoing leader involvement and support. One way that leaders can get involved in the PPR process is by appointing an administrative sponsor or a steering committee that keeps other senior staff informed about the status and results of the PPR.

As previously mentioned, one of the many benefits of the PPR process is that it offers an opportunity to involve different staff in evaluating standards compliance. This involvement can encourage familiarity with the standards and ultimately offer significant educational benefits as well as buy-in to improvement initiatives. In particular, the PPR can involve groups not traditionally a part of systems analysis, such as physicians. Although physicians have generally recognized the importance of the accreditation process, many have not found ways of contributing to it in a meaningful way. Sidebar 6, above, provides ideas for encouraging the medical director to participate in the PPR.

Educating Staff

To realize the full benefits of the PPR, your long term care organization should take time before staff members begin the PPR process to educate them on how it works. How prepared staff members are to conduct the review is ultimately more important than who is actually chosen to do the review. By knowing what to expect and what is expected of them, staff members can perform to the best of their abilities. Some specific topics to cover include the following:

- The goals of the PPR and how it relates to accreditation and quality improvement
- The role of the continuous PPR tool in ongoing performance improvement activities. By continuously entering information into the tool, you can identify performance issues throughout the year and address them before they become serious issues.
- How the PPR tool works
- What standards must be addressed
- What it means to comply with the standards
- How compliance should be assessed
- How to access information needed to assess compliance and to develop Plans of Action

Selecting the Appropriate Data

After your long term care organization decides on a staffing approach, it is important to consider the types of data that will be needed to verify standards compliance. In most cases, simply verifying the existence of policies and procedures is not enough to show compliance with an EP. Instead, your long term care organization must evaluate your performance in terms of the standards. To prove compliance, long term care organizations may have to gather evidence to answer a question, identify sample processes, and thoroughly review documents. The appropriate data will vary depending on the type of organization and the standard being examined. Again, the PPR process is not designed to make more work for your long term care organization. When possible, you should use existing data to help verify compliance. The following list provides suggestions on possible sources of such information:

- Clinical records. When such data are used, your long term care organization should select an appropriate sample and establish reasonable thresholds for compliance.
- Policies and procedures. Again, simply verifying their existence is not enough. The content of the policies and procedures and their implementation are also important.
- Human resources data. These data may include personnel files, performance reviews, and orientation surveys.
- Meeting minutes
- Interviews with key staff members, management, and leaders
- Surveys of staff, residents, and the community
- Building tours
- Exercises
- Planning documents
- Complaint data
- Error reports
- Performance improvement data
- Infection control data
- Electronic Statement of Conditions™ (e-SOC). This statement can help verify compliance with any applicable "Management of the Environment of Care" (EC) standards and identify any violations of the *Life Safety Code*®.*
- Mock surveys. Although a mock survey may result in slightly more work for your long term care organization, it will provide a true picture of standards compliance and highlight any issues that need to be addressed. As a part of this mock survey process, your long term care organization may choose to select individual tracers—those individuals who represent the clinical service groups identified through the PFP output for your organization—and follow them through the care process.
- Other information provided through the PFP output available on your extranet site

TIP *To ensure that data are collected for all applicable standards, your long term care organization may want to use a checklist of applicable standards and EPs for review. Make sure to include the APRs and National Patient Safety Goals in this checklist. Part 2 of this book may serve as a source for this checklist, and the "Reports by Chapter" section of the PPR tool offers an "All Standards" report that lists all the standards and EPs required for your long term care organization.* See *the "Generating Reports" section on pages 22–23 for more information.*

Developing a Time Line

If choosing the full PPR or Option 1, your long term care organization has three months to submit the PPR to The Joint Commission or attest that you have completed a PPR and that you have been advised by legal counsel not to participate in the full PPR. This time frame offers a reasonable period in which to thoroughly assess what compliance option to submit.

In planning for submitting your PPR, your long term care organization should set deadlines for completing the components of the projects planned. For example, because you have continuous access to the PPR tool, your organization may want to select the PPR team or individual to lead and train any participating staff well before the submission time frame begins. During this continuous access time frame, you may want to run through a mock PPR to discover any potential issues. Then, after the submission time frame begins, you may set a goal to review a third of the standards each month. However your long term care organization decides to divide the time, some thought should be given to how you will spend the time. All staff members should be aware of the time line and work toward meeting preset deadlines.

TIP *Your organization must make sure that staff members working on the PPR are given enough time during their schedule to complete any work relating to the process. The staff must have sufficient time to examine the long term care organization's practices, to verify implementation, and to assess compliance with each standard and APR (including any progress toward the National Patient Safety Goals, many of which are scored in the long term care standards).*

Periodically throughout the PPR process, the PPR team should report back to your long term care organization, outlining the status of the process and any issues uncovered. The frequency of these reports should be determined by your long term care organization prior to the start of the PPR. The PPR tool can help streamline this reporting process. More information on how to use the tool to help with reporting appears on pages 22–23.

* *Life Safety Code*® is a registered trademark of the National Fire Protection Association, Quincy, MA.

☑ Conducting the PPR

After your long term care organization decides on a strategy, determines the data needed, and sets deadlines for implementation, it is time to begin conducting your PPR.

When completing the PPR, a long term care organization may choose to put information directly into the PPR tool, or it may collect data, design plans on paper, and then transfer the plans to the electronic tool. You may want to use Part 2 of this book as a PPR workbook in concert with the use of the electronic tool. You can more easily enter your data into the tool directly from the workbook and use your time more effectively to help implement Plans of Action, rather than worry about charting your compliance. The amount of space for text to be entered in the PPR tool is unlimited, but it is a good idea to limit yourself. The workbook can provide a place to edit your information.

The following section is an overview of how to conduct a PPR. These are just suggestions, not requirements, on how to conduct your PPR. Most sections apply to the full PPR and to Options 1, 2, and 3, but those sections specifically about using the PPR extranet tool apply only to the full PPR.

TIP *The staff in the SIG at The Joint Commission offer the following pointers on getting the most out of your PPR experience:*

- *Do not wait until the last minute. Give yourself enough time to do a thorough job.*
- *Read the user guide and follow the instructions for writing the Plan of Action and MOS.*
- *If you are unsure about anything while completing the PPR, call your account representative.*
- *Get the staff involved in the process. This will encourage ownership and understanding of the standards, EPs, and on-site survey.*
- *Take full advantage of the conference call with the SIG. They have experience in your accreditation program.*
- *For Option 1, submit a list of standards-related issues or topics so the appropriate staff will be available for the phone call. You will be notified in advance via e-mail of the date and time for your call.*
- *Understand that if your organization decides not to participate in the conference call, its Plans of Action and MOS are only reviewed, not* approved. *When SIG approves Plans of Action and MOS, they cannot be challenged by the surveyors on site. If your organization wants The Joint Commission to approve its Plans of Action and MOS, it must schedule and participate in the conference call.*

Used well, the PPR tool can foster a creative brainstorm among your staff members and give them a feeling of accomplishment.

Evaluating Compliance

Ideally, you should be evaluating compliance on a regular basis throughout your accreditation cycle, not just during the three-month PPR submission time frame. Continually assessing yourself against the standards will allow you to not only get the most benefit from your PPR but also promote continuous standards compliance, which helps ensure safe, quality care. Evaluating your compliance involves more than just checking a box in the PPR tool or verifying the existence of a policy. Reviewers must assess the process or system discussed, determine how it is implemented, and analyze the resulting outcomes.

The first step in determining whether or not your long term care organization is compliant with a standard involves examining each EP for that standard. The EPs provide performance expectations about the standard and detail specific structures, processes, or systems that must be in place for a long term care organization to provide quality care, treatment, or services.

The advantage of having a list of all EPs is that they clearly outline the scored requirements of the standards. Both the surveyor and the long term care organization have access to the EPs, so everyone is on the same page and knows what the requirements are. Standards compliance is based on these EPs, and every organization is evaluated against them.

When assessing compliance with the various EPs, the staff should collect the relevant data that will help determine the level of compliance. These data should then be interpreted and summarized as needed for internal use. Helpful questions to ask when reviewing the data include the following:

- Is this EP applicable to our organization or to this service?
- Is the EP's requirement present?
- If the requirement must be performed or accomplished within a particular time frame, is it being met?
- Is the requirement being met completely, effectively, and appropriately?

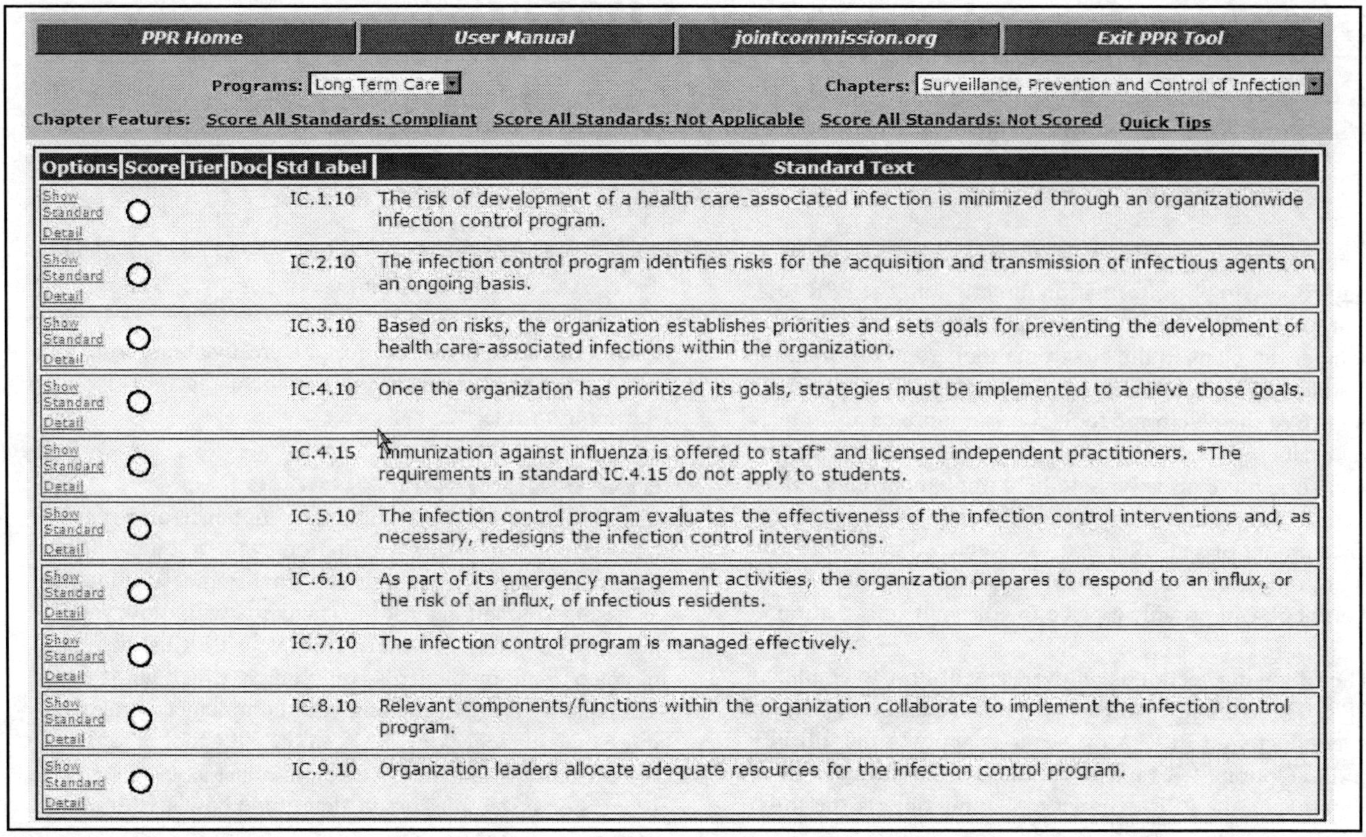

Figure 6. *Sample standards list screen.*

After you answer these questions and your organization reviews and assesses compliance, the staff should be prepared to score your long term care organization's compliance.

Note: *To find out how to score EPs,* see *pages 338–340.*

Getting Started Accessing the PPR

Accredited organizations can continually access the PPR through The Joint Commission Web site (http://www.jointcommission.org). Click *The Joint Commission Connect* link on the far right side under "search box." The login window will appear, displaying the words "Connect To www.jointcommissionconnect.org." Click this phrase to get to the login window. To log in, use your user name and password, per instructions from The Joint Commission. Your *The Joint Commission Connect* extranet home page will display. Locate and click on the link for the PPR tool to open a general information screen.

Clicking through, the next window you will access in the PPR tool is a historical screen. Here you can access previously submitted PPR data and work in an open PPR tool. You open the desired PPR tool by clicking the "Select" link, which displays the "Reviewer Information Page." After either filling out this page or just clicking on a name, you can open the "Standards Data Page." (*See* Figure 6, above, for a sample standards list screen.) Prominent on the page is a list of standards for the chapter selected. Above this list of standards are two drop-down menus that allow you to choose a different health care program or a different standards chapter. To access a particular standards chapter, simply click on the arrow to view the drop-down list and select the standard.

Note: *An organization undergoing initial accreditation will have access to the PPR tool after The Joint Commission receives its e-App and deposit and after the account representative reviews the e-App.*

Getting Help

To aid in assessing compliance using the PPR tool, the "Standards Data Page" has a number of options. There are four buttons near the top of the screen, and within the navigation bar, five sections containing various links. You will find some of these links helpful as you use the tool.

On the navigation bar you will find the "References" section. This section may be particularly helpful because it provides a scoring guideline that will help your organization determine the level of compliance for a particular EP. The scoring guideline defines the quantitative measures that constitute full compliance, partial compliance, and noncompliance. What defines compliance will vary depending on the scoring criteria categories mentioned

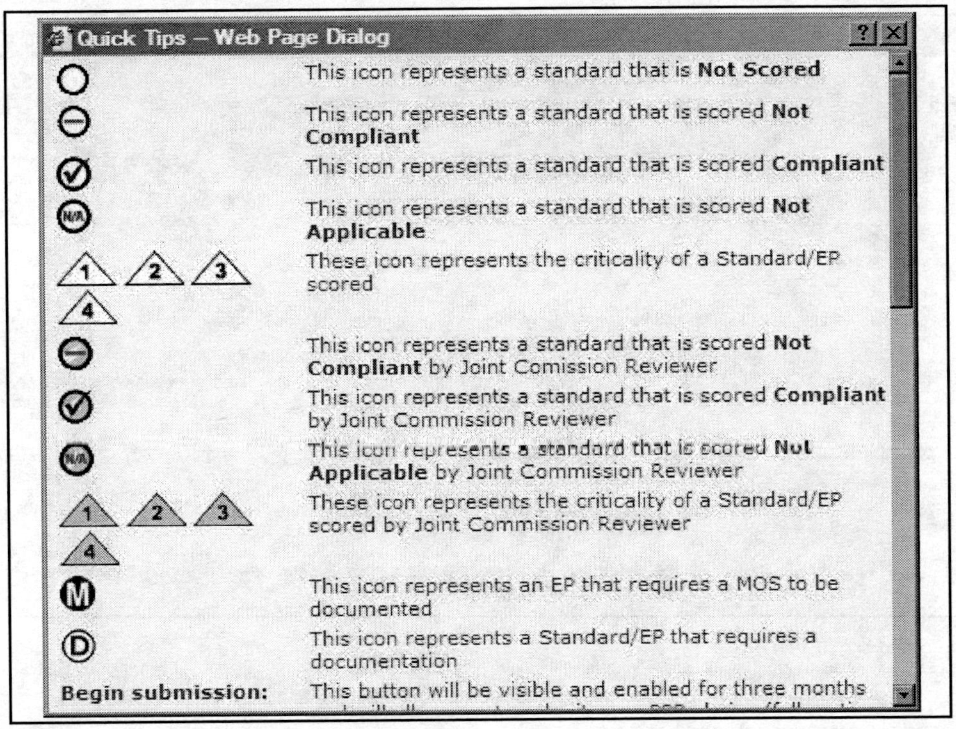

Figure 7. *Standard compliance legend for the PPR.*

later in this book, beginning on page 338. To view the scoring guidelines, select the appropriate link under the "References" section. This section also includes a link containing instructions on effectively writing Plans of Action.

One of the large buttons near the top of the "Standards Data Page" allows access to a manual. To access it, click the "User Manual" button near the top of the screen. This full-color document takes you through every step of accessing, using, and submitting the electronic tool. You may view and print this manual as needed.

Still another source of help on the screen is "Quick Tips" that follows the links after the "Chapter Features" heading. This heading is located immediately below the two drop-down menus near the top of the page. This link contains a short list (a legend) describing the circular and triangular scoring icons used in the PPR tool. (*See* Figure 7, above.)

In addition to the resources in the electronic PPR tool, several other tools may help your organization with its compliance goals. For example, The Joint Commission Web site (http://wwwjointcommission.org) is an excellent source of standards compliance information. Specifically, the "Standards FAQ" and "Accreditation Process for Long Term Care Organizations" sections of the Web site may address compliance issues. If your question is not addressed within these sections, you may submit your question online using the " Standards Online Question Form." Your organization may also contact The Joint Commission's SIG directly with any standards-related questions.

Entering Compliance in the PPR

Your organization should focus on updating any new standards or EPs and the previously scored not compliant standards and EPs to reflect any progress you have made as a result of implementing the Plans of Action and to accurately reflect your current level of compliance. In addition, you should update any other standards and EPs for which you have assessed that your level of compliance, as previously submitted, might have changed.

To enter data for a specific standard on the "Standards Data Page," click a "Show Standard Detail" link to the left of a listed standard. This action expands that standard to show all its EPs. Under the heading "EP Scores," a drop-down menu allows you to choose your organization's self-assessed level of compliance with each EP. Your choices in this area are as follows:

- Satisfactory compliance
- Partial compliance
- Insufficient compliance
- Not applicable

See Figure 8, on page 22, for a sample standard and EP screen in the PPR tool.

All EPs associated with a standard require an entry. To ease the data-entry process, you may elect to score all the

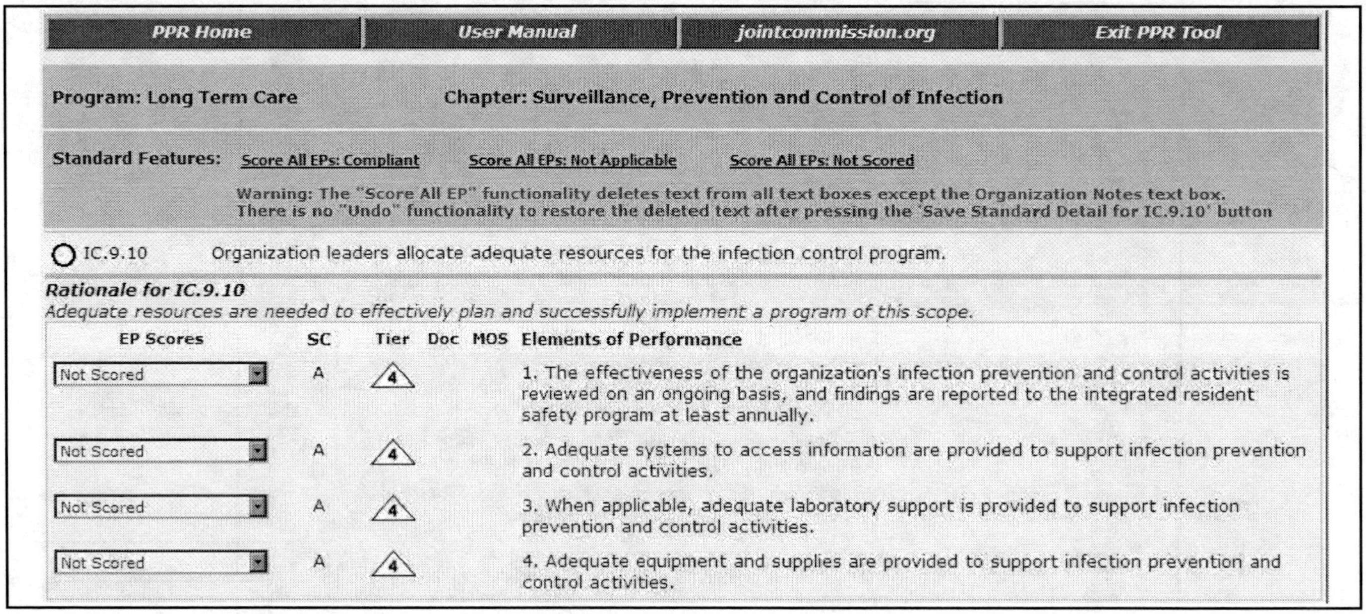

Figure 8. *Sample standard and EPs screen.*

EPs for a standard as compliant, not applicable (N/A), or not scored. You can also "score all" in the EP functionality at the standard detail level. If you should change the compliance determination of an EP, you can change the level of compliance of the EP or return it to unscored at any time.

TIP *When using the PPR extranet tool, remember to save data regularly. You must click "Save" before leaving the scoring screen. Frequently clicking "Save" helps ensure that no information is lost.*

After you enter a compliance score for every EP, you need to save your work. The computer then aggregates the results to reach a standards-level compliance rating. This aggregation happens only after every EP for that standard has been evaluated and scored. The standards are scored one of three ways: compliant, not compliant, or not applicable. When the standard score is determined, a symbol appears next to the standard indicating its score. A check appears next to all compliant standards, while a horizontal line will appear next to all not compliant standards. An icon with an exclamation point will appear beside a standard that has at least one EP scored partially compliant.

TIP *As you enter scores for each EP, it may be helpful to use the "Organization Findings" section of the PPR tool. This window allows you to enter specific comments on a particular EP. For example, you may want to note in this area the data used to determine compliance or noncompliance for the EPs. If the standard is found not compliant, it can be helpful to know which data were used so that they can be easily accessed when developing the Plan of Action and determining MOS. Using the same data source for both assessment and correction makes improvement easier to track. In addition, if a question about compliance arises, it is helpful to know what information was used to make the determination.*

Any information entered in the "Organization Notes" window is solely for the benefit of your organization and is not viewable by The Joint Commission with the standards compliance information. It may be helpful to identify possible causes of a compliance problem. Causes might relate to staffing effectiveness, resource allocation, lack of policies, or insufficient leader support. By identifying these possible causes, you may reveal a larger problem that should be addressed. Several areas of noncompliance around a particular issue may point to a system or organizational problem. See *Figure 9, on page 23,* *for an example of the entire documentation fields screen.*

Generating Reports

The Joint Commission's PPR tool offers a section devoted to reports, which can be helpful as you do the following:

- Complete the PPR
- Identify areas of noncompliance
- Generate written reports for leaders and staff on the status and outcome of the PPR

Locate the "Chapter Reports" section in the left navigation bar (use the back arrow button on your browser toolbar to

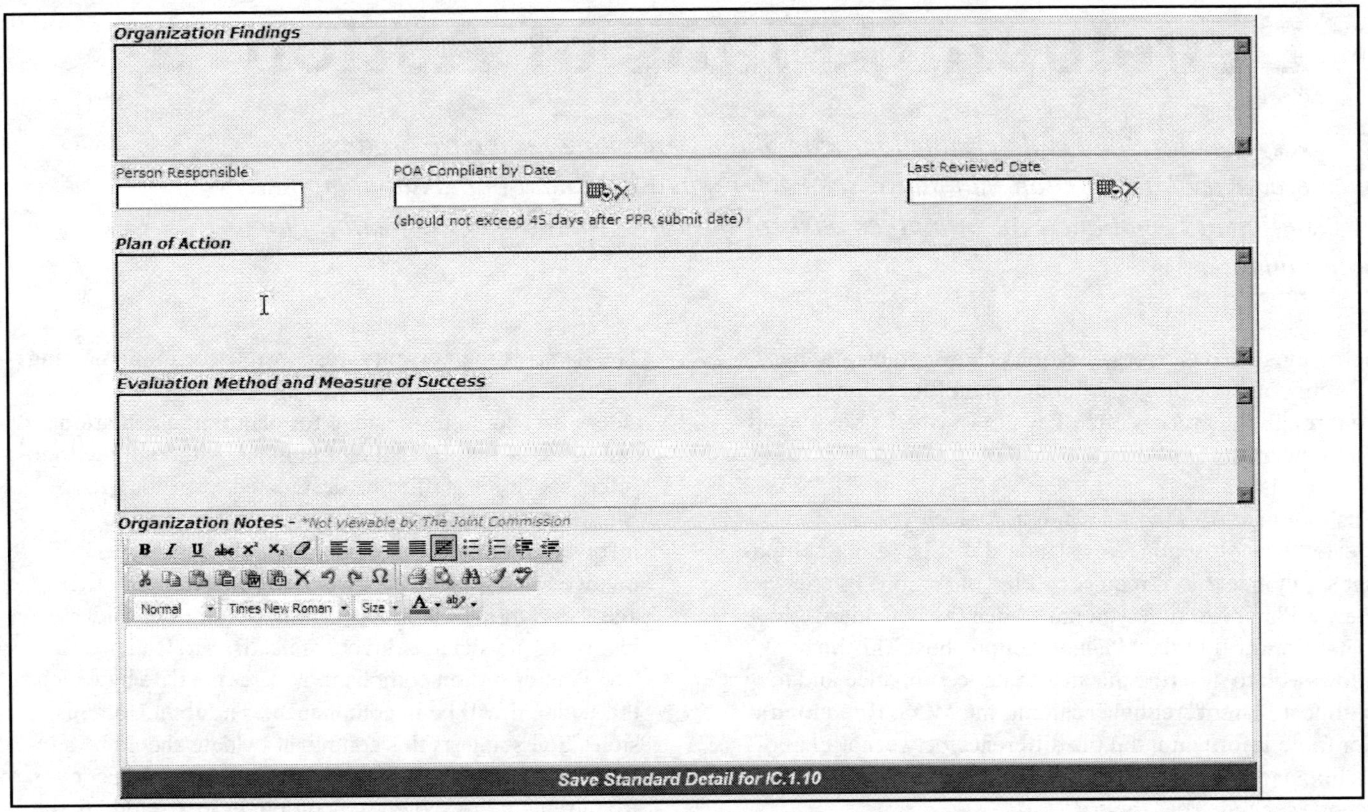

Figure 9. *Documentation fields in the PPR tool.*

return to the PPR tool). Clicking on "All Standards" allows you to review a copy of all the standards within the selected chapter. You may also print this report. The following section, "Program Reports," provides you with access to the following additional reports:

- *Scored standards.* This report details all standards and EPs in the selected chapter that have been scored to date. Your long term care organization may want to use this report as a periodic status report that keeps the PPR team and leader on track and on time.
- *Not compliant standards.* These reports list all the standards in the selected chapter that your long term care organization has assessed as not compliant. It also includes the associated out-of-compliance EPs, a brief description of the noncompliance problem, your Plan of Action, the due date, the person responsible, and Joint Commission staff comments. This report can be very helpful in easily communicating to staff and leaders the nature of the problems that need to be fixed and the plans to fix them.
- *Compliant standards with EPs scored partial.* These reports identify all the standards in the selected chapter that have been found compliant but have EPs scored partial. Long term care organizations may want to use this report to help communicate standards that require attention in the future.
- *Standards not scored.* This report details all the standards in the selected chapter that are not yet scored by the long term care organization.

Still another report appears in the left navigation bar under "Organization Data." The link called "Scoring Summary" outlines your long term care organization's overall progress toward PPR completion as seen through aggregate data. For example, you can view the number of standards you have scored versus the number of total standards. This comparison will help you track progress toward completion and assess whether the PPR process is running on schedule. In this report, you can view the following:

- Required update standards
- Not compliant standards
- Not scored standards
- Not applicable standards
- Partially compliant standards
- Compliant standards
- Total standards

Although generating reports is not required in the PPR process, your organization should maintain some type of communication regarding the status and outcomes of the process with leaders and staff. These tools provide an easy way to generate written reports. Some organizations may choose to communicate status through verbal reports instead.

☑ Developing Plans of Action

For every standard that is determined not compliant, your long term care organization must create a Plan of Action that addresses each related EP found in partial compliance or insufficient compliance. As with other parts of the PPR, you have some flexibility in doing this.

Some long term care organizations choose to create Plans of Action as they progress through the PPR tool, but others go through the process after they are finished assessing all the standards.

The tool identifies the standards for which you need to create Plans of Action. Any standard that has a not compliant symbol next to it requires a Plan of Action. To complete a Plan of Action, you must open the "Standard Detail" and fill in the "Plan of Action" box. This box allows you to describe the area of noncompliance and to outline a Plan of Action (including the MOS, if required). For more information on the difference between a Plan of Action and Evidence of Standards Compliance (ESC) report, *see* Sidebar 7, below.

Writing a Plan of Action

To ensure that organizations write their Plans of Action as efficiently as possible, the PPR tool has limited space for the Plan of Action description. Therefore, your long term care organization must be succinct in its descriptions, but still contain some detail or provide a thorough outline. Although it is possible to include large amounts of data and information in the plan, simply stating that a policy or procedure will be created is not sufficient. Each plan should include the facts and consider the who, when, and how of the Plan of Action. Several elements may make up a Plan of Action, including the following:

- The name of the person(s) responsible for implementing the plan. The PPR tool accepts alpha and numeric characters, so people responsible for plan implementation can be identified by name or number. Although the tool offers space for staff to be designated, your long term care organization should consider all who will be involved in implementation. Although the persons involved will depend on the long term care standard, and the Plan(s) of Action, it is important to consider involving physicians, direct care staff, and leaders.
- The Plan of Action compliant by date (the date by which the standard will be in compliance). The Joint Commission's SIG suggests this compliant by date should be similar to an ESC. If any EPs related to a Direct Impact Requirement are scored noncompliant in a standard, the standard should be brought into compliance within 45 days. If any EPs related to an Indirect Impact Requirement are scored noncompliant in a standard, then the standard should be brought into compliance within 60 days.
- The nature and scope of the compliance issue. Each EP that is identified as partially compliant or insufficiently compliant should be addressed.
- How the long term care organization will resolve the issue. This element can be determined by asking two questions: (1) What actions can bring the EP into compliance? (2) How will these actions bring the EP into compliance? These actions need not be complex or sup-

Sidebar 7. Compliance Reports Defined

There are major differences between a Plan of Action and an Evidence of Standards Compliance (ESC) report. The Plan of Action is a plan a long term care organization uses to come into compliance. The ESC report is a report on what has already been done to come into compliance. The following are more detailed descriptions of both:

- **Plan of Action.** For every standard self-identified as out of compliance, an organization will develop and submit a Plan of Action addressing related EPs that were scored partially compliant or insufficiently compliant. The Plan of Action details the problem, the solution, the time frame, the person responsible for implementation, and an MOS, if necessary.
- **ESC report.** This report requires long term care organizations to describe actions taken to achieve compliance with a not compliant standard, identify how ongoing compliance will be identified, and set a goal (as a percentage) for compliance in the form of an MOS. For more information on the ESC report, please *see* "The Accreditation Process" (ACC) chapter of the *CAMLTC*.

Sidebar 8. One Approach to Writing a Plan of Action

Standard MM.3.10
Only medications needed to treat the resident's condition are ordered, provided, or administered.

Element of Performance:
1. There is a documented diagnosis, condition, or indication-for-use for each medication ordered.

Organization Findings:
Clinical record reviews show that there is a documented diagnosis, condition, or indication-for-use only 65% of the time.

Plan of Action:
Re-educate medical staff and nursing staff on the need to document the diagnosis, condition, or indication-for-use for each medication. The information must be located in the order for as-needed medications as per our policy. For all other medications, the information can be located in the order, the history and physical, physician progress notes, nursing assessment, or nursing notes. Clinical staff need to be able to locate the information and will be educated. Pharmacy review will include verifying this information is present.

Plan of Action Compliant by Date:
8/1/09

Person or Department Responsible for Ensuring Standards Compliance: ____________

Measure of Success:
Monthly clinical record audits will demonstrate a minimum of 90% compliance with documentation of diagnosis, condition, or indication-for-use for each medication. Sample sizes will be defined in the *CAMLTC*.

ported by research, but they should fit the problem identified and be appropriate for the long term care organization.

- How the proposed actions will be implemented
- An MOS that will show the standard in compliance (if required). An MOS is a measurable, objective criterion that shows that the long term care organization has achieved and maintained compliance with an EP. An EP requires an MOS if the "Ⓜ" symbol is next to it. Typically, an MOS is related to some type of audit that determines whether an action is effective and sustained. Long term care organizations can determine appropriate MOS by asking, "What measurable, objective criteria can show that the EP is in compliance?" Appropriate data to use may include clinical records, staff interviews, building inspections, or performance improvement (PI) data—any data that can show a track record of compliance. If possible, it is most efficient to use existing data sources for MOS.

The data used as an MOS must show at least a 90% compliance rate for a Category C EP to be scored 2. (For more information about scoring categories, *see* pages 338–340.) For example, if your long term care organization chooses to take a random sample of 25 clinical records and use them as an MOS, then 90% of those records should reflect compliance with the EP. For Category A EPs requiring an MOS, 100% compliance must be demonstrated.

Sidebar 8, above, illustrates one approach to writing a Plan of Action. This sample provides a written plan that is detailed yet brief. Some long term care organizations may want to simplify the plan even further by using bullet points and shorter phrases.

TIP *Only those standards identified as not compliant will require a Plan of Action. However, staff should, at the very least, investigate and monitor those compliant standards with any partially compliant EPs.*

☑ Submitting the PPR and Following Up

When you have completed assessing the EPs, documenting compliance, creating Plans of Action, and identifying MOS, you are ready to submit the PPR to The Joint Commission.

The PPR tool does not allow you to submit until all EPs are scored and all necessary Plans of Action are entered. (The CEO or another designee typically completes the submission process.) If you are allowed to submit your PPR information, the "Begin Submission" link appears in the left navigation bar on the PPR tool. Clicking it takes you to a screen that explains the full PPR and Options 1, 2, and 3. Here you can select the method that best fits your organization.

If you select the full PPR, the next screen allows you to either continue your submission or click an attestation box if you want a conference call with SIG staff. The latter requires you to identify a main and a backup contact person for the PPR conference call. (It is crucial that you keep this information as up to date as possible. If the information changes after you submit your PPR, you should notify your account representative.)

Another screen allows you to identify up to five avoid dates for your Joint Commission phone call. A field called "Topics for Discussion during Conference Call with Joint Commission Staff" allows you to describe those areas you would like to discuss during the conference call. After you enter this information, you must read the attestation, verify that you understand it, and click "Complete Submission."

After the full PPR is submitted, the CEO or other designee receives an e-mail confirming that The Joint Commission has successfully received the PPR. You may not make changes to the PPR data submitted; however, you may continue entering data into the open PPR tool.

If you choose Option 1, you are taken to an attestation screen as well. There you also have the option of requesting a conference call to discuss general standards-related issues with Joint Commission staff. You will then have to follow the same steps explained previously (if submitting a full PPR). However, you are required to attest to the following as well:

- Your organization has self-assessed its compliance, developed Plans of Action, and identified MOS, if required.
- Your organization, for substantive reasons, has been advised by legal counsel not to participate in the full PPR.

Submitting Option 2 or Option 3 automatically triggers The Joint Commission to schedule an on-site survey. If you select Option 2 or Option 3, you attest that your organization, after careful consideration with legal counsel, has decided not to participate in the full PPR. You can also select avoid dates for your limited on-site survey. The surveyor reviews the results of the on-site visit with you at the end of that visit.

When the surveyor submits the findings for Option 2 surveys, the historical PPR tool reopens data to the health care organization. If the surveyor identified not compliant standards, you then have 30 days to write and submit your Plans of Action, including MOS, if required. A conference call follows the same format as the one for the full PPR. However, if the surveyor did not identify any not compliant standards, you may submit a request for a conference call to review general topics for discussion.

For Option 3 surveys, the historical PPR tool reopens to the health care organization. You have 30 days to request a conference call with SIG and submit any general topics for discussion.

Checking the Status

The "Messages" section of the PPR tool appears on the "Standards Data Page," in the left navigation bar. This section provides your organization with an area in which to check the current status of your submitted PPR. You may print this page and show it to the survey team at the time of your next full survey as evidence of your compliance with APR.03.01.01.

The Conference Call

After your PPR is finished, a SIG representative reviews your information. The representative specifically looks at the Plans of Action to make sure that they are complete, realistic, specific, appropriate, timely, and measurable.

Sidebar 9. Getting the Most Out of The Joint Commission Conference Call

- Schedule a three-hour block of time on the identified date.
- Commit staff to participate in the call who are knowledgeable about the PPR's contents. Only two organization representatives may participate in the call at any given time.
- Print out a copy of your PPR and, if applicable, Plans of Action to have as a reference during the call.
- Plan ahead because you cannot take breaks during the conference call, although participants may step out as long as it does not disrupt the call. If a call is running particularly long, a short break in the call may be feasible.
- Understand that if your organization decides not to participate in the conference call, its Plans of Action and MOS are only reviewed, not approved. When SIG approves Plans of Action and MOS, they cannot be challenged by the surveyors on site. If your organization wants The Joint Commission to approve its Plans of Action and MOS, it must schedule and participate in the conference call.

He or she reviews the following required elements of each plan:
- Actions
- Implementation date
- MOS

If they have comments, the reviewers note them in "The Joint Commission Comments" section of the PPR tool after the call is complete. The review of your PPR does not affect your accreditation decision.

SIG staff members will have familiarized themselves with your long term care organization's PPR before the conference call. No preparation on the part of your organization is required, although staff participants should have a printout of the PPR and associated Plans of Action for reference. In particular, you should print out a conference call report to refer to during the call.

Two people who are knowledgeable about the PPR and its information should be selected as representatives to speak with the SIG staff member during the call, although others involved in the PPR process are encouraged to listen in. If you choose, you may switch staff depending on the topics being covered. However, no more than two people should actively participate in the call at one time. The length of the call varies depending on the results of the PPR and the complexity of the Plans of Action. To help plan the day, your long term care organization should set aside approximately three hours for the staff to participate in the call. *See* Sidebar 9, above, for tips for a productive conference call.

During the phone call, the SIG representative reviews with you your organization's areas of noncompliance, Plans of Action, and any MOS. He or she discusses these elements with you and offers other ideas or additional suggestions. Your long term care organization should raise any questions about the PPR, standards, or Plans of Action at this time.

In some cases, The Joint Commission may determine that your organization is compliant with a standard that you assessed as not compliant and vice versa. If that occurs, the reviewer will note it on the PPR tool to be submitted to The Joint Commission and no Plan of Action is required (or a Plan of Action is required if the standard is found not compliant).

Implementing Your Plan of Action

After your call with The Joint Commission, you must address the issues identified in the PPR. A first step in this process should be revising your Plans of Action based on comments and feedback from The Joint Commission. Individuals in charge of implementing the plans should review the notes taken during the conference call and the notes provided by Joint Commission staff in the PPR. You may choose to add them to your long term care organization's open PPR tool.

TIP *One way to make sure that Plans of Action are sustained is to periodically audit performance. This audit reveals whether a plan is being implemented and performance is improving. If the audit reveals that a plan is not working, your organization should refocus its efforts. However, if the audit shows that a plan is on track and improvement is being realized and sustained, it serves as evidence of successful implementation.*

Sidebar 10. Can My Periodic Performance Review Affect My Accreditation Decision?

The PPR itself cannot affect your accreditation decision. However, failure to participate in the full PPR or an approved option can affect a long term care organization's accreditation decision. When an accredited organization does not participate in the PPR, its decision is changed to Provisional Accreditation 31 days after the PPR due date. After 61 days, this becomes Conditional Accreditation, and after 91 days, the situation is reviewed by The Joint Commission's Accreditation Committee for possible Denial of Accreditation.

Addressing the PPR During the Full On-Site Survey

Typically, this review is done during the Team Planning Meeting on the first day of survey. The surveyors may look for further ESC through discussions with staff, reviews of documents, and observations during tracers. Any MOS data resulting from your PPR should be shared with the surveyor(s) during this meeting.

For those long term care organizations that choose Option 3, because no MOS data is required, surveyors focus only on compliance with all standards at the time of the full survey.

If your long term care organization has not completed the Plans of Action approved by SIG, or if you fail to maintain compliance with all standards, a Requirement for Improvement might require that you outline a resolution in an ESC due within 45 days. (*See* Sidebar 10, above, for more information on how the PPR can affect your accreditation status.)

The Importance of a Thorough PPR

Any time an individual or long term care organization is asked to assess itself, a question arises as to whether it will do a thorough and comprehensive job. Some critics of the PPR process have expressed concern that organizations will complete only a cursory review that indicates full or significant compliance with the standards and APRs instead of performing the suggested thorough review.

In the case of the PPR, it is to your organization's benefit to identify problem areas, work with The Joint Commission on plans for improvement, and address issues in the months before your next on-site survey. The most significant benefit of doing so is that it fully supports continuous standards compliance and the improvement of safety and quality of care in your organization. In addition, if your organization does not identify compliance issues in the PPR and these issues are discovered during the on-site survey, you have only 45 days to correct EPs related to Direct Impact Requirements and 60 days to correct EPs related to Indirect Impact Requirements. If your organization is not compliant with a standard, it is evident at the on-site survey. At that point, you must correct the problem quickly or face a change to your accreditation decision.

Not only is it beneficial for your organization to perform a comprehensive PPR, but your organization is required by Joint Commission policy to be truthful in the assessment process. If false information is provided, The Joint Commission's Information Accuracy and Truthfulness Policy would apply. For more information on this policy, *see* "The Accreditation Process" (ACC) chapter of the *CAMLTC*.

When you thoroughly assess compliance with standards during the PPR process, your organization has time to implement any Plans of Action and create a track record thus reducing the need to "fix" issues right before survey. Instead of using costly ramp-up activities to assess and prove compliance at the last minute before survey, becoming aware of compliance issues and addressing them can happen at a more relaxed pace. By spreading out the compliance process over time, your organization can also move toward continuous standards compliance, thus improving the quality and safety of resident care.

Part 2
Compliance Assessment Checklist

- ☑ National Patient Safety Goals (NPSG)
- ☑ Accreditation Participation Requirements (APR)
- ☑ Ethics, Rights, and Responsibilities (RI)
- ☑ Provision of Care, Treatment, and Services (PC)
- ☑ Medication Management (MM)
- ☑ Surveillance, Prevention, and Control of Infection (IC)
- ☑ Improving Organization Performance (PI)
- ☑ Leadership (LD)
- ☑ Management of the Environment of Care (EC)
- ☑ Life Safety (LS)
- ☑ Management of Human Resources (HR)
- ☑ Management of Information (IM)

The following information is provided after each assessment question:

A or **C** indicates scoring category*

(EP #) indicates the Element of Performance (EP) number as it appears in the *Comprehensive Accreditation Manual for Long Term Care (CAMLTC)*

Ⓜ indicates the requirement for a Measure of Success, if applicable†

▲(2) indicates situational decision rules apply‡

△(3) indicates direct impact requirements apply‡

☆ indicates this standard also applies to organizations seeking Joint Commission's Medicare/Medicaid certification-based long term care accreditation

Please consult the *CAMLTC* to determine which standards and EPs are applicable or not applicable to your organization.

---

* See Part 3 for more information on the scoring categories.

† See Part 3 for more information on the measures of success.

‡ See Part 3 for more information on the criticality of survey findings.

National Patient Safety Goals (NPSG)

This chapter addresses the 2009 National Patient Safety Goals, requirements, and elements of performance for long term care organizations. This chapter has been reformatted to make it consistent with the structure of the standards in this checklist as well as in the CAMLTC. *EPs have been added to each requirement.*

All National Patient Safety Goals also apply to organizations seeking Joint Commission's Medicare/Medicaid Certification–based long term care accreditation and are indicated with a ☆

NPSG.01.01.01 ★

Use at least two resident identifiers when providing care, treatment, or services.

Assessment Question	Level of Compliance	Evidence of Compliance	Action Needed/ Measure of Success (if needed)	Due Date
1. Prior to any specimen collection, medication administration, or treatment, is the resident and family actively involved in the identification and matching process? When active resident involvement is not possible or the resident's reliability is in question, does the organization designate the caregiver responsible for identity verification? **Note:** *The involvement of a single caregiver is acceptable as long as the other components of resident identification are satisfied.* **C (EP 1)** Ⓜ △3				
2. Does the organization use two resident identifiers when administering medications, blood, or blood components? **C (EP 2)** Ⓜ △3				
3. Does the organization use two resident identifiers when collecting blood samples or other specimens for clinical testing? **A (EP 3)** Ⓜ △3				
4. Does the organization use two resident identifiers when providing other treatments or procedures? **C (EP 4)** Ⓜ △3				
5. Is neither the resident's room number nor physical location used as an identifier? **A (EP 5)** △3				
6. Are containers used for blood and other specimens labeled in the presence of the resident? **A (EP 6)** Ⓜ △3				

NPSG.01.02.01 ★

Prior to the start of any surgical or invasive procedure, individuals involved in the procedure conduct a final verification process, such as a time-out, to confirm the correct resident, procedure and site, using active, not passive, communication techniques.

Assessment Question	Level of Compliance	Evidence of Compliance	Action Needed/ Measure of Success (if needed)	Due Date
1. Does the organization conduct a final verification process in the location where the procedure will be done, just before starting the procedure? **A (EP 1)** △3				

Key: 0 = Insufficient compliance; 1 = Partial compliance; 2 = Satisfactory compliance; NA = Not applicable; **A** indicates scoring category A; **C** indicates scoring category C; ▲2 indicates situational decision rules apply; △3 indicates direct impact requirements apply; Ⓜ indicates Measure of success is needed; ☆ indicates this standard also applies to organizations seeking Joint Commission's Medicare/Medicaid certification–based long term care accreditation

NPSG.01.02.01 ★				
Assessment Question	**Level of Compliance**	**Evidence of Compliance**	**Action Needed/ Measure of Success (if needed)**	**Due Date**
2. Does the final verification process involve the entire team, use active communication, and include the following: • Correct resident identity • Correct side and site • Agreement on the procedure to be done • Correct resident position • Availability of correct implants and any special equipment or special requirements? **A (EP 2)** Ⓜ ⚠3				
3. Is the verification process briefly documented in a checklist or other type of documentation determined by the organization? **A (EP 3)** ⚠3				
4. Does the organization have processes and systems in place for reconciling differences in staff responses during the final verification process? **A (EP 4)** ⚠3				

NPSG.02.01.01 ★	For verbal or telephone orders or for telephone reporting of critical test results, the individual giving the order or test result verifies the complete order or test result by having the person receiving the information record and "read back" the complete order or test result.			
Assessment Question	**Level of Compliance**	**Evidence of Compliance**	**Action Needed/ Measure of Success (if needed)**	**Due Date**
1. Does the receiver of the information **write** down the complete order or test result or enter it into a computer? **C (EP 1)** Ⓜ ⚠3				
2. Does the receiver of the information **read** back the complete order or test result? **C (EP 2)** Ⓜ ⚠3				
3. Does the individual who gave the order or test result confirm the information that was read back? **C (EP 3)** Ⓜ ⚠3				

Key: 0 = Insufficient compliance; 1 = Partial compliance; 2 = Satisfactory compliance; NA = Not applicable; **A** indicates scoring category A; **C** indicates scoring category C; ▲ indicates situational decision rules apply; ⚠3 indicates direct impact requirements apply; Ⓜ indicates Measure of success is needed; ☆ indicates this standard also applies to organizations seeking Joint Commission's Medicare/Medicaid certification–based long term care accreditation

NPSG.02.02.01 ★	There is a standardized list of abbreviations, acronyms, symbols, and dose designations that are not to be used throughout the long term care organization.			
Assessment Question	**Level of Compliance**	**Evidence of Compliance**	**Action Needed/ Measure of Success (if needed)**	**Due Date**
1. Has the organization developed a standardized list of abbreviations, acronyms, symbols, and dose designations that are not to be used throughout the organization? **A (EP 1)**				
2. Does the list of abbreviations, acronyms, symbols, and dose designations not to be used include the following: • U,u • IU • Q.D., QD, q.d., qd • Q.O.D., QOD, q.o.d., qod • Trailing zero (X.0 mg)* • Lack of leading zero (.X mg) • MS • MSO_4 • $MgSO_4$? **A (EP 2)** ⚠3				
3. Does the organization implement the "do not use" list and apply this list to all orders and all medication-related documentation when handwritten or entered as free text into a computer? **C (EP 3)** Ⓜ ⚠3				
4. Does the organization ensure that preprinted forms do not include any abbreviations identified as not to be used? **A (EP 4)** ⚠3				

NPSG.02.03.01 ★	The organization measures, assesses, and, if needed, takes action to improve the timeliness of reporting, and the timeliness of receipt of critical tests and critical test results and values by the responsible licensed caregiver.			
Assessment Question	**Level of Compliance**	**Evidence of Compliance**	**Action Needed/ Measure of Success (if needed)**	**Due Date**
1. Does the organization define critical tests and critical results and values? **A (EP 1)**				

* **Exception** A "trailing zero" may be used only where required to demonstrate the level of precision of the value being reported, such as for laboratory results, imaging studies that report size of lesions, or catheter/tube sizes. It may not be used in medication orders or other medication-related documentation.

Key: 0 = Insufficient compliance; 1 = Partial compliance; 2 = Satisfactory compliance; NA = Not applicable; **A** indicates scoring category A; **C** indicates scoring category C; ▲2 indicates situational decision rules apply; ⚠3 indicates direct impact requirements apply; Ⓜ indicates Measure of success is needed; ☆ indicates this standard also applies to organizations seeking Joint Commission's Medicare/Medicaid certification–based long term care accreditation

NPSG.02.03.01 ★

Assessment Question	Level of Compliance	Evidence of Compliance	Plan of Action/ Measure of Success (if needed)	Due Date
2. Does the organization define the acceptable length of time between the ordering of critical tests and reporting the results of these tests whether normal or abnormal? **A (EP 2)**				
3. Does the organization define the acceptable length of time for reporting the results of routine tests with critical abnormal values or findings? **A (EP 3)**				
4. Does the organization define the acceptable length of time between the availability of critical tests and critical results and values and receipt by the responsible licensed caregiver? **A (EP 4)**				
5. Does the organization collect data on the timeliness of reporting critical test results and critical results and values from routine tests? **A (EP 5)**				
6. Does the organization assess the data on the timeliness of reporting critical test results and critical results and values from routine tests and determine whether a need for improvement exists? **A (EP 6)**				
7. Does the organization take appropriate action to improve the timeliness of reporting critical test results and critical results and values from routine tests and measure the effectiveness of those actions? **A (EP 7)**				

NPSG.02.05.01 ★

The organization implements a standardized approach to hand-off communications, including an opportunity to ask and respond to questions.

Assessment Question	Level of Compliance	Evidence of Compliance	Plan of Action/ Measure of Success (if needed)	Due Date
1. Does the organization's process for effective "hand-off" communication include interactive communications allowing for the opportunity for questioning between the giver and receiver of resident information? **C (EP 1)** Ⓜ ⚠3				

Key: 0 = Insufficient compliance; 1 = Partial compliance; 2 = Satisfactory compliance; NA = Not applicable; **A** indicates scoring category A; **C** indicates scoring category C; ▲2 indicates situational decision rules apply; △3 indicates direct impact requirements apply; Ⓜ indicates Measure of success is needed; ☆ indicates this standard also applies to organizations seeking Joint Commission's Medicare/Medicaid certification–based long term care accreditation

NPSG.02.05.01 ★

Assessment Question	Level of Compliance	Evidence of Compliance	Action Needed/ Measure of Success (if needed)	Due Date
2. Does the organization's process for effective hand-off communication include up-to-date information regarding the resident's condition, care, treatment, medications, services, and any recent or anticipated changes? (*See also* NPSG.08.01.01, EP 4) **C (EP 2)** Ⓜ ⚠3				
3. Does the organization's process for effective "hand-off" communication include a process for verification of the received information, including repeat-back or read-back techniques? **C (EP 3)** Ⓜ ⚠3				
4. Does the organization's process for effective "hand-off" communication include an opportunity for the receiver of the hand off information to review relevant resident historical data, which may include previous care, treatment, and services? **A (EP 4)** ⚠3				
5. Are interruptions during handoffs limited to minimize the possibility that information would fail to be conveyed or would be forgotten? **C (EP 5)** Ⓜ ⚠3				

NPSG.03.03.01 ★

The organization identifies and, at a minimum, annually reviews a list of look-alike/sound-alike medications used by the organization and takes action to prevent errors involving the interchange of these medications.

Assessment Question	Level of Compliance	Evidence of Compliance	Plan of Action/ Measure of Success (if needed)	Due Date
1. Has the organization identified a list of look-alike/sound-alike (LASA) drugs used by the organization (the list must include a minimum of 10 LASA drug combinations selected from the tables of LASA drugs posted on The Joint Commission Web site)? **A (EP 1)**				
2. Does the organization review the list of LASA drugs used by the organization at least annually? **A (EP 2)**				
3. Does the organization take action to prevent errors involving the interchange of these drugs? **A (EP 3)** ⚠3				

Key: 0 = Insufficient compliance; 1 = Partial compliance; 2 = Satisfactory compliance; NA = Not applicable; **A** indicates scoring category A; **C** indicates scoring category C; ▲ indicates situational decision rules apply; ⚠3 indicates direct impact requirements apply; Ⓜ indicates Measure of success is needed; ☆ indicates this standard also applies to organizations seeking Joint Commission's Medicare/Medicaid certification–based long term care accreditation

NPSG.03.05.01 ★	Reduce the likelihood of resident harm associated with the use of anticoagulant therapy.			
Assessment Question	**Level of Compliance**	**Evidence of Compliance**	**Action Needed/ Measure of Success (if needed)**	**Due Date**
1. Has the organization implemented a defined anticoagulation management program to individualize the care provided to each resident receiving anticoagulant therapy? **A (EP 1)** △3				
2. To reduce compounding and labeling errors, does the organization use only oral unit-dose products, pre-filled syringes, or pre-mixed infusion bags when these products are available? **Note:** *For pediatric patients, pre-loaded syringe products should only be used if specifically designed for children.* **A (EP 2)** △3				
3. Does the organization use approved protocols for the initiation and maintenance of anticoagulant therapy appropriate to the medication used, to the condition being treated, and to the potential for medication interactions? **C (EP 3)** Ⓜ △3				
4. For residents being started on warfarin, is a baseline International Normalized Ratio (INR) available? For all residents receiving warfarin therapy, is a current INR available and used to monitor and adjust this therapy? **A (EP 4)** △3				
5. When dietary services are provided by the organization, is the service notified of all residents receiving warfarin, and does the service respond according to its established food/medication interaction program? **C (EP 5)** Ⓜ △3				
6. When heparin is administered intravenously and continuously, does the organization use programmable infusion pumps in order to provide consistent and accurate dosing? **A (EP 6)** △3				
7. Does the organization have a written policy that addresses baseline and ongoing laboratory tests that are required for heparin and low molecular weight heparin therapies? **A (EP 7)** △3				

Key: 0 = Insufficient compliance; 1 = Partial compliance; 2 = Satisfactory compliance; NA = Not applicable; **A** indicates scoring category A; **C** indicates scoring category C; ▲2 indicates situational decision rules apply; △3 indicates direct impact requirements apply; Ⓜ indicates Measure of success is needed; ☆ indicates this standard also applies to organizations seeking Joint Commission's Medicare/Medicaid certification–based long term care accreditation

NPSG.03.05.01 ★

Assessment Question	Level of Compliance	Evidence of Compliance	Action Needed/ Measure of Success (if needed)	Due Date
8. Does the organization provide education regarding anticoagulation therapy to staff, residents, and families? **Note:** *Resident/family education includes the importance of follow-up monitoring, compliance issues, dietary restrictions, and potential for adverse drug reactions and interactions.* **C (EP 8)** Ⓜ △3				
9. Does the organization evaluate its anticoagulation safety practices, take appropriate action to improve its practices, and measure the effectiveness of those actions on a regular basis? **A (EP 9)**				

NPSG.07.01.01 ★

Comply with current World Health Organization (WHO) Hand Hygiene Guidelines or Centers for Disease Control and Prevention (CDC) hand hygiene guidelines.

Assessment Question	Level of Compliance	Evidence of Compliance	Action Needed/ Measure of Success (if needed)	Due Date
1. Does the organization comply with current World Health Organization (WHO) hand hygiene guidelines or Centers for Disease Control and Prevention (CDC) hand hygiene guidelines?* **C (EP 1)** Ⓜ △3				

NPSG.07.02.01 ★

Manage as sentinel events all identified cases of unanticipated death or major permanent loss of function related to a health care-associated infection.

Assessment Question	Level of Compliance	Evidence of Compliance	Plan of Action/ Measure of Success (if needed)	Due Date
1. Does the organization manage all identified cases of unanticipated death or major permanent loss of function associated with a health care–associated infection as sentinel events (that is, conduct a root cause analysis)? **C (EP 1)** Ⓜ △3				
2. Does the root cause analysis address the management of the resident before and after the identification of infection? **A (EP 2)**				

* Organizations are required to comply with all 1A, 1B, and 1C CDC or WHO guidelines.

Key: 0 = Insufficient compliance; 1 = Partial compliance; 2 = Satisfactory compliance; NA = Not applicable; **A** indicates scoring category A; **C** indicates scoring category C; ▲2 indicates situational decision rules apply; △3 indicates direct impact requirements apply; Ⓜ indicates Measure of success is needed; ☆ indicates this standard also applies to organizations seeking Joint Commission's Medicare/Medicaid certification–based long term care accreditation

NPSG.07.04.01 ★	Implement best practices or evidence-based guidelines to prevent central line-associated bloodstream infections. **Note:** *This requirement covers short- and long-term central venous catheters and peripherally inserted central catheter (PICC) lines.* **Note:** *This requirement has a one-year phase-in period that includes defined expectations for planning, development, and testing ("milestones") at three, six, and nine months in 2009, with the expectation of full implementation by January 1, 2010.*			
Assessment Question	**Level of Compliance**	**Evidence of Compliance**	**Plan of Action/ Measure of Success (if needed)**	**Due Date**
1. As of April 1, 2009, does the organization's leadership assign responsibility for oversight and coordination of the development, testing, and implementation of NPSG.07.04.01? **A (EP 1)**				
2. As of July 1, 2009, is an implementation work plan in place that identifies adequate resources, assigned accountabilities, and a time line for full implementation of NPSG.07.04.01 by January 1, 2010? **A (EP 2)**				
3. As of October 1, 2009, is pilot testing in at least one clinical unit under way for the requirements in NPSG.07.04.01? **A (EP 3)**				
4. As of January 1, 2010, are the elements of performance in NPSG.07.04.01 fully implemented across the organization? **A (EP 4)** △3				
5. As of January 1, 2010, does the organization educate health care workers who are involved in these procedures about health care–associated infections, central line–associated bloodstream infections, and the importance of prevention? Does the education occur upon hire, annually thereafter, and when involvement in these procedures is added to an individual's job responsibilities? **C (EP 5)** Ⓜ				
6. As of January 1, 2010, does the organization educate residents, and their families as needed, about central line–associated bloodstream infection prevention prior to insertion of a central venous catheter? **C (EP 6)** Ⓜ				

Key: 0 = Insufficient compliance; 1 = Partial compliance; 2 = Satisfactory compliance; NA = Not applicable; **A** indicates scoring category A; **C** indicates scoring category C; ▲2 indicates situational decision rules apply; △3 indicates direct impact requirements apply; Ⓜ indicates Measure of success is needed; ☆ indicates this standard also applies to organizations seeking Joint Commission's Medicare/Medicaid certification–based long term care accreditation

NPSG.07.04.01

Assessment Question	Level of Compliance	Evidence of Compliance	Plan of Action/ Measure of Success (if needed)	Due Date
7. As of January 1, 2010, does the organization implement policies and practices aimed at reducing the risk of central line–associated bloodstream infections that meet regulatory requirements and are aligned with evidence-based standards (for example, the Centers for Disease Control and Prevention (CDC) and/or professional organization guidelines)? **C (EP 7)** Ⓜ ⚠3				
8. As of January 1, 2010, does the organization conduct periodic risk assessment for surgical site infections, measure central line–associated bloodstream infection rates, monitor compliance with best practices or evidence-based guidelines, and evaluate the effectiveness of prevention efforts? **A (EP 8)**				
9. As of January 1, 2010, does the organization provide central line–associated bloodstream infections rate data and prevention outcome measures to key stakeholders including leaders, licensed independent practitioners, nursing staff, and other clinicians? **A (EP 9)**				
10. As of January 1, 2010, does the organization use a standardized protocol to disinfect catheter hubs and injection ports before accessing the ports? **A (EP 16)** ⚠3				
11. As of January 1, 2010, does the organization evaluate all central venous catheters routinely and remove nonessential catheters? **A (EP 17)** ⚠3				

NPSG.08.01.01 ★

There is a process for comparing the resident's current medications with those ordered for the resident while under the care of the organization.

Assessment Question	Level of Compliance	Evidence of Compliance	Plan of Action/ Measure of Success (if needed)	Due Date
1. At the time the resident enters the organization or is admitted, does the organization create and document a complete list of the medications the resident is taking at home (including dose, route, and frequency)? Is the resident, and family as needed, involved in creating this list? **C (EP 1)** Ⓜ ⚠3				

Key: 0 = Insufficient compliance; 1 = Partial compliance; 2 = Satisfactory compliance; NA = Not applicable; **A** indicates scoring category A; **C** indicates scoring category C; ▲2 indicates situational decision rules apply; ⚠3 indicates direct impact requirements apply; Ⓜ indicates Measure of success is needed; ☆ indicates this standard also applies to organizations seeking Joint Commission's Medicare/Medicaid certification–based long term care accreditation

NPSG.08.01.01 ★

Assessment Question	Level of Compliance	Evidence of Compliance	Plan of Action/ Measure of Success (if needed)	Due Date
2. Are the medications ordered for the resident while under the care of the organization compared to those on the list created at the time of entry to the organization or admission? **C (EP 2)** Ⓜ △3				
3. Are any discrepancies (that is, omissions, duplications, adjustments, deletions, additions) reconciled and documented while the resident is under the care of the organization? **C (EP 3)** Ⓜ △3				
4. When the resident's care is transferred within the organization, does the current provider(s) inform the receiving provider(s) about the up-to-date reconciled medication list and document the communication? **Note:** *Updating the status of a resident's medications is also an important component of all resident care hand-offs.* (See also *NPSG.02.05.01, EP 2*) **C (EP 4)** Ⓜ △3				

NPSG.08.02.01 ★

When a resident is referred to or transferred from one organization to another, the complete and reconciled list of medications is communicated to the next provider of service, and the communication is documented. Alternatively, when a resident leaves the organization's care to go directly to his or her home, the complete and reconciled list of medications is provided to the resident's known primary care provider, original referring provider, or a known next provider of service.

Note: *When the next provider of service is unknown or when no known formal relationship is planned with a next provider, giving the resident and, as needed, the family the list of reconciled medications is sufficient.*

Assessment Question	Level of Compliance	Evidence of Compliance	Plan of Action/ Measure of Success (if needed)	Due Date
1. Is the resident's most current reconciled medication list communicated to the next provider of service, either within or outside the organization? Is the communication between providers documented? **C (EP 1)** Ⓜ △3				
2. At the time of transfer, does the transferring organization inform the next provider of service how to obtain clarification on the list of reconciled medications? **C (EP 2)** Ⓜ				

Key: 0 = Insufficient compliance; 1 = Partial compliance; 2 = Satisfactory compliance; NA = Not applicable; **A** indicates scoring category A; **C** indicates scoring category C; ▲2 indicates situational decision rules apply; △3 indicates direct impact requirements apply; Ⓜ indicates Measure of success is needed; ☆ indicates this standard also applies to organizations seeking Joint Commission's Medicare/Medicaid certification–based long term care accreditation

NPSG.08.03.01 ★	When a resident leaves the organization's care, a complete and reconciled list of the resident's medications is provided directly to the resident and, as needed, the family and the list is explained to the resident and/or family.			
Assessment Question	**Level of Compliance**	**Evidence of Compliance**	**Plan of Action/ Measure of Success (if needed)**	**Due Date**
1. When the resident leaves the organization's care, is the current list of reconciled medications provided to the resident, and family as needed? Is the list explained to the resident and/or family? Is the interaction documented? **Note:** *Residents and families are reminded to discard old lists and to update any records with all medication providers or retail pharmacies.* **C (EP 1) Ⓜ**				

NPSG.08.04.01 ★	In settings where medications are used minimally or prescribed for a short duration, modified medication reconciliation processes are performed. **Note:** *This requirement does not apply to organizations that do not administer medications. However, it may be important for health care organizations to know which types of medications their residents are taking because these medications could affect the care, treatment, or services provided.*			
Assessment Question	**Level of Compliance**	**Evidence of Compliance**	**Plan of Action/ Measure of Success (if needed)**	**Due Date**
1. Does the organization obtain and document an accurate list of the resident's current medications and known allergies in order to safely prescribe any setting–specific medications (for example, local anesthesia, antibiotics) and to assess for potential allergic or adverse drug reactions? **C (EP 1) Ⓜ ⚠3**				
2. When only short-term medications (for example., a pre-procedure medication or a short-term course of an antibiotic) will be prescribed and no changes are made to the resident's current medication list, is the resident and family as needed, provided with a list containing the short-term medication additions that the resident will continue after leaving the organization? **Note:** *This list of new short-term medications is not considered to be part of the original, known and current medication list. When residents leave these settings, a list of the original, known, and current medications does not need to be provided unless the resident is assessed to be confused or unable to comprehend adequately. In this case, the resident's family is provided both medication lists, and the circumstances are documented.* **C (EP 2) Ⓜ**				

Key: 0 = Insufficient compliance; 1 = Partial compliance; 2 = Satisfactory compliance; NA = Not applicable; **A** indicates scoring category A; **C** indicates scoring category C; ▲2 indicates situational decision rules apply; ⚠3 indicates direct impact requirements apply; Ⓜ indicates Measure of success is needed; ☆ indicates this standard also applies to organizations seeking Joint Commission's Medicare/Medicaid certification–based long term care accreditation

NPSG.08.04.01 ★

Assessment Question	Level of Compliance	Evidence of Compliance	Plan of Action/ Measure of Success (if needed)	Due Date
3. Is there a complete, documented medication reconciliation process used when any new long-term (chronic) medications are prescribed? **C (EP 3)** Ⓜ △3				
4. Is there a complete, documented medication reconciliation process used when there is a prescription change for any of the resident's current known long-term medications? **C (EP 4)** Ⓜ △3				
5. Is there a complete, documented medication reconciliation process used when the resident is required to be subsequently admitted to an organization from these settings for ongoing care? **C (EP 5)** Ⓜ △3				
6. When a complete documented, medication reconciliation is required in any of these settings, is the complete list of reconciled medications provided to the resident and the resident's family as needed, and to the resident's known primary care provider or original referring provider, or a known next provider of service? **C (EP 6)** Ⓜ △3				

NPSG.09.02.01 ★

The organization implements a fall reduction program that includes an evaluation of the effectiveness of the program.

Assessment Question	Level of Compliance	Evidence of Compliance	Plan of Action/ Measure of Success (if needed)	Due Date
1. Has the organization established a fall reduction program? **A (EP 1)**				
2. Does the fall reduction program include an evaluation appropriate to the resident populations, settings, and services provided? **C (EP 2)** Ⓜ △3				
3. Does the fall reduction program include interventions to reduce the resident's fall risk factors? **A (EP 3)** △3				
4. Do staff members receive education and training for the fall reduction program? **C (EP 4)** Ⓜ				

Key: 0 = Insufficient compliance; 1 = Partial compliance; 2 = Satisfactory compliance; NA = Not applicable; **A** indicates scoring category A; **C** indicates scoring category C; ▲2 indicates situational decision rules apply; △3 indicates direct impact requirements apply; Ⓜ indicates Measure of success is needed; ☆ indicates this standard also applies to organizations seeking Joint Commission's Medicare/Medicaid certification–based long term care accreditation

NPSG.09.02.01 ★				
Assessment Question	**Level of Compliance**	**Evidence of Compliance**	**Action Needed/ Measure of Success (if needed)**	**Due Date**
5. Is the resident and resident's family educated on the fall reduction program and any individualized fall reduction strategies? **C (EP 5) Ⓜ**				
6. Is the fall reduction program evaluated to determine the effectiveness of the program? (Outcome indicators such as decreased number of falls and decreased number and severity of fall-related injuries could be used.) **A (EP 6)**				

NPSG.10.01.01 ★	The organization develops and implements protocols for administration of the influenza vaccine.			
Assessment Question	**Level of Compliance**	**Evidence of Compliance**	**Action Needed/ Measure of Success (if needed)**	**Due Date**
1. Does the organization develop appropriate protocols to determine whether or not to administer the influenza vaccine to residents? **A (EP 1) △3**				
2. Is there evidence that protocols were implemented to identify residents as high risk for influenza? **C (EP 2) Ⓜ △3**				

NPSG.10.02.01 ★	The organization develops and implements protocols for administration of the pneumococcus vaccine.			
Assessment Question	**Level of Compliance**	**Evidence of Compliance**	**Action Needed/ Measure of Success (if needed)**	**Due Date**
1. Did the organization develop appropriate protocols to determine whether or not to administer the pneumococcus vaccine to residents? **A (EP 1) △3**				
2. Is there evidence that protocols were implemented to identify residents as high risk for pneumococcus? **C (EP 2) Ⓜ △3**				

Key: 0 = Insufficient compliance; 1 = Partial compliance; 2 = Satisfactory compliance; NA = Not applicable; **A** indicates scoring category A; **C** indicates scoring category C; ▲2 indicates situational decision rules apply; △3 indicates direct impact requirements apply; Ⓜ indicates Measure of success is needed; ☆ indicates this standard also applies to organizations seeking Joint Commission's Medicare/Medicaid certification–based long term care accreditation

NPSG.10.03.01 ★	The organization develops and implements protocols to identify new cases of influenza and to manage outbreaks.			
Assessment Question	**Level of Compliance**	**Evidence of Compliance**	**Action Needed/ Measure of Success (if needed)**	**Due Date**
1. Has the organization developed protocols to identify new cases of influenza and to manage an outbreak? **A (EP 1)** ⚠3				
2. Are protocols implemented for residents displaying signs and symptoms of influenza? **C (EP 2)** Ⓜ ⚠3				
3. Is there evidence that the organization managed (or identified) and tracked any influenza outbreaks? **A (EP 3)**				

NPSG.13.01.01 ★	Identify the ways in which the resident and his or her family can report concerns about safety and encourage them to do so.			
Assessment Question	**Level of Compliance**	**Evidence of Compliance**	**Action Needed/ Measure of Success (if needed)**	**Due Date**
1. Are residents and families educated on methods available to report concerns related to care, treatment, services, and resident safety issues? **C (EP 1)** Ⓜ				
2. Does the organization provide the resident with information regarding infection control measures for hand hygiene practices, respiratory hygiene practices, and contact precautions according to the resident's condition? Is the information discussed with the resident and family members on the day the resident enters the organization? Is the resident's understanding evaluated and documented? **Note:** *The information provided to the resident may be in any form of media.* **C (EP 2)** Ⓜ				
3. Does the organization encourage residents and their families to report concerns about safety? **C (EP 4)** Ⓜ				

Key: 0 = Insufficient compliance; 1 = Partial compliance; 2 = Satisfactory compliance; NA = Not applicable; **A** indicates scoring category A; **C** indicates scoring category C; ▲2 indicates situational decision rules apply; ⚠3 indicates direct impact requirements apply; Ⓜ indicates Measure of success is needed; ☆ indicates this standard also applies to organizations seeking Joint Commission's Medicare/Medicaid certification–based long term care accreditation

NPSG.14.01.01 ★	Assess and periodically reassess each resident's risk for developing a pressure ulcer (decubitus ulcer) and take action to address any identified risks.			
Assessment Question	**Level of Compliance**	**Evidence of Compliance**	**Action Needed/ Measure of Success (if needed)**	**Due Date**
1. Does the organization have a written plan for the prediction, prevention, and early treatment of pressure ulcers, which addresses: • Identifying individuals at risk for pressure ulcers and the specific factors placing them at risk • Maintaining and improving tissue tolerance to pressure in order to prevent injury • Protecting against the adverse effects of external mechanical forces • Reducing the incidence of pressure ulcers through staff educational programs? **A (EP 1)**				
2. Does the organization perform an initial assessment for the risk of pressure ulcers for each resident at admission? **C (EP 2)** Ⓜ ⚠3				
3. Does the organization conduct systematic risk assessments for pressure ulcers using a validated risk assessment tool such as the Braden Scale or Norton Scale? **C (EP 3)** Ⓜ ⚠3				
4. Does the organization reassess pressure ulcers at periodic intervals? **C (EP 4)** Ⓜ ⚠3				
5. Does the organization take action to address any identified pressure ulcer risks? **C (EP 5)** Ⓜ ⚠3				

Key: 0 = Insufficient compliance; 1 = Partial compliance; 2 = Satisfactory compliance; NA = Not applicable; **A** indicates scoring category A; **C** indicates scoring category C; ▲2 indicates situational decision rules apply; ⚠3 indicates direct impact requirements apply; Ⓜ indicates Measure of success is needed; ☆ indicates this standard also applies to organizations seeking Joint Commission's Medicare/Medicaid certification–based long term care accreditation

Accreditation Participation Requirements (APR)

APR.01.01.01 ★	The organization submits information to The Joint Commission as required.			
Assessment Question	**Level of Compliance**	**Evidence of Compliance**	**Plan of Action/ Measure of Success (if needed)**	**Due Date**
1. Does the organization meet all requirements for timely submissions of data and information to The Joint Commission? **Note:** *The Joint Commission will impose the following consequences for failure to comply with this APR:* • *If the organization does not comply with this requirement after 31 days, the organization will be placed in Provisional Accreditation.* • *If the organization does not comply with the requirement after 61 days, the organization's accreditation decision will be changed from Provisional Accreditation to Conditional Accreditation.* • *If the organization does not comply with the requirement after 91 days, the organization's accreditation decision will be changed from Conditional Accreditation to Denial of Accreditation. In accordance with the Accreditation Committee policy, such organizations will not be afforded any appeal.* *The proposed consequences address only compliance with the requirement itself. They do not address the content of the organization's submissions to The Joint Commission. For example, if information in an organization's electronic application for accreditation (e-App) leads to inaccuracies in the appropriate length of the survey and a longer survey is required, the organization will incur the additional costs of the longer survey. In addition, if there is evidence that the organization has intentionally falsified the information submitted to The Joint Commission, the requirement at APR.01.02.01, EP 1, and its consequences will apply.* (See also *APR.01.02.01, EP 1)* **A (EP 1)** ▲2				

Key: 0 = Insufficient compliance; 1 = Partial compliance; 2 = Satisfactory compliance; NA = Not applicable; **A** indicates scoring category A; **C** indicates scoring category C; ▲2 indicates situational decision rules apply; △3 indicates direct impact requirements apply; Ⓜ indicates Measure of success is needed; ☆ indicates this APR also applies to organizations seeking Joint Commission's Medicare/Medicaid certification–based long term care accreditation

APR.01.02.01 ★	The organization provides accurate information throughout the accreditation process.			
Assessment Question	**Level of Compliance**	**Evidence of Compliance**	**Plan of Action/ Measure of Success (if needed)**	**Due Date**
1. Does the organization provide accurate information throughout the accreditation process? (*See also* APR.01.01.01, EP 1) **Note 1:** *Information may be received in any of the following ways:* • *Provided verbally* • *Obtained through direct observation by, or in an interview or any other type of communication with, a Joint Commission employee* • *Derived from documents supplied by the organization to The Joint Commission* • *Submitted electronically by the organization through a performance measurement system to The Joint Commission* **Note 2:** *For the purpose of this requirement, falsification is defined as the fabrication, in whole or in part, of any information provided by an applicant or accredited organization to The Joint Commission. This includes redrafting, reformatting, or deleting document content. However, the organization may submit supporting material that explains the original information submitted to The Joint Commission. These additional materials must be properly identified, dated, and accompanied by the original documents.* **A (EP 1)** ▲2				

APR.01.03.01 ★	The organization reports any changes in the information provided in the application for accreditation and any changes made between surveys.			
Assessment Question	**Level of Compliance**	**Evidence of Compliance**	**Plan of Action/ Measure of Success (if needed)**	**Due Date**
1. Does the organization notify The Joint Commission in writing within 30 days of a change in ownership, control, location, capacity, or services offered? **Note:** *When the organization changes ownership, control, location, capacity or services offered, it may be necessary for The Joint Commission to survey the organization again. If the organization does not provide written notification to The Joint Commission within 30 days of these changes, the organization could lose its accreditation.* **A (EP 1)**				

Key: 0 = Insufficient compliance; 1 = Partial compliance; 2 = Satisfactory compliance; NA = Not applicable; **A** indicates scoring category A; **C** indicates scoring category C; ▲2 indicates situational decision rules apply; △3 indicates direct impact requirements apply; Ⓜ indicates Measure of success is needed; ☆ indicates this APR also applies to organizations seeking Joint Commission's Medicare/Medicaid certification–based long term care accreditation

APR.02.01.01 ★	The organization permits the performance of a survey at The Joint Commission's discretion.			
Assessment Question	**Level of Compliance**	**Evidence of Compliance**	**Plan of Action/ Measure of Success (if needed)**	**Due Date**
1. Does the organization permit the performance of a survey? **A (EP 1)** ▲2				

APR.03.01.01	The organization fulfills requirements for Periodic Performance Review.			
Assessment Question	**Level of Compliance**	**Evidence of Compliance**	**Plan of Action/ Measure of Success (if needed)**	**Due Date**
1. Does the organization annually update and transmit to The Joint Commission the full Periodic Performance Review (PPR) and its plan of action on any recommendations cited? (Refer also to "PPR Options" in "The Accreditation Process" chapter of the *CAMLTC*) **Note:** *For organizations that select Options 1, 2, or 3, the requirement to transmit the PPR and its plan of action to The Joint Commission may not apply in part or in whole.* **A (EP 1)** ▲2				
2. Does the organization exercising Option 1, 2, or 3 for the Periodic Performance Review (PPR) annually attest that, after careful consideration with legal counsel, the organization has decided not to participate in the full PPR and instead intends to undergo a limited survey? **A (EP 3)**				
3. Does the organization exercising Option 1 for the Periodic Performance Review (PPR) complete a PPR and plan of action? **Note:** *The organization does not submit this information to The Joint Commission.* **A (EP 4)**				
4. Does organization exercising Option 2 for the Periodic Performance Review agree to undergo a limited survey and submit a plan of action for recommendations cited as a result of the survey? **A (EP 6)**				
5. Does the organization exercising Option 3 for the Periodic Performance Review agree to undergo a limited survey? **Note:** *The organization does not receive a written report after the survey.* **A (EP 7)**				

Key: 0 = Insufficient compliance; 1 = Partial compliance; 2 = Satisfactory compliance; NA = Not applicable; **A** indicates scoring category A; **C** indicates scoring category C; ▲2 indicates situational decision rules apply; △3 indicates direct impact requirements apply; Ⓜ indicates Measure of success is needed; ☆ indicates this APR also applies to organizations seeking Joint Commission's Medicare/Medicaid certification–based long term care accreditation

APR.04.01.01 ★	The organization selects and uses core performance measures relevant to the services it provides and population(s) it serves.			
Assessment Question	**Level of Compliance**	**Evidence of Compliance**	**Plan of Action/ Measure of Success (if needed)**	**Due Date**
1. Does the Medicare/Medicaid-certified organization required to collect and submit Minimum Data Set data to a state agency provide surveyors with Monthly Facility Quality Indicator reports? **A (EP 6)**				
2. Does the Medicare/Medicaid-certified organization required to collect and submit Minimum Data Set data to a state agency provide surveyors with Quality Measure reports? **A (EP 7)**				
3. Does the Medicare/Medicaid-certified organization required to collect and submit Minimum Data Set data to a state agency provide surveyors with CMS Form 2567 reports? **A (EP 8)**				
4. Does the Medicare/Medicaid-certified organization required to collect and submit Minimum Data Set data to a state agency provide surveyors with Plans of Correction? **A (EP 9)**				
5. Does the Medicare/Medicaid-certified organization required to collect and submit Minimum Data Set data to a state agency provide surveyors with publicly reported Quality Measure reports? **A (EP 10)**				
6. Does the organization not collecting Minimum Data Set data select a sufficient number of measures from an approved performance measurement system to meet current ORYX requirements? **A (EP 11)**				
7. Does the organization notify The Joint Commission of its performance measures selections by the required date? **A (EP 12)**				
8. Does the organization discuss with the surveyor how the data are used to identify, prioritize, and monitor performance improvement activities? **A (EP 17)**				

Key: 0 = Insufficient compliance; 1 = Partial compliance; 2 = Satisfactory compliance; NA = Not applicable; **A** indicates scoring category A; **C** indicates scoring category C; ▲(2) indicates situational decision rules apply; △(3) indicates direct impact requirements apply; Ⓜ indicates Measure of success is needed; ☆ indicates this APR also applies to organizations seeking Joint Commission's Medicare/Medicaid certification–based long term care accreditation

APR.04.01.01

Assessment Question	Level of Compliance	Evidence of Compliance	Plan of Action/ Measure of Success (if needed)	Due Date
9. Does the organization use an individual measure for at least four consecutive quarters before replacing it? **A (EP 18)**				
10. Does the organization continue to use a measure if the data suggest an unstable pattern of performance or otherwise identify an opportunity for improvement? **A (EP 19)**				
11. Does the organization select a new measure if the data reflect stable and satisfactory performance? **A (EP 20)**				
12. Does the organization participating in a performance measurement system notify The Joint Commission of any changes in its measure selection? **A (EP 21)**				
13. Does the organization participating in a performance measurement system submit aggregate data to The Joint Commission at least quarterly? **A (EP 25)**				

APR.05.01.01 ★

The organization allows The Joint Commission to review the results of external evaluations from publicly recognized bodies.

Assessment Question	Level of Compliance	Evidence of Compliance	Plan of Action/ Measure of Success (if needed)	Due Date
1. When requested, does the organization provide The Joint Commission with all official record and report of licensing, examining, reviewing, or planning bodies? **A (EP 1)**				
2. Does the organization notify The Joint Commission when it is designated by the Centers for Medicare & Medicaid Services (CMS) as a Special Focus Facility prior to public announcement of its designation by CMS? **Note:** *If the organization fails to notify The Joint Commission, a recommendation will be made to the Accreditation Committee to place the organization in Conditional Accreditation.* **A (EP 3)** ▲2				

Key: 0 = Insufficient compliance; 1 = Partial compliance; 2 = Satisfactory compliance; NA = Not applicable; **A** indicates scoring category A; **C** indicates scoring category C; ▲2 indicates situational decision rules apply; △3 indicates direct impact requirements apply; Ⓜ indicates Measure of success is needed; ☆ indicates this APR also applies to organizations seeking Joint Commission's Medicare/Medicaid certification–based long term care accreditation

APR.06.01.01 ★	Applicant or accredited organizations do not use Joint Commission employees to provide accreditation-related consulting services.			
Assessment Question	**Level of Compliance**	**Evidence of Compliance**	**Plan of Action/ Measure of Success (if needed)**	**Due Date**
1. Does the organization not use Joint Commission employees to provide any accreditation-related consulting services? **Note:** *Consulting services include, but are not limited to, the following:* • *Helping the organization to meet Joint Commission standards* • *Helping the organization to complete its Periodic Performance Review (PPR)* • *Assisting the organization in remedying areas identified in its PPR as needing improvement* • *Conducting mock surveys* • *Providing the organization with consultation to address Priority Focus Process information* **A (EP 1)** ▲2				

APR.07.01.01 ★	The organization accepts the presence of Joint Commission surveyor management staff or a Board of Commissioners member in the role of observer of an on-site survey.			
Assessment Question	**Level of Compliance**	**Evidence of Compliance**	**Plan of Action/ Measure of Success (if needed)**	**Due Date**
1. Does the organization allow Joint Commission surveyor management staff or a member of the Board of Commissioners to observe the on-site survey? **Note:** *The observer will not participate in the on-site survey process, including the scoring of standards compliance. The organization will not incur any additional survey fees because an observer(s) is present.* **A (EP 1)**				

APR.08.01.01 ★	The organization accurately represents its accreditation status and the facilities and services to which Joint Commission accreditation applies.			
Assessment Question	**Level of Compliance**	**Evidence of Compliance**	**Plan of Action/ Measure of Success (if needed)**	**Due Date**
1. Does the organization's advertising accurately reflect the scope of facilities and services that are accredited by The Joint Commission? **A (EP 1)**				
2. Does the organization not engage in any false or misleading advertising about its accreditation award? **A (EP 2)**				

Key: 0 = Insufficient compliance; 1 = Partial compliance; 2 = Satisfactory compliance; NA = Not applicable; **A** indicates scoring category A; **C** indicates scoring category C; ▲2 indicates situational decision rules apply; △3 indicates direct impact requirements apply; Ⓜ indicates Measure of success is needed; ☆ indicates this APR also applies to organizations seeking Joint Commission's Medicare/Medicaid certification–based long term care accreditation

APR.09.01.01 ★	The organization notifies its public about how to contact its organization management or The Joint Commission to report concerns about resident safety and quality of care. **Note:** *Methods of notice may include, but are not limited to, distribution of information about The Joint Commission, including contact information in published materials such as brochures and/or posting this information on the organization's web site.*			
Assessment Question	**Level of Compliance**	**Evidence of Compliance**	**Plan of Action/ Measure of Success (if needed)**	**Due Date**
1. Does the organization inform the public it serves about how to contact its management to report concerns about resident safety and quality of care? **A (EP 1)**				
2. Does the organization inform the public it serves about how to contact The Joint Commission to report concerns about resident safety and quality of care? **A (EP 2)**				

APR.09.02.01 ★	Any individual who provides care, treatment, or services can report concerns about safety or the quality of care to The Joint Commission without retaliatory action from the organization.			
Assessment Question	**Level of Compliance**	**Evidence of Compliance**	**Plan of Action/ Measure of Success (if needed)**	**Due Date**
1. Does the organization educate its staff that any employee or other individual who provides care, treatment, or services or who has concerns about the safety or quality of care provided in the organization may report these concerns to The Joint Commission? **A (EP 1)**				
2. Does the organization inform its staff that it will take no disciplinary or punitive action because an employee or other individual who provides care, treatment, or services reports safety or quality-of-care concerns to The Joint Commission? **A (EP 2)**				
3. Does the organization take no disciplinary or punitive action against employees or other individuals who provide care, treatment, or services when they report safety or quality-of-care concerns to The Joint Commission? **A (EP 3)**				

Key: 0 = Insufficient compliance; 1 = Partial compliance; 2 = Satisfactory compliance; NA = Not applicable; **A** indicates scoring category A; **C** indicates scoring category C; ▲ indicates situational decision rules apply; △ indicates direct impact requirements apply; Ⓜ indicates Measure of success is needed; ☆ indicates this APR also applies to organizations seeking Joint Commission's Medicare/Medicaid certification–based long term care accreditation

APR.09.03.01 ★	The organization is truthful and accurate when describing information in its Quality Report to the public.			
Assessment Question	**Level of Compliance**	**Evidence of Compliance**	**Plan of Action/ Measure of Success (if needed)**	**Due Date**
1. Does the organization adhere to The Joint Commission's published guidelines for how it describes information in its Quality Report? **A (EP 1)**				

APR.10.01.01 ★	The organization notifies The Joint Commission if it has been terminated from the Medicare/Medicaid program.			
Assessment Question	**Level of Compliance**	**Evidence of Compliance**	**Plan of Action/ Measure of Success (if needed)**	**Due Date**
1. Does the organization notify The Joint Commission within 24 hours of learning that its Medicare/ Medicaid certification has been terminated? **A (EP 1)** ▲2				

APR.10.02.01 ★	The organization implements and maintains plans of correction that are required by state and federal inspections.			
Assessment Question	**Level of Compliance**	**Evidence of Compliance**	**Plan of Action/ Measure of Success (if needed)**	**Due Date**
1. Does the organization implement and maintain plans of correction from its most recent state or federal inspection? **A (EP 1)**				

Key: 0 = Insufficient compliance; 1 = Partial compliance; 2 = Satisfactory compliance; NA = Not applicable; **A** indicates scoring category A; **C** indicates scoring category C; ▲2 indicates situational decision rules apply; △3 indicates direct impact requirements apply; Ⓜ indicates Measure of success is needed; ☆ indicates this APR also applies to organizations seeking Joint Commission's Medicare/Medicaid certification–based long term care accreditation

Ethics, Rights, and Responsibilities (RI)

Standard RI.2.10	**Standard Score:** ❑ Compliant ❑ Not Compliant			
Assessment Question	**Level of Compliance**	**Evidence of Compliance**	**Plan of Action/ Measure of Success (if needed)**	**Due Date**
1. Do the organization's policies and practices address the rights of residents to care, treatment, and services within its capability and mission and in compliance with law and regulation? **A (EP 1)**				
2. Does each resident have a right to have his or her cultural, psychosocial, spiritual, and personal values, beliefs, and preferences respected? **C (EP 2) Ⓜ**				
3. Does the organization support the right of each resident to personal dignity? **C (EP 3) Ⓜ**				
4. Does the organization accommodate the right to pastoral and other spiritual services for residents? **C (EP 4) Ⓜ**				

Standard RI.2.20	**Standard Score:** ❑ Compliant ❑ Not Compliant			
Assessment Question	**Level of Compliance**	**Evidence of Compliance**	**Plan of Action/ Measure of Success (if needed)**	**Due Date**
1. Is information on rights given and explained to each resident upon admission and when any rights are changed? **C (EP 3) Ⓜ**				
2. Does the resident acknowledge in writing receipt of rights information and any changes to it as appropriate to the populations served or residents? **C (EP 4) Ⓜ**				
3. Is information on the extent to which the organization is able, unable, or unwilling to honor advance directives given upon admission if the resident has an advance directive? **C (EP 5) Ⓜ**				
4. Does the resident have the right to access, request amendment to, and receive an accounting of disclosures regarding his or her own health information as permitted under applicable law? **C (EP 6) Ⓜ**				

Key: 0 = Insufficient compliance; 1 = Partial compliance; 2 = Satisfactory compliance; NA = Not applicable; **A** indicates scoring category A; **C** indicates scoring category C; ▲ indicates situational decision rules apply; △ indicates direct impact requirements apply; Ⓜ indicates Measure of success is needed; ☆ indicates this standard also applies to organizations seeking Joint Commission's Medicare/Medicaid certification–based long term care accreditation

Standard RI.2.20

Assessment Question	Level of Compliance	Evidence of Compliance	Plan of Action/ Measure of Success (if needed)	Due Date
5. Regardless of payment method, do residents have access to at least appropriate and timely care; their attending physician; all staff, including administrative staff; care-planning and discharge-planning processes; uniform policies and practices for providing care throughout the organization; and comparable provision of care, treatment, and services to all residents under applicable state plan or other payer source? **A (EP 7)**				
6. Does the organization have policies and practices about transfers, including room-to-room transfers; discharges; and providing services consistent with the applicable state plan or other payer source? **A (EP 8)**				
7. Upon admission, are residents informed about the organization's policies and procedures regarding the handling of life-threatening emergencies (*see* Standard PC.9.20 regarding policies and procedures for life-threatening emergencies)? **C (EP 9) Ⓜ**				

Standard RI.2.30

Standard Score: ❑ Compliant ❑ Not Compliant

Assessment Question	Level of Compliance	Evidence of Compliance	Plan of Action/ Measure of Success (if needed)	Due Date
1. Are residents involved in decisions about their care, treatment, and services? **C (EP 1) Ⓜ △3**				
2. Are residents involved in resolving dilemmas about care, treatment, and services? **C (EP 2) Ⓜ △3**				
3. Is a surrogate decision maker, as allowed by law, identified when a resident cannot make decisions about his or her care, treatment, and services? **C (EP 3) Ⓜ △3**				
4. Does the legally responsible representative approve care, treatment, and services decisions?* **C (EP 4) Ⓜ △3**				

* In some states, law dictates that urgent care, family planning, and/or behavioral health services can be provided to a minor without the approval or consent of a parent or guardian.

Key: 0 = Insufficient compliance; 1 = Partial compliance; 2 = Satisfactory compliance; NA = Not applicable; **A** indicates scoring category A; **C** indicates scoring category C; ▲2 indicates situational decision rules apply; △3 indicates direct impact requirements apply; Ⓜ indicates Measure of success is needed; ☆ indicates this standard also applies to organizations seeking Joint Commission's Medicare/Medicaid certification–based long term care accreditation

Standard RI.2.30

Assessment Question	Level of Compliance	Evidence of Compliance	Plan of Action/ Measure of Success (if needed)	Due Date
5. Is the family, as appropriate and as allowed by law, with permission of the resident or surrogate decision maker, involved in care, treatment, and services decisions? **C (EP 5) Ⓜ**				
6. Are family or surrogate decision makers, as allowed by law, actively involved under the following circumstances: • When the resident has been legally judged incompetent • When the resident's physician determines he or she is medically incapable of understanding or making decisions? **A (EP 10)**				
7. Does the organization help in the process of assigning a legal guardian to a resident for health decision making, when necessary? **C (EP 11) Ⓜ**				
8. Does the organization identify those authorized for resolving conflicts related to transfer and discharge? **C (EP 12) Ⓜ**				
9. Does the organization identify those authorized for resolving conflicts related to room and roommate assignments? **C (EP 13) Ⓜ**				

Key: 0 = Insufficient compliance; 1 = Partial compliance; 2 = Satisfactory compliance; NA = Not applicable; **A** indicates scoring category A; **C** indicates scoring category C; ▲ indicates situational decision rules apply; △ indicates direct impact requirements apply; Ⓜ indicates Measure of success is needed; ☆ indicates this standard also applies to organizations seeking Joint Commission's Medicare/Medicaid certification–based long term care accreditation

Standard RI.2.40	**Standard Score:** ❑ Compliant ❑ Not Compliant			
Assessment Question	**Level of Compliance**	**Evidence of Compliance**	**Plan of Action/ Measure of Success (if needed)**	**Due Date**
1. Do the organization's policies describe the following: • Which, if any, procedures or care, treatment, and services provided require informed consent • What is the process used to obtain informed consent • How informed consent is to be documented in the record including informed consent gathered by other providers, if required • When a surrogate decision maker, rather than the resident, may give informed consent • When procedures or care, treatment, and services normally requiring informed consent may be given without informed consent? **A (EP 1)**				
2. Is informed consent obtained and documented in accordance with the organization's policy? **C (EP 2)** Ⓜ ⚠3				
3. Does a complete informed consent process include a discussion of the following elements: • The nature of the proposed care, treatment, services, medications, interventions, or procedures • Potential benefits, risks, or side effects, including potential problems that might occur during recuperation • The likelihood of achieving goals • Reasonable alternatives • The relevant risks, benefits, and side effects related to alternatives, including the possible results of not receiving care, treatment, and services • When indicated, any limitations on the confidentiality of information learned from or about the resident? **A (EP 3)** ⚠3				

Key: 0 = Insufficient compliance; 1 = Partial compliance; 2 = Satisfactory compliance; NA = Not applicable; **A** indicates scoring category A; **C** indicates scoring category C; ▲2 indicates situational decision rules apply; ⚠3 indicates direct impact requirements apply; Ⓜ indicates Measure of success is needed; ☆ indicates this standard also applies to organizations seeking Joint Commission's Medicare/Medicaid certification–based long term care accreditation

Standard RI.2.50	Standard Score: ❑ Compliant ❑ Not Compliant			
Assessment Question	**Level of Compliance**	**Evidence of Compliance**	**Plan of Action/ Measure of Success (if needed)**	**Due Date**
1. When recording or filming* are to be used only for internal organizational purposes (for example, performance improvement, education), is there documentation of consent, which may be obtained as part of general consent to treatment or another form, if a statement is included in the form regarding the use of recordings or filming for such internal purposes? **C (EP 1) Ⓜ**				
2. When recordings or films are made for external purposes that will be heard or seen by the public (for example, commercial filming, television programs, marketing), is there documentation of a specific, separate consent that includes the circumstances of the use of the recording or film? **C (EP 2) Ⓜ**				
3. Except for the circumstances set forth in EP 4 (below), is there documentation of consent before recording or filming? **C (EP 3) Ⓜ**				
4. Does the following occur in situations in which the resident is unable to give informed consent before recording or filming: • The recording or filming may occur before consent, provided it is within the established policy of the organization and the policy is established through an appropriate ethical mechanism (for example, an ethics committee) that includes community input • The recording or film remains in the organization's possession and is not used for any purpose until and unless consent is obtained • If consent for use cannot subsequently be obtained, the recording or film is either destroyed or the nonconsenting resident must be removed from the recording or film? **C (EP 4) Ⓜ**				
5. Do residents have the right to request cessation of recording or filming? **A (EP 5)**				
6. Do residents have the right to rescind consent for use up until a reasonable time before the recording or film is used? **A (EP 6)**				

* Recording or filming refers to photographic, video, electronic, or audio media.

Key: 0 = Insufficient compliance; 1 = Partial compliance; 2 = Satisfactory compliance; NA = Not applicable; **A** indicates scoring category A; **C** indicates scoring category C; ❷ indicates situational decision rules apply; ⚠3 indicates direct impact requirements apply; Ⓜ indicates Measure of success is needed; ☆ indicates this standard also applies to organizations seeking Joint Commission's Medicare/Medicaid certification–based long term care accreditation

Standard RI.2.50

Assessment Question	Level of Compliance	Evidence of Compliance	Plan of Action/ Measure of Success (if needed)	Due Date
7. Does anyone who engages in recording or filming (who is not already bound by the organization's confidentiality policy) sign a confidentiality statement to protect the resident's identity and confidential information? **C (EP 7)** Ⓜ				

Standard RI.2.70

Standard Score: ❑ Compliant ❑ Not Compliant

Assessment Question	Level of Compliance	Evidence of Compliance	Plan of Action/ Measure of Success (if needed)	Due Date
1. Do residents have the right to refuse care, treatment, and services in accordance with law and regulation? **A (EP 1)** △3				
2. When the resident is not legally responsible, does the surrogate decision maker, as allowed by law, have the right to refuse care, treatment, and services on the resident's behalf? **A (EP 2)** △3				
3. Is the resident's right to refuse care, treatment, and services consistent with the most current advance directive information obtained from the resident or family upon admission? **C (EP 4)** Ⓜ				

Standard RI.2.80

Standard Score: ❑ Compliant ❑ Not Compliant

Assessment Question	Level of Compliance	Evidence of Compliance	Plan of Action/ Measure of Success (if needed)	Due Date
1. Do policies, in accordance with law and regulation, address advance directives and the framework for forgoing or withdrawing life-sustaining treatment and withholding resuscitative services? **A (EP 1)**				
2. Are adults given written information about their right to accept or refuse medical or surgical treatment, including forgoing or withdrawing life-sustaining treatment or withholding resuscitative services? **C (EP 2)** Ⓜ				

Key: 0 = Insufficient compliance; 1 = Partial compliance; 2 = Satisfactory compliance; NA = Not applicable; **A** indicates scoring category A; **C** indicates scoring category C; ▲2 indicates situational decision rules apply; △3 indicates direct impact requirements apply; Ⓜ indicates Measure of success is needed; ☆ indicates this standard also applies to organizations seeking Joint Commission's Medicare/Medicaid certification–based long term care accreditation

Standard RI.2.80

Assessment Question	Level of Compliance	Evidence of Compliance	Plan of Action/ Measure of Success (if needed)	Due Date
3. Does the organization ensure that the existence or lack of an advance directive does not determine an individual's access to care, treatment, and services? **A (EP 3)**				
4. Does documentation indicate whether or not the resident has signed an advance directive? **C (EP 4)** Ⓜ				
5. Does the resident have the option to review and revise advance directives? **A (EP 5)**				
6. Are appropriate staff members aware of the advance directive if one exists? **C (EP 6)** Ⓜ				
7. Does the organization help or refer the residents for assistance in formulating advance directives upon request? **C (EP 7)** Ⓜ				
8. Does the organization have a mechanism for health care professionals and designated representatives to honor advance directives within the limits of the law and the organization's capabilities? **A (EP 8)**				
9. Does the organization document and honor the resident's wishes concerning organ donation within the limits of the law or organization capacity? **C (EP 9)** Ⓜ				
10. Does organization policy require residents to be informed about the laws governing advance directives, including "do not hospitalize" orders; "do-not-resuscitate" orders; and organ-donation request procedures? **A (EP 19)**				
11. Does the organization determine residents' wishes about organ donation when they are admitted? **C (EP 20)** Ⓜ				
12. Are the policies consistently implemented? **C (EP 21)** Ⓜ △3				

Key: 0 = Insufficient compliance; 1 = Partial compliance; 2 = Satisfactory compliance; NA = Not applicable; **A** indicates scoring category A; **C** indicates scoring category C; ▲2 indicates situational decision rules apply; △3 indicates direct impact requirements apply; Ⓜ indicates Measure of success is needed; ☆ indicates this standard also applies to organizations seeking Joint Commission's Medicare/Medicaid certification–based long term care accreditation

Standard RI.2.90 ★	**Standard Score:** ❑ Compliant ❑ Not Compliant			
Assessment Question	**Level of Compliance**	**Evidence of Compliance**	**Plan of Action/ Measure of Success (if needed)**	**Due Date**
1. At a minimum, is the resident and, when appropriate, his or her family, informed about outcomes of care, treatment, and services that have been provided that the resident (or family) must be knowledgeable about to participate in current and future decisions affecting the resident's care, treatment, and services? **C (EP 1) Ⓜ**				
2. At a minimum, is the resident and, when appropriate, his or her family, informed about unanticipated outcomes of care, treatment, and services that relate to sentinel events considered reviewable* by the Joint Commission? **C (EP 2) Ⓜ**				
3. Does the responsible licensed independent practitioner or his or her designee inform the resident (and when appropriate, his or her family) about those unanticipated outcomes of care, treatment, and services related to sentinel events, when the resident is not already aware of the occurrence, or further discussion is needed (*see* EP 2)†? **C (EP 3) Ⓜ**				

Standard RI.2.100	**Standard Score:** ❑ Compliant ❑ Not Compliant			
Assessment Question	**Level of Compliance**	**Evidence of Compliance**	**Plan of Action/ Measure of Success (if needed)**	**Due Date**
1. Does the organization respect the right and need of residents for effective communication? **A (EP 1)**				
2. Is written information provided appropriate to the age; understanding; and, as appropriate, to the population served, the language of the resident? **A (EP 2)** △3				
3. Does the organization provide interpretation (including translation) services as necessary? **C (EP 3) Ⓜ** △3				
4. Does the organization address the needs of those with vision, speech, hearing, language, and cognitive impairments? **C (EP 4) Ⓜ** △3				

* *See* the "Sentinel Events" (SE) chapter of the *CAMLTC* for a definition of reviewable sentinel events.

† In settings where there is no licensed independent practitioner, the staff member responsible for the care of the resident is responsible for sharing information about such outcomes.

Key: 0 = Insufficient compliance; 1 = Partial compliance; 2 = Satisfactory compliance; NA = Not applicable; **A** indicates scoring category A; **C** indicates scoring category C; ▲2 indicates situational decision rules apply; △3 indicates direct impact requirements apply; Ⓜ indicates Measure of success is needed; ☆ indicates this standard also applies to organizations seeking Joint Commission's Medicare/Medicaid certification–based long term care accreditation

Standard RI.2.100

Assessment Question	Level of Compliance	Evidence of Compliance	Plan of Action/ Measure of Success (if needed)	Due Date
5. Does the organization offer telephone and mail service as appropriate to the setting and population? **A (EP 5)**				

Standard RI.2.110

Standard Score: ❑ Compliant ❑ Not Compliant

Assessment Question	Level of Compliance	Evidence of Compliance	Plan of Action/ Measure of Success (if needed)	Due Date
1. Does the organization establish liberal visiting hours that are limited only by the residents' personal preferences? **A (EP 1)**				
2. Does the organization clearly communicate rules and regulations about visitors and visiting hours? **C (EP 2)** Ⓜ				
3. Are residents provided space to receive visitors in comfort and privacy? **A (EP 3)**				
4. Does the organization support the right of residents to choose with whom they want to talk? **C (EP 4)** Ⓜ				
5. Does the organization comply with law and regulation for visitors allowed immediate access to residents and exempted from normal visiting hours? **C (EP 5)** Ⓜ				
6. Can residents refuse to talk to persons not associated with the organization or not directly involved in his or her care? (Such persons include visitors, vendors, accreditation surveyors, and representatives of community organizations.) **C (EP 6)** Ⓜ				
7. Does the organization ensure that residents' privacy and security are considered in all interactions? **C (EP 7)** Ⓜ				

Key: 0 = Insufficient compliance; 1 = Partial compliance; 2 = Satisfactory compliance; NA = Not applicable; **A** indicates scoring category A; **C** indicates scoring category C; ▲ indicates situational decision rules apply; △ indicates direct impact requirements apply; Ⓜ indicates Measure of success is needed; ☆ indicates this standard also applies to organizations seeking Joint Commission's Medicare/Medicaid certification–based long term care accreditation

Standard RI.2.120	**Standard Score:** ❑ Compliant ❑ Not Compliant			
Assessment Question	**Level of Compliance**	**Evidence of Compliance**	**Plan of Action/ Measure of Success (if needed)**	**Due Date**
1. Does the organization inform residents, families, and staff about the internal complaint/grievance resolution process upon admission? **C (EP 1) Ⓜ**				
2. Does the organization receive; review; and, when possible, resolve complaints from residents and their families? **C (EP 2) Ⓜ**				
3. Does the organization respond to individuals making a significant (as defined by the organization) or recurring complaint? **C (EP 3) Ⓜ**				
4. Does the organization inform residents about their right to file a complaint with the state authority? **C (EP 4) Ⓜ**				
5. Can residents freely voice complaints and recommend changes without being subject to coercion; discrimination; reprisal; or unreasonable interruption of care, treatment, and services? **C (EP 5) Ⓜ**				
6. Does the organization prominently post a description of the complaint/grievance process in the facility? **A (EP 6)**				
7. If the organization does not resolve the complaint/grievance to the resident's or family's satisfaction, does it refer them to other sources of assistance, such as ombudsman, legal services, or adult protective services programs? **C (EP 7) Ⓜ**				
8. Do the organization's written admission guidelines list other sources of assistance, including ombudsman, legal services, or adult protective services programs, for complaint resolution? **A (EP 8)**				
9. Does the organization provide these guidelines to residents and families on admission? **C (EP 9) Ⓜ**				

Key: 0 = Insufficient compliance; 1 = Partial compliance; 2 = Satisfactory compliance; NA = Not applicable; **A** indicates scoring category A; **C** indicates scoring category C; ▲ indicates situational decision rules apply; △ indicates direct impact requirements apply; Ⓜ indicates Measure of success is needed; ☆ indicates this standard also applies to organizations seeking Joint Commission's Medicare/Medicaid certification–based long term care accreditation

Standard RI.2.130	**Standard Score: ❑ Compliant ❑ Not Compliant**			
Assessment Question	**Level of Compliance**	**Evidence of Compliance**	**Plan of Action/ Measure of Success (if needed)**	**Due Date**
1. Does the organization protect confidentiality of information about residents? **C (EP 1) Ⓜ**				
2. Does the organization respect the privacy of residents? **C (EP 2) Ⓜ**				
3. Do residents who desire private telephone conversations have access to space and telephones appropriate to their needs and the care, treatment, and services provided? **C (EP 3) Ⓜ**				
4. Does the organization provide for the safety and security of residents and their property? **C (EP 4) Ⓜ ⚠3**				
5. Are residents who are married or have significant others given a reasonable degree of privacy? **C (EP 5) Ⓜ**				
6. Does the organization obtain documented resident/family consent when confidential information needs to be posted in the organization? **C (EP 6) Ⓜ**				

Standard RI.2.140	**Standard Score: ❑ Compliant ❑ Not Compliant**			
Assessment Question	**Level of Compliance**	**Evidence of Compliance**	**Plan of Action/ Measure of Success (if needed)**	**Due Date**
1. Does the environment of care support the positive self-image of residents and preserve their human dignity? **A (EP 1)**				
2. Does the organization provide sufficient storage space to meet the personal needs of the residents? **A (EP 2)**				
3. Does the organization allow residents to keep and use personal clothing and possessions, unless this infringes on others' rights or is medically or therapeutically contraindicated (as appropriate to the setting or service)? **A (EP 3)**				

Key: 0 = Insufficient compliance; 1 = Partial compliance; 2 = Satisfactory compliance; NA = Not applicable; **A** indicates scoring category A; **C** indicates scoring category C; ▲2 indicates situational decision rules apply; ⚠3 indicates direct impact requirements apply; Ⓜ indicates Measure of success is needed; ☆ indicates this standard also applies to organizations seeking Joint Commission's Medicare/Medicaid certification–based long term care accreditation

Standard RI.2.140

Assessment Question	Level of Compliance	Evidence of Compliance	Plan of Action/ Measure of Success (if needed)	Due Date
4. Do the environment's essential components include the following: • Homelike surroundings • Sufficient space with access to personal living space • Appropriate communication about room and roommate assignments or changes • Environmental adaptations to help those with dementia, cognitive impairment, or temporary confusion • Appropriate accommodations for married couples and clients with significant others regardless of sexual orientation, unless any limitations consistent with the organization's mission and philosophy have been disclosed to the resident at the time of or before admission? **A (EP 4)**				

Standard RI.2.150

Standard Score: ❑ Compliant ❑ Not Compliant

Assessment Question	Level of Compliance	Evidence of Compliance	Plan of Action/ Measure of Success (if needed)	Due Date
1. Does the organization address how it will, to the best of its ability, protect residents from real or perceived abuse; neglect, including involuntary seclusion; or exploitation from anyone, including staff members, students, volunteers, other residents, visitors, or family mombors? **A (EP 1)** △3				
2. Are all allegations, observations, or suspected cases of abuse, neglect, or exploitation that occur in the organization explored by the organization and, based on the type of event, referred to the appropriate authorities for investigation? **C (EP 2)** Ⓜ △3				

Key: 0 = Insufficient compliance; 1 = Partial compliance; 2 = Satisfactory compliance; NA = Not applicable; **A** indicates scoring category A; **C** indicates scoring category C; ▲2 indicates situational decision rules apply; △3 indicates direct impact requirements apply; Ⓜ indicates Measure of success is needed; ☆ indicates this standard also applies to organizations seeking Joint Commission's Medicare/Medicaid certification–based long term care accreditation

Standard RI.2.160 ★	Standard Score: ❑ Compliant ❑ Not Compliant			
Assessment Question	**Level of Compliance**	**Evidence of Compliance**	**Plan of Action/ Measure of Success (if needed)**	**Due Date**
1. Does the organization plan, support, and coordinate activities and resources to ensure that pain is recognized and addressed appropriately and in accordance with the care, treatment, and services provided, including the following: • Assessing for pain • Educating all relevant providers about assessing and managing pain • Educating residents and families, when appropriate, about their roles in managing pain and the potential limitations and side effects of pain treatments? **A (EP 1)** △3				

Standard RI.2.170	Standard Score: ❑ Compliant ❑ Not Compliant			
Assessment Question	**Level of Compliance**	**Evidence of Compliance**	**Plan of Action/ Measure of Success (if needed)**	**Due Date**
1. When the organization serves a population of residents who often need protective services (that is, guardianship and advocacy services, conservatorship, and child or adult protective services), does it provide resources to help the family and the courts determine the resident's needs for such services? **C (EP 1)** Ⓜ				
2. When appropriate, does the organization maintain a list of names, addresses, and telephone numbers of pertinent state client advocacy groups such as the state authority and the protection and advocacy network? **A (EP 2)**				
3. Is the list given to residents when requested? **C (EP 3)** Ⓜ				
4. Does the organization develop and implement policies and procedures for the above requirements? **A (EP 4)**				

Key: 0 = Insufficient compliance; 1 = Partial compliance; 2 = Satisfactory compliance; NA = Not applicable; **A** indicates scoring category A; **C** indicates scoring category C; ▲2 indicates situational decision rules apply; △3 indicates direct impact requirements apply; Ⓜ indicates Measure of success is needed; ☆ indicates this standard also applies to organizations seeking Joint Commission's Medicare/Medicaid certification–based long term care accreditation

Standard RI.2.180*	**Standard Score:** ❑ Compliant ❑ Not Compliant			
Assessment Question	**Level of Compliance**	**Evidence of Compliance**	**Plan of Action/ Measure of Success (if needed)**	**Due Date**
1. Does the organization review all research protocols in relation to its mission, values, and other guidelines and weigh the relative risks and benefits to the research subjects? **C (EP 1) Ⓜ**				
2. Does the organization provide residents who are potential subjects in research, investigation, and clinical trials with adequate information† to participate or refuse to participate in research? **C (EP 2) Ⓜ**				
3. Are residents informed that refusal to participate or discontinuing participation at any time will not compromise their access to care, treatment, and services not related to the research? **C (EP 3) Ⓜ**				
4. Do consent forms address the above EPs; indicate the name of the person who provided the information and the date the form was signed; and address the participant's right to privacy, confidentiality, and safety? **C (EP 4) Ⓜ**				
5. Are subjects told the extent to which their personally identifiable private information will be held in confidence? **C (EP 5) Ⓜ**				
6. Is all information given to subjects in the medical record or research file along with the consent forms? **C (EP 6) Ⓜ**				
7. If a research-related injury (that is, physical, psychological, social, financial, or otherwise) occurs, does the principal investigator attempt to address any harmful consequences the subject may have experienced as a result of research procedures? **C (EP 7) Ⓜ**				
8. Does the organization obtain and maintain a copy of the consent form? **C (EP 8) Ⓜ**				

* Applicable to long term care programs participating in research.

† Adequate information includes an explanation of the purpose of the research and expected duration of the subject's participation; a description of expected benefits, potential discomforts, and risks; alternative services that might prove advantageous to the resident; and a full explanation of the procedures to be followed.

Key: 0 = Insufficient compliance; 1 = Partial compliance; 2 = Satisfactory compliance; NA = Not applicable; **A** indicates scoring category A; **C** indicates scoring category C; ▲(2) indicates situational decision rules apply; △(3) indicates direct impact requirements apply; Ⓜ indicates Measure of success is needed; ☆ indicates this standard also applies to organizations seeking Joint Commission's Medicare/Medicaid certification–based long term care accreditation

Standard RI.2.190	Standard Score: ❑ Compliant ❑ Not Compliant			
Assessment Question	**Level of Compliance**	**Evidence of Compliance**	**Plan of Action/ Measure of Success (if needed)**	**Due Date**
1. Do policies and procedures address situations in which residents work? **A (EP 1)**				
2. Are policies and procedures implemented? **C (EP 2) Ⓜ**				
3. Are wages paid to residents in accordance with applicable law and regulation? **C (EP 3) Ⓜ**				
4. Is work addressed in the care, treatment, and services plan? **C (EP 4) Ⓜ**				
5. Is work performed voluntarily? **C (EP 5) Ⓜ**				

Standard RI.2.200	Standard Score: ❑ Compliant ❑ Not Compliant			
Assessment Question	**Level of Compliance**	**Evidence of Compliance**	**Plan of Action/ Measure of Success (if needed)**	**Due Date**
1. Does the organization help residents with citizenship privileges to exercise their citizenship privileges, including arranging for them to vote? **C (EP 1) Ⓜ**				

Standard RI.2.210	Standard Score: ❑ Compliant ❑ Not Compliant			
Assessment Question	**Level of Compliance**	**Evidence of Compliance**	**Plan of Action/ Measure of Success (if needed)**	**Due Date**
1. Do residents receive care that respects their independence, expression of choice, and decision making? **A (EP 1)**				
2. Are residents' choices about their planned course of care, treatment, and services supported by the organization? **C (EP 2) Ⓜ**				
3. Are residents' health beliefs and expectations honored by the organization? **C (EP 3) Ⓜ**				

Key: 0 = Insufficient compliance; 1 = Partial compliance; 2 = Satisfactory compliance; NA = Not applicable; **A** indicates scoring category A; **C** indicates scoring category C; ▲ indicates situational decision rules apply; △ indicates direct impact requirements apply; Ⓜ indicates Measure of success is needed; ☆ indicates this standard also applies to organizations seeking Joint Commission's Medicare/Medicaid certification–based long term care accreditation

Standard RI.2.220	**Standard Score:** ❑ Compliant ❑ Not Compliant			
Assessment Question	**Level of Compliance**	**Evidence of Compliance**	**Plan of Action/ Measure of Success (if needed)**	**Due Date**
1. Are residents' personal values, beliefs, and cultural and spiritual preferences respected by the organization? **C (EP 1) Ⓜ**				
2. Are residents' life-long patterns of living, including lifestyle choices related to sexual orientation respected by the organization? **C (EP 2) Ⓜ**				

Standard RI.2.230	**Standard Score:** ❑ Compliant ❑ Not Compliant			
Assessment Question	**Level of Compliance**	**Evidence of Compliance**	**Plan of Action/ Measure of Success (if needed)**	**Due Date**
1. Do organization policies and procedures support the resident's right to be free from restraints? **A (EP 1)**				

Standard RI.2.240	**Standard Score:** ❑ Compliant ❑ Not Compliant			
Assessment Question	**Level of Compliance**	**Evidence of Compliance**	**Plan of Action/ Measure of Success (if needed)**	**Due Date**
1. Is each resident's choice to participate or refuse to participate in social, spiritual, or community activities and groups supported by the organization? **C (EP 1) Ⓜ**				

Standard RI.2.250	**Standard Score:** ❑ Compliant ❑ Not Compliant			
Assessment Question	**Level of Compliance**	**Evidence of Compliance**	**Plan of Action/ Measure of Success (if needed)**	**Due Date**
1. Does the organization arrange transportation for residents to and from physician or dentist appointments and other activities identified in their care or service plan? **C (EP 1) Ⓜ**				
2. Does the organization arrange for an appropriate attendant, as necessary, when transporting residents? **C (EP 2) Ⓜ**				

Key: 0 = Insufficient compliance; 1 = Partial compliance; 2 = Satisfactory compliance; NA = Not applicable; **A** indicates scoring category A; **C** indicates scoring category C; ▲(2) indicates situational decision rules apply; △(3) indicates direct impact requirements apply; Ⓜ indicates Measure of success is needed; ☆ indicates this standard also applies to organizations seeking Joint Commission's Medicare/Medicaid certification–based long term care accreditation

Standard RI.2.260	Standard Score: ❑ Compliant ❑ Not Compliant			
Assessment Question	**Level of Compliance**	**Evidence of Compliance**	**Plan of Action/ Measure of Success (if needed)**	**Due Date**
1. Does the organization establish a resident council? **A (EP 1)**				
2. Are residents involved in planning and running the resident council? **A (EP 2)**				
3. Are residents informed of council meetings and invited to attend? **C (EP 3) Ⓜ**				
4. When a resident cannot attend or chooses not to attend the resident council, does the organization have a way to send that resident's concerns to the council and provide feedback to the residents? **C (EP 4) Ⓜ**				
5. When a resident council is not a suitable forum for resolving particular complaints or addressing certain cases, does the organization provide a resident representative or advocate? **C (EP 5) Ⓜ**				

Standard RI.2.270	Standard Score: ❑ Compliant ❑ Not Compliant			
Assessment Question	**Level of Compliance**	**Evidence of Compliance**	**Plan of Action/ Measure of Success (if needed)**	**Due Date**
1. Does the organization support each resident's right to choose an attending physician, dentist, and other licensed independent practitioner? **C (EP 1) Ⓜ**				
2. Does the organization support resident requests for a different licensed independent practitioner both on admission and throughout the course of care? **C (EP 2) Ⓜ**				
3. Does the organization make reasonable attempts to respond to these requests? **C (EP 3) Ⓜ**				

Key: 0 = Insufficient compliance; 1 = Partial compliance; 2 = Satisfactory compliance; NA = Not applicable; **A** indicates scoring category A; **C** indicates scoring category C; ▲ indicates situational decision rules apply; △ indicates direct impact requirements apply; Ⓜ indicates Measure of success is needed; ☆ indicates this standard also applies to organizations seeking Joint Commission's Medicare/Medicaid certification–based long term care accreditation

Standard RI.2.280	**Standard Score:** ❑ Compliant ❑ Not Compliant			
Assessment Question	**Level of Compliance**	**Evidence of Compliance**	**Plan of Action/ Measure of Success (if needed)**	**Due Date**
1. Does the organization support the residents' right to know their medical, dental, and other licensed independent practitioner care providers? C (EP 1) Ⓜ				
2. Does the organization provide residents and families with names and telephone numbers of the physician or other practitioner primarily responsible for their care? C (EP 2) Ⓜ				
3. Does the organization provide residents and families with names and professional status of individuals responsible for authorizing and performing procedures and treatments, when appropriate? C (EP 3) Ⓜ				
4. Does the organization help residents make and keep appointments? C (EP 4) Ⓜ				
5. Does the organization consider residents' possible impairments when providing information? C (EP 5) Ⓜ				

Standard RI.2.290	**Standard Score:** ❑ Compliant ❑ Not Compliant			
Assessment Question	**Level of Compliance**	**Evidence of Compliance**	**Plan of Action/ Measure of Success (if needed)**	**Due Date**
1. Can residents access and use available funds? C (EP 1) Ⓜ				
2. Do residents authorize the organization to manage their funds in writing? C (EP 2) Ⓜ				
3. When the organization manages a resident's personal funds, does the resident have ready and reasonable access to those funds? C (EP 3) Ⓜ				
4. When the organization manages a resident's personal funds, does it give the resident at least quarterly an accurate accounting of all financial transactions on the resident's behalf? C (EP 4) Ⓜ				

Key: 0 = Insufficient compliance; 1 = Partial compliance; 2 = Satisfactory compliance; NA = Not applicable; **A** indicates scoring category A; **C** indicates scoring category C; ▲2 indicates situational decision rules apply; △3 indicates direct impact requirements apply; Ⓜ indicates Measure of success is needed; ☆ indicates this standard also applies to organizations seeking Joint Commission's Medicare/Medicaid certification–based long term care accreditation

Standard RI.2.290

Assessment Question	Level of Compliance	Evidence of Compliance	Plan of Action/ Measure of Success (if needed)	Due Date
5. Does the organization involve the legal guardian, durable power of attorney, or family, as appropriate? **C (EP 5) Ⓜ**				

Standard RI.3.10

Standard Score: ❑ Compliant ❑ Not Compliant

Assessment Question	Level of Compliance	Evidence of Compliance	Plan of Action/ Measure of Success (if needed)	Due Date
1. Does the organization have a policy that defines the mechanism for communicating responsibilities of residents? **A (EP 1)**				
2. Does the policy include the responsibilities for providing information, asking questions, following instructions, accepting consequences, following rules and regulations, showing respect and consideration, and meeting financial commitments? **A (EP 2)**				
3. Are residents informed about their responsibilities verbally, in writing, or both, based on organization policy? **C (EP 3) Ⓜ**				
4. Are residents informed about their responsibilities initially and as needed thereafter? **C (EP 4) Ⓜ**				

Key: 0 = Insufficient compliance; 1 = Partial compliance; 2 = Satisfactory compliance; NA = Not applicable; **A** indicates scoring category A; **C** indicates scoring category C; ▲ indicates situational decision rules apply; △ indicates direct impact requirements apply; Ⓜ indicates Measure of success is needed; ☆ indicates this standard also applies to organizations seeking Joint Commission's Medicare/Medicaid certification–based long term care accreditation

Provision of Care, Treatment, and Services (PC)

Standard PC.1.10	Standard Score: ❑ Compliant ❑ Not Compliant			
Assessment Question	**Level of Compliance**	**Evidence of Compliance**	**Plan of Action/ Measure of Success (if needed)**	**Due Date**
1. Does the organization have a defined written process that includes the following: • Information to be gathered to determine eligibility for entrance into the organization • Populations of residents accepted or not accepted by the organization (for example, programs designed to treat adults, that do not treat young children) • Criteria to determine eligibility for entry into the system • Procedures for accepting referrals? **A (EP 1)**				
2. Are residents screened for appropriateness at the point of first contact (including contact by telephone) with the organization? **C (EP 2) Ⓜ**				
3. Is the interdisciplinary team consulted when necessary to determine whether or not a prospective resident meets admission criteria? **A (EP 3)**				
4. If a resident is not accepted after referral and preadmission screening, are the reasons for denying admission stated? **C (EP 4) Ⓜ**				
5. Do the staff members make reasonable efforts to refer the resident to another appropriate organization? **A (EP 5)**				
6. Do the staff members explain to the referring organization the reason for not accepting the resident, and when possible, suggest a more appropriate organization? **A (EP 6)**				
7. When warranted by need, are separate specialized screening, assessment, and reassessment processes identified for the various populations served? **A (EP 7)**				
8. Does the organization accept residents for care, treatment, and services according to established processes? **C (EP 9) Ⓜ**				

Key: 0 = Insufficient compliance; 1 = Partial compliance; 2 = Satisfactory compliance; NA = Not applicable; **A** indicates scoring category A; **C** indicates scoring category C; ▲ indicates situational decision rules apply; △ indicates direct impact requirements apply; Ⓜ indicates Measure of success is needed; ☆ indicates this standard also applies to organizations seeking Joint Commission's Medicare/Medicaid certification–based long term care accreditation

Standard PC.2.20	**Standard Score:** ❑ Compliant ❑ Not Compliant			
Assessment Question	**Level of Compliance**	**Evidence of Compliance**	**Plan of Action/ Measure of Success (if needed)**	**Due Date**
1. Does the organization's written definition of the data and information gathered during assessment and reassessment include the following: • The scope of assessment and reassessment activities by each discipline • The content of the assessment and reassessment • The criteria for when an additional or more in-depth assessment is done by each discipline?* **A (EP 1)**				
2. Are the screening, assessment, and reassessment activities described within the scope of practice, state licensure, laws, applicable regulations, or certification of the discipline doing the assessment? **A (EP 2)**				
3. If applicable, is separate specialized assessment and reassessment information identified for the various populations served? **A (EP 3)**				
4. Does the information defined by the organization to be gathered during the initial assessment(s) include the following, as relevant to the care, treatment, and services: • Current diagnosis(es) • Pertinent history • Medication history including drug allergies and sensitivities • Current medications including prescribed and over-the-counter medications • Current treatments? **A (EP 12)**				
5. Does the information defined by the organization to be gathered during the initial assessment(s) for the resident's physical and neuropsychiatric status include the following: • Musculoskeletal status • Cardiorespiratory status • Gastrointestinal status • Integumentary status • Foot care needs • Mental, affective, and cognitive status and needs? **A (EP 13)**				

* For example, nutritional or functional risk assessments may be defined for at-risk residents. In such cases, nutritional risk criteria should be developed by dietitians or other qualified individuals, and functional risk criteria should be developed by rehabilitation specialists or other qualified individuals.

Key: 0 = Insufficient compliance; 1 = Partial compliance; 2 = Satisfactory compliance; NA = Not applicable; **A** indicates scoring category A; **C** indicates scoring category C; ▲ indicates situational decision rules apply; △ indicates direct impact requirements apply; Ⓜ indicates Measure of success is needed; ☆ indicates this standard also applies to organizations seeking Joint Commission's Medicare/Medicaid certification–based long term care accreditation

Standard PC.2.20

Assessment Question	Level of Compliance	Evidence of Compliance	Plan of Action/ Measure of Success (if needed)	Due Date
6. Does the information defined by the organization to be gathered during the initial assessment(s) for the resident's communication status include the following: • Ability to hear • Ability to speak • Predominant language(s) • Modes of expression? **A (EP 14)**				
7. Does the information defined by the organization to be gathered during the initial assessment(s) for the resident's functional status include the following: • Ability to perform activities of daily living • Mobility, balance, and strength • Ability to swallow • Physical limitations and precautions • Rehabilitation status, needs, and potential • Orientation? **A (EP 15)**				
8. Does the information defined by the organization to be gathered during the initial assessment(s) for the resident's activity status, needs, and potential, include the following: • Personal preferences regarding schedules and grooming • The resident's activity and recreational skills, based on his or her cognitive abilities and limitations of his or her illness or treatment • Hobbies, recreational interests, associated needs, and potential • Ability to participate in structured and group activities? **A (EP 16)**				

Key: 0 = Insufficient compliance; 1 = Partial compliance; 2 = Satisfactory compliance; NA = Not applicable; **A** indicates scoring category A; **C** indicates scoring category C; ▲ indicates situational decision rules apply; △ indicates direct impact requirements apply; Ⓜ indicates Measure of success is needed; ☆ indicates this standard also applies to organizations seeking Joint Commission's Medicare/Medicaid certification–based long term care accreditation

Standard PC.2.20

Assessment Question	Level of Compliance	Evidence of Compliance	Plan of Action/ Measure of Success (if needed)	Due Date
9. Does the information defined by the organization to be gathered during the initial assessment(s) for the resident's nutritional* and hydration status and needs include the following: • Potential nutritional risk, deficiencies, and needs • Cultural, religious, and ethnic food preferences • Nutrient-intake patterns and special dietary requirements • Dietary/food allergies • Food and fluid consumption • Bowel and urinary output • Skin integrity • Swallowing problems • Appropriate laboratory tests • Weight (at least monthly) • Criteria used to evaluate weight gain and loss to determine the need for further assessment? **A (EP 17)**				
10. Does the information defined by the organization to be gathered during the initial assessment(s) for the resident's dental status and oral health include the following: • Dental status and oral health, including the condition of the oral cavity, teeth, and tooth-supporting structures • The presence or absence of natural teeth or dentures, and the ability to function with or without teeth or dentures? **A (EP 18)**				
11. Does the information defined by the organization to be gathered during the initial assessment(s) for the resident's pain include the following: • Pain status, including its origin, location, severity, and alleviating and exacerbating factors • Current treatment for pain and response to current treatment? **A (EP 19)**				

* The content of the nutritional screening criteria that the organization develops (which may include the Minimum Data Set [MDS]), is at the discretion of the organization, but should be contained in an approved policy. The standards also reflect that, based on the results of the nutrition screen, further nutrition assessment is completed when indicated and the resident is reassessed at determined intervals.

Key: 0 = Insufficient compliance; 1 = Partial compliance; 2 = Satisfactory compliance; NA = Not applicable; **A** indicates scoring category A; **C** indicates scoring category C; ▲ indicates situational decision rules apply; △ indicates direct impact requirements apply; Ⓜ indicates Measure of success is needed; ☆ indicates this standard also applies to organizations seeking Joint Commission's Medicare/Medicaid certification–based long term care accreditation

Standard PC.2.20

Assessment Question	Level of Compliance	Evidence of Compliance	Plan of Action/ Measure of Success (if needed)	Due Date
12. Does the information defined by the organization to be gathered during the initial assessment(s) for the resident's psychosocial and spiritual status include the following: • Cultural and ethnic factors which influence care, treatment, and services • Current emotional status • Social skills • Current living situation • Family relationships and circumstances • Relevant past history of roles • Response to stress caused by the illness and required treatment • Spiritual orientation, status, and needs • The dying resident's concerns related to hope, despair, guilt, or forgiveness? **A (EP 20)**				
13. When the bereavement process is a significant factor, does the psychosocial assessment include the social, spiritual, and cultural variables that influence the perceptions and expressions of grief by the resident or family? **A (EP 21)**				

Standard PC.2.120

Standard Score: ❑ Compliant ❑ Not Compliant

Assessment Question	Level of Compliance	Evidence of Compliance	Plan of Action/ Measure of Success (if needed)	Due Date
1. Does the organization define the time frame(s) for conducting the initial assessment(s)? **A (EP 1)**				
2. At a minimum, does the organization specify that each resident's Minimum Data Set/interdisciplinary assessment is completed within 14 days of admission as required by law and regulation? **A (EP 8) Ⓜ**				

Key: 0 = Insufficient compliance; 1 = Partial compliance; 2 = Satisfactory compliance; NA = Not applicable; **A** indicates scoring category A; **C** indicates scoring category C; ▲ indicates situational decision rules apply; △ indicates direct impact requirements apply; Ⓜ indicates Measure of success is needed; ☆ indicates this standard also applies to organizations seeking Joint Commission's Medicare/Medicaid certification–based long term care accreditation

Standard PC.2.120

Assessment Question	Level of Compliance	Evidence of Compliance	Plan of Action/ Measure of Success (if needed)	Due Date
3. At a minimum, does the attending physician or licensed independent practitioner perform a medical assessment for all admissions and readmissions and meet the following criteria: • A previous medical history does not have to be completely redone if it is updated with information about the most recent illness and hospitalization since the date the last history was taken within a time frame appropriate to the resident's condition which does not exceed 24 hours before admission and 72 hours after admission • Durable, legible originals or reproductions of a medical history and physical examination obtained by the attending physician or licensed independent practitioner and completed within 30 days before admission or readmission provided there is a summary of the resident's condition and course of care during the interim period and the summary includes the current physical/psychosocial status? **A (EP 10)**				
4. If the attending physician or licensed independent practitioner other than the attending physician performed the medical assessment that is being transferred, and that assessment was performed within 30 days before admission, then within 24 hours of admission or 72 hours after admission, does the attending physician or licensed independent practitioner do the following: • Review the physical examination • Conduct a second medical assessment to confirm the information and findings • Update any information and findings as necessary, including a summary of the resident's condition and course of care during the interim period and the current physical/psychosocial status • Sign and date the additional information to attest its currency? **A (EP 11)**				
5. At a minimum, does the organization record the assessment findings recorded in the medical record on admission within the time frames noted in EP 11? **A (EP 12)**				
6. At a minimum, does the organization access and document each resident's oral health within 90 days before admission or within 14 days after admission? **A (EP 13)**				

Key: 0 = Insufficient compliance; 1 = Partial compliance; 2 = Satisfactory compliance; NA = Not applicable; **A** indicates scoring category A; **C** indicates scoring category C; ▲ indicates situational decision rules apply; △ indicates direct impact requirements apply; Ⓜ indicates Measure of success is needed; ☆ indicates this standard also applies to organizations seeking Joint Commission's Medicare/Medicaid certification–based long term care accreditation

Standard PC.2.120

Assessment Question	Level of Compliance	Evidence of Compliance	Plan of Action/ Measure of Success (if needed)	Due Date
7. For residents with complex needs or who require short lengths of stay, does the organization complete assessments within five calendar days after admission for all disciplines pertinent to the reason for admission or as required by law and regulation? **C (EP 17) Ⓜ**				

Standard PC.2.130

Standard Score: ❑ Compliant ❑ Not Compliant

Assessment Question	Level of Compliance	Evidence of Compliance	Plan of Action/ Measure of Success (if needed)	Due Date
1. Are initial assessments performed per organization policy? **C (EP 1) Ⓜ △3**				
2. Is each resident's initial assessment conducted within the time frame specified by the needs of the resident, organization policy, and law and regulation? **C (EP 2) Ⓜ △3**				
3. Does a registered nurse assess the resident's need for nursing care in all settings, as required by law, regulation, or organization policy? **A (EP 3) △3**				
4. Are residents who exhibit symptoms of dementia evaluated, and is a differential diagnosis established? **C (EP 4) Ⓜ △3**				
5. Is the evaluation* of residents who exhibit symptoms of dementia performed by a neurologist, a psychiatrist, or a geriatrician, if available, or another qualified physician? **C (EP 5) Ⓜ △3**				

Standard PC 2.150

Standard Score: ❑ Compliant ❑ Not Compliant

Assessment Question	Level of Compliance	Evidence of Compliance	Plan of Action/ Measure of Success (if needed)	Due Date
1. Is each resident reassessed as needed? **C (EP 1) Ⓜ △3**				

* Guidelines for conducting such an evaluation are available from the "Guidelines for Dignity" from the Alzheimer's Association. The guidelines include a history and physical examination; a mental status evaluation; a neurologic examination; blood workup; a psychiatric evaluation; a neuropsychiatric assessment; a psychological assessment; CT/MRI, as indicated; and any reversible causes for the presenting symptoms.

Key: 0 = Insufficient compliance; 1 = Partial compliance; 2 = Satisfactory compliance; NA = Not applicable; **A** indicates scoring category A; **C** indicates scoring category C; ▲ indicates situational decision rules apply; △3 indicates direct impact requirements apply; Ⓜ indicates Measure of success is needed; ☆ indicates this standard also applies to organizations seeking Joint Commission's Medicare/Medicaid certification–based long term care accreditation

Standard PC 2.150

Assessment Question	Level of Compliance	Evidence of Compliance	Plan of Action/ Measure of Success (if needed)	Due Date
2. Does reassessment occur in conjunction with the interdisciplinary care plan schedule or in response to changes in the resident's condition as required by law and regulation? **C (EP 2)** Ⓜ ⚠3				

Standard PC.3.10

Standard Score: ❑ Compliant ❑ Not Compliant

Assessment Question	Level of Compliance	Evidence of Compliance	Plan of Action/ Measure of Success (if needed)	Due Date
1. Does the organization develop or adopt criteria* for identifying victims in each of the following situations: • Physical assault • Rape • Sexual molestation • Domestic abuse • Elder neglect or abuse • Child neglect or abuse • Exploitation? **A (EP 1)**				
2. Are appropriate staff† members educated about abuse, neglect, or exploitation and how to refer as appropriate? **A (EP 2)**				
3. Is a list of private and public community agencies that provide and arrange for assessment and care of abuse victims maintained to facilitate appropriate referrals? **A (EP 3)**				
4. Are victims of abuse, neglect, and exploitation identified using the criteria developed or adopted by the organization at entry into the system and on an ongoing basis? **A (EP 4)** ⚠3				
5. Do the organization's staff members refer appropriately or conduct the assessment of victims of abuse, neglect, or exploitation? **A (EP 5)** ⚠3				

* The Family Violence Prevention Fund is one resource that can be contacted for further information at http://www.fvpf.org.

† Staff members should be able to screen for abuse and neglect as indicated by the resident's needs or conditions. The organization may define who conducts the full assessment for alleged or suspected abuse or neglect or refer to another organization.

Key: 0 = Insufficient compliance; 1 = Partial compliance; 2 = Satisfactory compliance; NA = Not applicable; **A** indicates scoring category A; **C** indicates scoring category C; ▲2 indicates situational decision rules apply; ⚠3 indicates direct impact requirements apply; Ⓜ indicates Measure of success is needed; ☆ indicates this standard also applies to organizations seeking Joint Commission's Medicare/Medicaid certification–based long term care accreditation

Standard PC.3.10				
Assessment Question	Level of Compliance	Evidence of Compliance	Plan of Action/ Measure of Success (if needed)	Due Date
6. Are all cases of abuse, neglect, or exploitation reported to appropriate agencies according to organization policy and law and regulation? **A (EP 6)** △3				
7. Are all cases of abuse, neglect, or exploitation immediately reported in the organization? **A (EP 7)** △3				

Standard PC.3.230	Standard Score: ❑ Compliant ❑ Not Compliant			
Assessment Question	Level of Compliance	Evidence of Compliance	Plan of Action/ Measure of Success (if needed)	Due Date
1. Are diagnostic testing and procedures performed as ordered? **C (EP 1)** Ⓜ △3				
2. Are diagnostic testing and procedures performed in a timely manner as defined by the organization? **C (EP 2)** Ⓜ △3				
3. When a test report requires clinical interpretation, is there relevant information provided with the request? **C (EP 3)** Ⓜ △3				
4. Are radiologic and other diagnostic services, including pathology and clinical laboratory services, available 24 hours a day, 7 days a week? **A (EP 5)** △3				

Key: 0 = Insufficient compliance; 1 = Partial compliance; 2 = Satisfactory compliance; NA = Not applicable; **A** indicates scoring category A; **C** indicates scoring category C; ▲2 indicates situational decision rules apply; △3 indicates direct impact requirements apply; Ⓜ indicates Measure of success is needed; ☆ indicates this standard also applies to organizations seeking Joint Commission's Medicare/Medicaid certification–based long term care accreditation

Standard PC.4.10

Assessment Question	Level of Compliance	Evidence of Compliance	Plan of Action/ Measure of Success (if needed)	Due Date
1. Are care, treatment, and services planned to ensure that they are individualized to the resident's needs? **A (EP 1)**				
2. Does the interdisciplinary team identify and prioritize each resident's care needs based on the analysis of assessment data? **A (EP 3)**				
3. Is an individualized, interdisciplinary plan of care, treatment, and services developed by an interdisciplinary team representing all appropriate health care professionals, as soon as possible after admission, but no later than seven calendar days after comprehensive assessments are completed? **C (EP 4)** Ⓜ △3				
4. Does the plan identify the following: • The care, treatment, and settings • The frequency at which care, services, treatments, and interventions will occur • The team members responsible for providing care, treatment, and services • The financial implications of care, treatment, and services • Interventions to facilitate the resident's return to the community or discharge to an appropriate level of care? **A (EP 7)**				
5. Is an interim plan for care, treatment, or services developed for each resident immediately after the resident is admitted? **C (EP 8)** Ⓜ △3				
6. Is there a process in place for gathering input, collaborating on care plan development, and reporting the final plan to team members not available to participate in care planning? **A (EP 9)**				
7. Do policies and procedures define how care plans can be modified between team meetings? **A (EP 10)**				

Key: 0 = Insufficient compliance; 1 = Partial compliance; 2 = Satisfactory compliance; NA = Not applicable; **A** indicates scoring category A; **C** indicates scoring category C; ▲2 indicates situational decision rules apply; △3 indicates direct impact requirements apply; Ⓜ indicates Measure of success is needed; ☆ indicates this standard also applies to organizations seeking Joint Commission's Medicare/Medicaid certification–based long term care accreditation

Standard PC.4.10

Assessment Question	Level of Compliance	Evidence of Compliance	Plan of Action/ Measure of Success (if needed)	Due Date
8. Does the organization implement a process for evaluating the plan for care, treatment, and services and its effectiveness, which includes the following: • 90-day evaluation intervals or more frequent intervals in response to a significant change in the resident's physical, communicative, psychosocial, functional, or emotional status • Care plan revisions that reflect the resident's current needs, problems, goals, care, treatment, and service • Review and revision by the interdisciplinary team of all components of care, treatment, and services needed by the resident? **A (EP 11)**				
9. Is the evaluation of the resident based on the resident care goals and the resident's plan for care, treatment, and services? **C (EP 12)** Ⓜ ⚠3				
10. Are the goals of care, treatment, and services revised when necessary? **C (EP 13)** Ⓜ				
11. Are the plans for care, treatment, and services revised when necessary? **A (EP 14)**				
12. Does the interdisciplinary team revise the care plan in collaboration with residents, families, and the individual responsible for financial resource monitoring? **A (EP 15)**				
13. Does the care plan review occur quarterly, or more frequently when indicated by a change in the resident's condition or as required by law and regulation? **C (EP 16)** Ⓜ				

Key: 0 = Insufficient compliance; 1 = Partial compliance; 2 = Satisfactory compliance; NA = Not applicable; **A** indicates scoring category A; **C** indicates scoring category C; ▲2 indicates situational decision rules apply; ⚠3 indicates direct impact requirements apply; Ⓜ indicates Measure of success is needed; ☆ indicates this standard also applies to organizations seeking Joint Commission's Medicare/Medicaid certification–based long term care accreditation

Standard PC.5.10 ★	Standard Score: ❑ Compliant ❑ Not Compliant			
Assessment Question	**Level of Compliance**	**Evidence of Compliance**	**Plan of Action/ Measure of Success (if needed)**	**Due Date**
1. Does the organization provide care, treatment, and services for each resident according to the plan for care, treatment, and services? **C (EP 1) Ⓜ ⚠3**				
2. Does the organization use at least two resident identifiers (neither to be the resident's room number) whenever administering medications or blood products; taking blood samples and other specimens for clinical testing, or providing any other treatments or procedures? (This requirement is not scored here. It is scored at NPSG.01.01.01.) **(EP 4)**				

Standard PC.5.30	Standard Score: ❑ Compliant ❑ Not Compliant			
Assessment Question	**Level of Compliance**	**Evidence of Compliance**	**Plan of Action/ Measure of Success (if needed)**	**Due Date**
1. Are orders* obtained from the physician or other authorized individuals according to law and regulation and professional practice acts before providing care, treatment, and services? **C (EP 1) Ⓜ ⚠3**				
2. Is the order tailored to each resident's needs and includes all elements required by law and regulation? **C (EP 2) Ⓜ ⚠3**				

* These orders may be verbal or written and include prescriptions.

Key: 0 = Insufficient compliance; 1 = Partial compliance; 2 = Satisfactory compliance; NA = Not applicable; **A** indicates scoring category A; **C** indicates scoring category C; ▲2 indicates situational decision rules apply; ⚠3 indicates direct impact requirements apply; Ⓜ indicates Measure of success is needed; ☆ indicates this standard also applies to organizations seeking Joint Commission's Medicare/Medicaid certification–based long term care accreditation

Standard PC.5.30				
Assessment Question	**Level of Compliance**	**Evidence of Compliance**	**Plan of Action/ Measure of Success (if needed)**	**Due Date**
3. Are all orders renewed or updated to reflect the following: • Changes in the care, treatment, or service being provided • Changes in the resident's physical or psychosocial condition • The resident's response to care, treatment, or services • The resident's outcome related to care, treatment, or services • Changes in diagnosis, treatment (including procedures and medications), and equipment • The minimum review time frame defined by the organization • Applicable law and regulation? **C (EP 3)** Ⓜ ⚠3				
4. Does the organization provide care, treatment, and services according to the most recent order? **C (EP 4)** Ⓜ ⚠3				
5. Does each attending physician designate an alternate physician whom the organization can contact to obtain regular or emergency care when the attending physician is not available? **C (EP 5)** Ⓜ				

Standard PC.5.40	Standard Score: ❑ Compliant ❑ Not Compliant			
Assessment Question	**Level of Compliance**	**Evidence of Compliance**	**Plan of Action/ Measure of Success (if needed)**	**Due Date**
1. Does the attending physician visit the resident in accordance with the resident's needs? **A (EP 1)** ⚠3				
2. Does the attending physician visit the resident at least once during the 30 days after admission? **C (EP 2)** Ⓜ				

Key: 0 = Insufficient compliance; 1 = Partial compliance; 2 = Satisfactory compliance; NA = Not applicable; **A** indicates scoring category A; **C** indicates scoring category C; ▲2 indicates situational decision rules apply; ⚠3 indicates direct impact requirements apply; Ⓜ indicates Measure of success is needed; ☆ indicates this standard also applies to organizations seeking Joint Commission's Medicare/Medicaid certification–based long term care accreditation

Standard PC.5.40

Assessment Question	Level of Compliance	Evidence of Compliance	Plan of Action/ Measure of Success (if needed)	Due Date
3. For planned stays of less than 30 days, does the resident's attending physician visit the resident at least once before discharge? **C (EP 3) Ⓜ**				
4. Is the resident seen within 72 hours of admission when the long term care physician is different from the resident's primary physician? **C (EP 4) Ⓜ**				
5. Do the physicians' visiting schedules comply with law, regulation, and organization policy regarding the following: • Frequency and timing of visits • Visits by physician assistants or advanced practice registered nurses instead of attending physicians? **C (EP 5)**				

Standard PC.5.50

Standard Score: ❑ Compliant ❑ Not Compliant

Assessment Question	Level of Compliance	Evidence of Compliance	Plan of Action/ Measure of Success (if needed)	Due Date
1. Are care, treatment, and services provided in an interdisciplinary, collaborative manner* as appropriate to the needs of the resident and the organization's scope of services? **A (EP 1)**				
2. Are changes in the resident's condition communicated to the physician or other authorized health care professionals, the resident, and his or her family? **A (EP 3)**				
3. Is information from consultation and evaluation reports communicated to the physician? **C (EP 4) Ⓜ**				
4. Does the organization provide this information on a timely basis as defined by the organization and required by law and regulation? **C (EP 5) Ⓜ**				

* The process is designed to ensure coordinated participation of all appropriate health care professionals from the appropriate settings and includes identifying interdisciplinary team members' responsibilities, holding interdisciplinary team meetings, providing for resolution of differences among interdisciplinary team members, documenting interdisciplinary team members' participation in the medical record, and discussing and modifying the resident's interdisciplinary care plan.

Key: 0 = Insufficient compliance; 1 = Partial compliance; 2 = Satisfactory compliance; NA = Not applicable; **A** indicates scoring category A; **C** indicates scoring category C; ▲(2) indicates situational decision rules apply; △(3) indicates direct impact requirements apply; Ⓜ indicates Measure of success is needed; ☆ indicates this standard also applies to organizations seeking Joint Commission's Medicare/Medicaid certification–based long term care accreditation

Standard PC.5.60	Standard Score: ❑ Compliant ❑ Not Compliant			
Assessment Question	**Level of Compliance**	**Evidence of Compliance**	**Plan of Action/ Measure of Success (if needed)**	**Due Date**
1. Does the organization coordinate the care, treatment, and services provided through internal resources to a resident? **A (EP 1)**				
2. When external resources are needed, does the organization participate in coordinating care, treatment, and services with these resources? **A (EP 2)**				
3. Does the organization have a process to receive or share relevant resident information to facilitate appropriate coordination and continuity when residents are referred to other care, treatment, or service providers? **A (EP 3)**				
4. Is there a process to resolve duplication or conflict with either internal or external resources? **A (EP 4)**				
5. Are the activities defined in the plan of care, treatment, and services provided in a time frame that meets the resident's health needs? **A (EP 5)**				
6. Are services made available directly or via arrangement to meet the following resident needs: • 24-hour emergency dental services • Spiritual services • Behavioral health services,* including counseling on a continuing basis in individual, family, and group services, as appropriate • Activity services for ambulatory and non-ambulatory residents at various functional levels as well as those who are unable to attend group activities • Assistance with guardianship and conservatorship, when indicated • Services to facilitate family support, social work, nursing care, dental care, rehabilitation, primary physician care, or discharge? **A (EP 7)**				

* These services may be provided by various disciplines (for instance, social workers, psychologists, clinical nurse specialists, or other appropriately educated consultants).

Key: 0 = Insufficient compliance; 1 = Partial compliance; 2 = Satisfactory compliance; NA = Not applicable; **A** indicates scoring category A; **C** indicates scoring category C; ▲ indicates situational decision rules apply; △ indicates direct impact requirements apply; Ⓜ indicates Measure of success is needed; ☆ indicates this standard also applies to organizations seeking Joint Commission's Medicare/Medicaid certification–based long term care accreditation

Standard PC.6.10 ★	**Standard Score: ❑ Compliant ❑ Not Compliant**			
Assessment Question	**Level of Compliance**	**Evidence of Compliance**	**Plan of Action/ Measure of Success (if needed)**	**Due Date**
1. Is education provided that is appropriate to the resident's needs? **A (EP 1)**				
2. Does the assessment of learning needs address cultural and religious beliefs, emotional barriers, desire and motivation to learn, physical or cognitive limitations, and barriers to communication as appropriate? **C (EP 2) Ⓜ**				
3. As appropriate to the resident's condition and assessed needs and the organization's scope of services, is the resident educated about the following: • The plan for care, treatment, and services • His or her condition or illness and preventive interventions • Basic health practices and safety • The safe and effective use of medications • Nutrition interventions, modified diets, or oral health • Safe and effective use of medical equipment or supplies when provided by the organization • Understanding pain, the risk for pain, the importance of effective pain management, the pain management process, and methods for pain management • Habilitation or rehabilitation techniques to help them reach maximum independence possible • Environmental and physical plant safety issues, such as fire safety, evacuation, storage of chemical agents, and so on • Use of nonmedical equipment, including but not limited to, operating call lights, beds, and personal appliances • How to carry out self-care • Transfer techniques • Personal safety and mobility • Bathroom safety • Available resources to meet identified needs and how to access such resources • When to seek and how to obtain follow-up or continuing care, treatment, and services? **A (EP 3)**				

Key: 0 = Insufficient compliance; 1 = Partial compliance; 2 = Satisfactory compliance; NA = Not applicable; **A** indicates scoring category A; **C** indicates scoring category C; ▲ indicates situational decision rules apply; △ indicates direct impact requirements apply; Ⓜ indicates Measure of success is needed; ☆ indicates this standard also applies to organizations seeking Joint Commission's Medicare/Medicaid certification–based long term care accreditation

Standard PC.6.30	**Standard Score:** ❑ Compliant ❑ Not Compliant			
Assessment Question	**Level of Compliance**	**Evidence of Compliance**	**Plan of Action/ Measure of Success (if needed)**	**Due Date**
1. Is the education provided appropriate to the resident's abilities? **A (EP 1)**				
2. Is education coordinated among the disciplines providing care, treatment, and services? **A (EP 2)**				
3. Is the content presented in an understandable manner? **A (EP 3)**				
4. Do teaching methods accommodate various learning styles? **A (EP 4)**				
5. Is comprehension evaluated? **C (EP 5)** Ⓜ				

Standard PC.6.50	**Standard Score:** ❑ Compliant ❑ Not Compliant			
Assessment Question	**Level of Compliance**	**Evidence of Compliance**	**Plan of Action/ Measure of Success (if needed)**	**Due Date**
1. Does the organization define the length of stay and absence from school that would require providing educational services in accordance with applicable law and regulation? **A (EP 1)**				
2. Are selected education resources based on the resident's identified needs? **A (EP 3)**				

Standard PC.7.10	**Standard Score:** ❑ Compliant ❑ Not Compliant			
Assessment Question	**Level of Compliance**	**Evidence of Compliance**	**Plan of Action/ Measure of Success (if needed)**	**Due Date**
1. Are food and nutrition products provided for the resident? **A (EP 1)** △3				
2. Are food and nutrition products stored under proper conditions of sanitation, temperature, light, moisture, ventilation, and security? **C (EP 2)** Ⓜ △3				

Key: 0 = Insufficient compliance; 1 = Partial compliance; 2 = Satisfactory compliance; NA = Not applicable; **A** indicates scoring category A; **C** indicates scoring category C; ▲2 indicates situational decision rules apply; △3 indicates direct impact requirements apply; Ⓜ indicates Measure of success is needed; ☆ indicates this standard also applies to organizations seeking Joint Commission's Medicare/Medicaid certification–based long term care accreditation

Standard PC.7.10

Assessment Question	Level of Compliance	Evidence of Compliance	Plan of Action/ Measure of Success (if needed)	Due Date
3. Are resident's cultural, religious, and ethnic food preferences honored when possible unless contraindicated? **C (EP 3) Ⓜ**				
4. Are substitutes of equal nutritional value offered when residents refuse the food served? **C (EP 4) Ⓜ**				
5. Do staff members assist residents when necessary? **C (EP 5) Ⓜ △3**				
6. Are resident communal dining areas adequately supervised? **A (EP 8)**				
7. Does a food service supervisor oversee general kitchen management? **A (EP 9)**				
8. Are menus planned in advance, dated, easy to read, and posted in conspicuous areas accessible to residents? **A (EP 10)**				
9. Are special diets and altered diet schedules accommodated? **C (EP 11) Ⓜ**				
10. Are cycled menus rotated over a period of at least three weeks? **A (EP 12)**				
11. Are food and nutrition products prepared under proper conditions of sanitation, temperature, light, moisture, ventilation, and security? **C (EP 17) Ⓜ △3**				

Key: 0 = Insufficient compliance; 1 = Partial compliance; 2 = Satisfactory compliance; NA = Not applicable; **A** indicates scoring category A; **C** indicates scoring category C; ▲2 indicates situational decision rules apply; △3 indicates direct impact requirements apply; Ⓜ indicates Measure of success is needed; ☆ indicates this standard also applies to organizations seeking Joint Commission's Medicare/Medicaid certification–based long term care accreditation

Standard PC.8.10	**Standard Score: ❑ Compliant ❑ Not Compliant**			
Assessment Question	**Level of Compliance**	**Evidence of Compliance**	**Plan of Action/ Measure of Success (if needed)**	**Due Date**
1. Is a comprehensive pain assessment conducted as appropriate to the resident's condition and the scope of care, treatment, and services provided? **C (EP 1)** Ⓜ ⚠3				
2. Does regular assessment and follow-up occur according to criteria developed by the organization? **C (EP 3)** Ⓜ ⚠3				
3. Are assessment methods appropriate to the resident's age and/or abilities? **C (EP 6)** Ⓜ ⚠3				
4. When pain is identified, is the resident treated by the organization or referred for treatment? **C (EP 7)** Ⓜ ⚠3				

Standard PC.8.20	**Standard Score: ❑ Compliant ❑ Not Compliant**			
Assessment Question	**Level of Compliance**	**Evidence of Compliance**	**Plan of Action/ Measure of Success (if needed)**	**Due Date**
1. Are appropriate supplies and equipment available to support self-care? **C (EP 1)** Ⓜ				
2. Are adaptive self-help devices provided when needed? **C (EP 2)** Ⓜ				
3. Are residents assisted with self-care activities when needed? **C (EP 3)** Ⓜ				
4. Are residents clean and well groomed? **C (EP 4)** Ⓜ				
5. Are oral prostheses clean? **C (EP 5)** Ⓜ				
6. Are residents free from discernible body odor? **C (EP 6)** Ⓜ				
7. Is skin clean and dry? **C (EP 7)** Ⓜ				
8. Are residents appropriately assisted with toileting activities? **C (EP 8)** Ⓜ				

Key: 0 = Insufficient compliance; 1 = Partial compliance; 2 = Satisfactory compliance; NA = Not applicable; **A** indicates scoring category A; **C** indicates scoring category C; ▲2 indicates situational decision rules apply; ⚠3 indicates direct impact requirements apply; Ⓜ indicates Measure of success is needed; ☆ indicates this standard also applies to organizations seeking Joint Commission's Medicare/Medicaid certification–based long term care accreditation

Standard PC.8.20

Assessment Question	Level of Compliance	Evidence of Compliance	Plan of Action/ Measure of Success (if needed)	Due Date
9. Are residents appropriately assisted with activities of daily living including the following: • Bathing • Dressing • Eating • Oral hygiene • Ambulation? **C (EP 9) Ⓜ**				
10. Are all reasonable steps taken to keep residents safe from accident and injury? **A (EP 10)**				

Standard PC.8.30

Standard Score: ❑ Compliant ❑ Not Compliant

Assessment Question	Level of Compliance	Evidence of Compliance	Plan of Action/ Measure of Success (if needed)	Due Date
1. Are preventive interventions performed according to the plan of care, treatment, and services to do the following: • Encourage and help residents to be out of bed, except when prohibited by a physician's order • Encourage and help chair-fast residents to leave their rooms for a change of environment • Maintain proper body position and alignment • Implement a skin integrity program • Implement a bowel management program • Implement a bladder management program • Assist with ambulation including maintenance of gait training • Provide active and passive range of motion exercises • Provide assistance to help prevent aspiration, dehydration, and malnutrition • Assist with coping with the effects of illness, disability, treatment, or stay in the facility? **C (EP 1) Ⓜ**				

Key: 0 = Insufficient compliance; 1 = Partial compliance; 2 = Satisfactory compliance; NA = Not applicable; **A** indicates scoring category A; **C** indicates scoring category C; ▲ indicates situational decision rules apply; △ indicates direct impact requirements apply; Ⓜ indicates Measure of success is needed; ☆ indicates this standard also applies to organizations seeking Joint Commission's Medicare/Medicaid certification–based long term care accreditation

Standard PC.8.40	Standard Score: ❑ Compliant ❑ Not Compliant			
Assessment Question	Level of Compliance	Evidence of Compliance	Plan of Action/ Measure of Success (if needed)	Due Date
1. Are residents assisted in participating in social and leisure activities according to their interests and needs? **C (EP 1) Ⓜ**				
2. Is an activity schedule made available to all residents, staff, and visitors? **A (EP 2)**				
3. Is the schedule of activities communicated to residents who have difficulty reading? **C (EP 3) Ⓜ**				
4. Do residents have access to a variety of activities based on their needs? **A (EP 4)**				

Standard PC.8.70	Standard Score: ❑ Compliant ❑ Not Compliant			
Assessment Question	Level of Compliance	Evidence of Compliance	Plan of Action/ Measure of Success (if needed)	Due Date
1. To the extent possible, as appropriate to the resident's and family's needs and the organization's services, do interventions address resident and family comfort, dignity, and psychosocial, emotional, and spiritual needs, as appropriate, about death and grief? **A (EP 1)**				
2. Is staff educated about the unique needs of dying residents and their families and caregivers? **C (EP 2) Ⓜ**				

Standard PC.9.10 ★	Standard Score: ❑ Compliant ❑ Not Compliant			
Assessment Question	Level of Compliance	Evidence of Compliance	Plan of Action/ Measure of Success (if needed)	Due Date
1. If the organization provides for the maintenance and transfusion of blood or blood components, does it meet all applicable law and regulation? **A (EP 10) Ⓜ**				

Key: 0 = Insufficient compliance; 1 = Partial compliance; 2 = Satisfactory compliance; NA = Not applicable; **A** indicates scoring category A; **C** indicates scoring category C; ▲(2) indicates situational decision rules apply; △(3) indicates direct impact requirements apply; Ⓜ indicates Measure of success is needed; ☆ indicates this standard also applies to organizations seeking Joint Commission's Medicare/Medicaid certification–based long term care accreditation

Standard PC.9.20	**Standard Score:** ❑ Compliant ❑ Not Compliant			
Assessment Question	**Level of Compliance**	**Evidence of Compliance**	**Plan of Action/ Measure of Success (if needed)**	**Due Date**
1. Does the organization develop policies and procedures for responding to life-threatening emergencies such as respiratory arrest and cardiac arrest? **A (EP 1)**				
2. Do policies and procedures that address life-threatening emergencies include the following: • Availability of first aid and Basic Life Support (CPR) services • Emergency transfer to another organization • Placing a telephone call to 911? **A (EP 2)**				
3. Does the organization respond to life-threatening emergencies according to organization policy and procedure? **A (EP 3)** ⚠3				

Standard PC.11.80	**Standard Score:** ❑ Compliant ❑ Not Compliant			
Assessment Question	**Level of Compliance**	**Evidence of Compliance**	**Plan of Action/ Measure of Success (if needed)**	**Due Date**
1. Is achieving a restraint-free environment a stated goal of the organization? **A (EP 1)**				
2. Are processes implemented to actively pursue this goal? **A (EP 2)**				
3. Is the use of physical or chemical restraints prohibited for discipline or staff convenience or to prevent wandering? **A (EP 3)** ⚠3				
4. Is the use of physical or chemical restraints prohibited except to facilitate or support treatment of a resident's medical symptoms? **A (EP 4)** ⚠3				
5. Are residents allowed to refuse restraints? **A (EP 5)** ⚠3				

Key: 0 = Insufficient compliance; 1 = Partial compliance; 2 = Satisfactory compliance; NA = Not applicable; **A** indicates scoring category A; **C** indicates scoring category C; ▲2 indicates situational decision rules apply; ⚠3 indicates direct impact requirements apply; Ⓜ indicates Measure of success is needed; ☆ indicates this standard also applies to organizations seeking Joint Commission's Medicare/Medicaid certification–based long term care accreditation

Standard PC.11.80

Assessment Question	Level of Compliance	Evidence of Compliance	Plan of Action/ Measure of Success (if needed)	Due Date
6. Is the decision to use restraints based on an assessment of the resident's needs and never based on a request from a resident's representative? **A (EP 6)** ⚠3				
7. Do the processes emphasize alternatives to restraint, including the following: • Restorative programs • Management of the resident's personal environment • Well-trained staff to support each resident • Support of resident's rights • Recognition and respect for the resident's past interests • Supportive devices and special equipment • Involvement of other people in each resident's care, such as nursing assistants, housekeeping staff, secretaries, and other administrative staff, who have been trained in resident-orientation techniques? **A (EP 7)**				

Standard PC.11.90

Standard Score: ❑ Compliant ❑ Not Compliant

Assessment Question	Level of Compliance	Evidence of Compliance	Plan of Action/ Measure of Success (if needed)	Due Date
1. Is the use of restraints based on the resident's assessed needs, including precipitating factors, and is this documented? **C (EP 1)** Ⓜ ⚠3				
2. Is a trial of alternatives before the use of restraints documented? **C (EP 2)** Ⓜ ⚠3				
3. Is there a licensed independent practitioner's written order for the use of restraints? **A (EP 3)** ⚠3				
4. Are time limitations determined for the use of restraints? **A (EP 4)** ⚠3				
5. Is the frequency of observing and assessing the resident determined? **A (EP 5)** ⚠3				

Key: 0 = Insufficient compliance; 1 = Partial compliance; 2 = Satisfactory compliance; NA = Not applicable; **A** indicates scoring category A; **C** indicates scoring category C; ▲2 indicates situational decision rules apply; ⚠3 indicates direct impact requirements apply; Ⓜ indicates Measure of success is needed; ☆ indicates this standard also applies to organizations seeking Joint Commission's Medicare/Medicaid certification–based long term care accreditation

Standard PC.11.90

Assessment Question	Level of Compliance	Evidence of Compliance	Plan of Action/ Measure of Success (if needed)	Due Date
6. Are restraint devices applied correctly? **A (EP 6)** ⚠3				
7. Are restraints periodically removed or released in accordance with law and regulation and the resident's needs? **A (EP 7)** ⚠3				
8. Is the competence of the staff applying such interventions determined? **A (EP 8)** ⚠3				
9. Is attention paid to the resident's needs while in restraint? **A (EP 9)** ⚠3				
10. Is informed consent obtained as appropriate? **A (EP 10)** ⚠3				
11. Is the use of restraint reviewed if frequent or prolonged? **A (EP 11)** ⚠3				
12. Are orders for restraint reviewed within time frames defined by the organization, not to exceed 30 days? **A (EP 12)** ⚠3				
13. Does the interdisciplinary team monitor the resident on an ongoing basis while in restraint and request a new physician order at any time within the 30 days due to changes in the resident's condition that require removing or modifying restraint? **A (EP 13)** ⚠3				
14. Are the resident and family educated about restraints and their alternatives? **C (EP 14)** Ⓜ				
15. Is the use of restraint measured, assessed, and reduced as part of the organization's quality improvement program, with the goal of becoming restraint free? **A (EP 15)**				

Key: 0 = Insufficient compliance; 1 = Partial compliance; 2 = Satisfactory compliance; NA = Not applicable; **A** indicates scoring category A; **C** indicates scoring category C; ▲2 indicates situational decision rules apply; ⚠3 indicates direct impact requirements apply; Ⓜ indicates Measure of success is needed; ☆ indicates this standard also applies to organizations seeking Joint Commission's Medicare/Medicaid certification–based long term care accreditation

Standard PC.11.90

Assessment Question	Level of Compliance	Evidence of Compliance	Plan of Action/ Measure of Success (if needed)	Due Date
16. Are restraints used only under the following circumstances: • When alternatives to restraint are not effective, as determined by the interdisciplinary team, with resident and family involvement as appropriate • When absolutely necessary to ensure safety of the resident, other residents, and staff? **A (EP 16)** ⚠3				
17. When restraints are used, does the following occur: • Staff interaction with the resident is positive and supportive in both verbal and nonverbal ways • Staff members interact regularly and appropriately with the resident so that the resident is not neglected? **C (EP 17)** Ⓜ ⚠3				
18. Are medications to control behavior used as part of a therapeutic plan only after appropriate assessment by professionals is performed? **A (EP 18)** ⚠3				

Standard PC.13.10

Standard Score: ❑ Compliant ❑ Not Compliant

Assessment Question	Level of Compliance	Evidence of Compliance	Plan of Action/ Measure of Success (if needed)	Due Date
1. Does the assessment include the following: • The resident's history • The resident's physical status • Diagnostic data • The risks and benefits of procedures • The possible need to administer blood or blood components? **A (EP 1)**				

Key: 0 = Insufficient compliance; 1 = Partial compliance; 2 = Satisfactory compliance; NA = Not applicable; **A** indicates scoring category A; **C** indicates scoring category C; ▲2 indicates situational decision rules apply; ⚠3 indicates direct impact requirements apply; Ⓜ indicates Measure of success is needed; ☆ indicates this standard also applies to organizations seeking Joint Commission's Medicare/Medicaid certification–based long term care accreditation

Standard PC.13.20	**Standard Score:** ❑ Compliant ❑ Not Compliant			
Assessment Question	**Level of Compliance**	**Evidence of Compliance**	**Plan of Action/ Measure of Success (if needed)**	**Due Date**
1. Are sufficient numbers of qualified staff members (in addition to the individual performing the procedure) present to evaluate the resident, help with the procedure, provide the sedation and/or anesthesia, monitor, and recover the resident? **A (EP 1)** ⚠3				
2. Are the individuals administering moderate or deep sedation and anesthesia qualified and do they have the appropriate credentials to manage residents at whatever level of sedation or anesthesia is achieved, either intentionally or unintentionally? **A (EP 2)** ⚠3				
3. Is appropriate equipment to monitor the resident's physiologic status available? **A (EP 4)** ⚠3				
4. Is appropriate equipment to administer intravenous fluids and drugs, including blood and blood components, available as needed? **A (EP 5)** ⚠3				
5. Are resuscitation capabilities available? **A (EP 6)** ⚠3				
6. Are the resident's anticipated needs assessed to plan for the appropriate level of postprocedure care before the operative and other procedures or the administration of moderate or deep sedation or anesthesia occurs? **C (EP 7)** Ⓜ ⚠3				
7. Are preprocedural education, treatments, and services according to the care, treatment, and services provided before the operative and other procedures or the administration of moderate or deep sedation or anesthesia occurs? **C (EP 8)** Ⓜ				
8. Prior to the start of any surgical or invasive procedure, is a final verification process, such as a "time out," conducted to confirm the correct resident, procedure and site, using active—not passive—communication techniques? (This requirement is not scored here. It is scored at NPSG.01.02.01.) **(EP 9)**				

Key: 0 = Insufficient compliance; 1 = Partial compliance; 2 = Satisfactory compliance; NA = Not applicable; **A** indicates scoring category A; **C** indicates scoring category C; ▲2 indicates situational decision rules apply; ⚠3 indicates direct impact requirements apply; Ⓜ indicates Measure of success is needed; ☆ indicates this standard also applies to organizations seeking Joint Commission's Medicare/Medicaid certification–based long term care accreditation

Standard PC.13.20				
Assessment Question	**Level of Compliance**	**Evidence of Compliance**	**Plan of Action/ Measure of Success (if needed)**	**Due Date**
9. Is a presedation or preanesthesia assessment conducted before the operative and other procedures or the administration of moderate or deep sedation or anesthesia occurs? **A (EP 10)** △3				
10. Does a licensed independent practitioner with appropriate clinical privileges plan or concur with the planned anesthesia, before sedating or anesthetizing a resident? **A (EP 11)** △3				
11. Is the resident reevaluated immediately before moderate or deep sedation and before anesthesia induction? **A (EP 12)** △3				

Standard PC.13.30	Standard Score: ❑ Compliant ❑ Not Compliant			
Assessment Question	**Level of Compliance**	**Evidence of Compliance**	**Plan of Action/ Measure of Success (if needed)**	**Due Date**
1. Are appropriate methods used to continuously monitor oxygenation, ventilation, and circulation during procedures that may affect the resident's physiological status? **A (EP 1)** △3				
2. Are the procedures and/or the administration of moderate or deep sedation or anesthesia for each resident documented in the medical record? **C (EP 2)** Ⓜ △3				

Standard PC.13.40	Standard Score: ❑ Compliant ❑ Not Compliant			
Assessment Question	**Level of Compliance**	**Evidence of Compliance**	**Plan of Action/ Measure of Success (if needed)**	**Due Date**
1. Is the resident's status assessed immediately after the procedure and/or administration of moderate or deep sedation or anesthesia? **A (EP 1)** △3				
2. Are each resident's physiological status, mental status, and pain level monitored? **C (EP 2)** Ⓜ △3				

Key: 0 = Insufficient compliance; 1 = Partial compliance; 2 = Satisfactory compliance; NA = Not applicable; **A** indicates scoring category A; **C** indicates scoring category C; ▲2 indicates situational decision rules apply; △3 indicates direct impact requirements apply; Ⓜ indicates Measure of success is needed; ☆ indicates this standard also applies to organizations seeking Joint Commission's Medicare/Medicaid certification–based long term care accreditation

Standard PC.13.40

Assessment Question	Level of Compliance	Evidence of Compliance	Plan of Action/ Measure of Success (if needed)	Due Date
3. Is monitoring at a level consistent with the potential effect of the procedure and/or sedation or anesthesia? **A (EP 3)** ⚠3				
4. Are residents discharged from the recovery area and organization by a qualified licensed independent practitioner according to rigorously applied criteria approved by the clinical leaders? **A (EP 4)** ⚠3				
5. Are residents who have received anesthesia discharged in the company of a responsible, designated adult? **C (EP 5)** Ⓜ ⚠3				

Standard PC.15.10

Standard Score: ❑ Compliant ❑ Not Compliant

Assessment Question	Level of Compliance	Evidence of Compliance	Plan of Action/ Measure of Success (if needed)	Due Date
1. Is there a process that addresses the needs for continuing care, treatment, and services after discharge or transfer that includes the following: • The reason for transfer or discharge • The conditions under which transfer or discharge can occur • Interdisciplinary team planning • The residents' and caregivers' knowledge of and demonstration of all necessary activities • Assessing the environment (home, hospital, other facility) to which the resident is being discharged • Identifying and indicating the involvement of supportive services* • Planning for providing necessary care, treatment, services, assistance, and instruction • Shifting responsibility for a resident's care from one clinician, organizational program, or service to another • Mechanisms for internal and external transfer • The accountability and responsibility for the resident's safety during transfer of both the organization initiating the transfer and the organization receiving the resident? **A (EP 1)**				

* Supportive services include community referral information and telephone numbers, needs for medical and adaptive equipment, specific instructions on medication administration and adverse effects, and follow-up appointments.

Key: 0 = Insufficient compliance; 1 = Partial compliance; 2 = Satisfactory compliance; NA = Not applicable; **A** indicates scoring category A; **C** indicates scoring category C; ▲2 indicates situational decision rules apply; ⚠3 indicates direct impact requirements apply; Ⓜ indicates Measure of success is needed; ☆ indicates this standard also applies to organizations seeking Joint Commission's Medicare/Medicaid certification–based long term care accreditation

Standard PC.15.10				
Assessment Question	Level of Compliance	Evidence of Compliance	Plan of Action/ Measure of Success (if needed)	Due Date
2. Are residents transferred or discharged by order of their attending physician? **C (EP 4)** Ⓜ				
3. Does the organization follow an established process for emergency discharge due to medical necessity? **A (EP 5)**				

Standard PC.15.20	Standard Score: ❑ Compliant ❑ Not Compliant			
Assessment Question	Level of Compliance	Evidence of Compliance	Plan of Action/ Measure of Success (if needed)	Due Date
1. Are the resident's needs for continuing care to meet physical and psychosocial needs identified? **C (EP 1)** Ⓜ ⚠3				
2. Are residents told in a timely manner of the need to plan for discharge or transfer to another organization or level of care? **C (EP 2)** Ⓜ				
3. Does planning for discharge involve the resident and all appropriate licensed independent practitioners, staff, and family members involved in the resident's care, treatment, and services? **C (EP 3)** Ⓜ				
4. When the resident is transferred, does information provided to the resident include the following: • The reason he or she is being transferred • Information on the facility or program to which the resident is being transferred • Alternatives to transfer, if any? **C (EP 4)** Ⓜ				
5. When the resident is discharged, is information provided that includes the following: • The reason he or she is being discharged • The anticipated need for continued care, treatment, and services* after discharge? **C (EP 6)** Ⓜ				

* Available services include, as appropriate, special education, adult day care, case management, home health services, hospice, long term care facilities, ambulatory care, support groups, rehabilitation services, and community mental health services.

Key: 0 = Insufficient compliance; 1 = Partial compliance; 2 = Satisfactory compliance; NA = Not applicable; **A** indicates scoring category A; **C** indicates scoring category C; ▲2 indicates situational decision rules apply; ⚠3 indicates direct impact requirements apply; Ⓜ indicates Measure of success is needed; ☆ indicates this standard also applies to organizations seeking Joint Commission's Medicare/Medicaid certification–based long term care accreditation

Standard PC.15.20

Assessment Question	Level of Compliance	Evidence of Compliance	Plan of Action/ Measure of Success (if needed)	Due Date
6. Is the resident educated about how to obtain further care, treatment, and services to meet his or her identified needs, when indicated? C (EP 7) Ⓜ				
7. Does the organization arrange for or help the family arrange for services needed to meet the resident's needs after discharge, when indicated and before discharge? C (EP 8) Ⓜ				
8. Are written discharge instructions in a form the resident can understand, given to the resident and/or those responsible for providing continuing care? C (EP 9) Ⓜ				
9. Does the organization notify the resident's family and encourage a family member to participate in the transfer whenever possible? C (EP 10) Ⓜ				

Standard PC.15.30

Standard Score: ❑ Compliant ❑ Not Compliant

Assessment Question	Level of Compliance	Evidence of Compliance	Plan of Action/ Measure of Success (if needed)	Due Date
1. Does the organization communicate appropriate information to any organization or provider to which the resident is transferred or discharged? C (EP 1) Ⓜ ⚠3				
2. Does the information shared include the following, as appropriate to the care, treatment, and services provided: • The reason for transfer or discharge • A summary of care, treatment, and services provided and progress toward goals • Community resources or referrals provided to the resident? C (EP 2) Ⓜ				

Key: 0 = Insufficient compliance; 1 = Partial compliance; 2 = Satisfactory compliance; NA = Not applicable; **A** indicates scoring category A; **C** indicates scoring category C; ▲ indicates situational decision rules apply; ⚠3 indicates direct impact requirements apply; Ⓜ indicates Measure of success is needed; ☆ indicates this standard also applies to organizations seeking Joint Commission's Medicare/Medicaid certification–based long term care accreditation

Standard PC.15.50	**Standard Score: ❑ Compliant ❑ Not Compliant**			
Assessment Question	**Level of Compliance**	**Evidence of Compliance**	**Plan of Action/ Measure of Success (if needed)**	**Due Date**
1. Does the organization explain in writing, the conditions of its bed-hold policy to the residents and a family member or legal guardian at the time of admission? **A (EP 1)**				

Standard PC.16.10 ★	**Standard Score: ❑ Compliant ❑ Not Compliant**			
Assessment Question	**Level of Compliance**	**Evidence of Compliance**	**Plan of Action/ Measure of Success (if needed)**	**Due Date**
1. Does the director named on the CLIA certificate determine the context in which waived tests are used? **A (EP 1)**				
2. Is the clinical use of results consistent with the organization's policies and the manufacturer's recommendations for waived tests? **C (EP 2)** Ⓜ △3				
3. Are the quantitative test result reports in the clinical record accompanied by reference ranges specific to the test method used and population served?* **A (EP 3)**				
4. Are criteria for confirmatory testing specified in the written procedures for qualitative and quantitative tests? **A (EP 4)**				
5. Are written procedures for confirmatory testing for qualitative and quantitative tests based on clinical usage and limitations of the test methodology? **A (EP 5)**				
6. Are criteria for confirmatory testing followed as specified in the written procedures? **C (EP 6)** Ⓜ △3				

* **Note:** *Semiquantitative results, such as urine macroscopic and urine dipsticks, are not required to comply with this EP.*

Key: 0 = Insufficient compliance; 1 = Partial compliance; 2 = Satisfactory compliance; NA = Not applicable; **A** indicates scoring category A; **C** indicates scoring category C; ▲2 indicates situational decision rules apply; △3 indicates direct impact requirements apply; Ⓜ indicates Measure of success is needed; ☆ indicates this standard also applies to organizations seeking Joint Commission's Medicare/Medicaid certification–based long term care accreditation

Standard PC.16.20 ★	**Standard Score:** ❑ Compliant ❑ Not Compliant			
Assessment Question	**Level of Compliance**	**Evidence of Compliance**	**Plan of Action/ Measure of Success (if needed)**	**Due Date**
1. Is the identity of staff members who perform waived testing documented?* **A (EP 1)**				
2. Is the identity of staff members who supervise waived testing documented?* **A (EP 2)**				

Standard PC.16.30 ★	**Standard Score:** ❑ Compliant ❑ Not Compliant			
Assessment Question	**Level of Compliance**	**Evidence of Compliance**	**Plan of Action/ Measure of Success (if needed)**	**Due Date**
1. Have staff members who perform testing been oriented according to the organization's specific services? **A (EP 1)**				
2. Have staff members who perform testing been trained for each test he or she is authorized to perform? **A (EP 2)**				
3. Have staff members who perform testing that requires the use of an instrument been trained on the use and maintenance of that instrument? **A (EP 3)**				
4. Has competence been assessed according to organization policy at defined intervals, but at least at the time of orientation and annually thereafter? **A (EP 4)**				
5. Is current competency assessed using at least two of the following methods per person per test: • Performing a test on a blind† specimen • Having a supervisor or qualified delegate periodically observe routine work • Monitoring each user's quality control performance • Having written testing that is specific to the method assessed? **A (EP 5)** ⚠3				

* **Note:** *These individuals may be employees of the organization, contracted staff, or employees of a contracted service.*

† **Blind specimen** A sample with known value tested by personnel who do not know the expected result.

Key: 0 = Insufficient compliance; 1 = Partial compliance; 2 = Satisfactory compliance; NA = Not applicable; **A** indicates scoring category A; **C** indicates scoring category C; ▲2 indicates situational decision rules apply; ⚠3 indicates direct impact requirements apply; Ⓜ indicates Measure of success is needed; ☆ indicates this standard also applies to organizations seeking Joint Commission's Medicare/Medicaid certification–based long term care accreditation

Standard PC.16.30 ★

Assessment Question	Level of Compliance	Evidence of Compliance	Plan of Action/ Measure of Success (if needed)	Due Date
6. Does the director named on the CLIA certificate or qualified designee evaluate and document evidence of orientation, training, and competency?* **A (EP 6)**				

Standard PC.16.40 ★

Standard Score: ❑ Compliant ❑ Not Compliant

Assessment Question	Level of Compliance	Evidence of Compliance	Plan of Action/ Measure of Success (if needed)	Due Date
1. Does the director named on the CLIA certificate or a qualified designee approve policies and procedures at the following times: • Before initial use of the test for patient testing • Periodically thereafter, defined by the director but at least once every three years • When there are changes in procedures?† **A (EP 1)**				
2. Do written policies and procedures address the following items: • Specimen type, collection, identification, and required labeling • Specimen preservation, as appropriate • Instrument maintenance and function checks, such as calibration • Storage conditions for test components **Note:** *No reagent is used after its expiration date.* • Quality control (including frequency and type) and remedial action • Result reporting‡ • Equipment performance evaluation • Test performance? **A (EP 2)**				
3. If manufacturers' manuals or package inserts are used as the policies or procedures for each test, are they enhanced to include specific operational policies (e.g., detailed quality control protocols and any other institution-specific procedures regarding the test or instrument)? **A (EP 3)**				

* **Note:** *Staff members who perform instrument-based testing, including but not limited to physicians, licensed independent practitioners, contracted staff, and RNs, participate in training and competence demonstrations.*

† **Changes in procedures** Manufacturer updates to package inserts can include procedural changes, or a different manufacturer is used.

‡ **Note:** *Individual patient results are not reported unless the quality control is acceptable.*

Key: 0 = Insufficient compliance; 1 = Partial compliance; 2 = Satisfactory compliance; NA = Not applicable; **A** indicates scoring category A; **C** indicates scoring category C; ▲ indicates situational decision rules apply; △ indicates direct impact requirements apply; Ⓜ indicates Measure of success is needed; ☆ indicates this standard also applies to organizations seeking Joint Commission's Medicare/Medicaid certification–based long term care accreditation

Standard PC.16.40 ★

Assessment Question	Level of Compliance	Evidence of Compliance	Plan of Action/ Measure of Success (if needed)	Due Date
4. Are current and complete policies and procedures readily available to the person performing the test? **A (EP 4)**				
5. Are written policies, procedures, and manufacturer's instructions followed? **A (EP 5)** △3				

Standard PC.16.50 ★

Standard Score: ❑ Compliant ❑ Not Compliant

Assessment Question	Level of Compliance	Evidence of Compliance	Plan of Action/ Measure of Success (if needed)	Due Date
1. Does the director named on the CLIA certificate establish a written quality control policy that specifies how procedures will be controlled for quality, establishes timetables, and explains the rationale for choice of procedures and timetables? **A (EP 1)**				
2. Is the documented quality control rationale based on the following: • How the test is used • Reagent stability • Manufacturers' recommendations • The organization's experience with the test • Currently accepted guidelines? **A (EP 2)**				
3. Are quality control procedures performed at least as frequently as recommended by the manufacturer, or defined by the organization's procedures?* **A (EP 3)** △3				
4. For instrument-based waived testing, do quality control requirements include two levels of control, if commercially available? **C (EP 4)** Ⓜ △3				
5. Are quality control procedures for instrument-based waived testing performed at least once each day on each instrument used that day for resident testing? **C (EP 5)** Ⓜ △3				

* If frequency of quality control is not defined by the manufacturer, the organization defines frequency of quality control.

Key: 0 = Insufficient compliance; 1 = Partial compliance; 2 = Satisfactory compliance; NA = Not applicable; **A** indicates scoring category A; **C** indicates scoring category C; ▲2 indicates situational decision rules apply; △3 indicates direct impact requirements apply; Ⓜ indicates Measure of success is needed; ☆ indicates this standard also applies to organizations seeking Joint Commission's Medicare/Medicaid certification–based long term care accreditation

Standard PC.16.60 ★	Standard Score: ❑ Compliant ❑ Not Compliant			
Assessment Question	**Level of Compliance**	**Evidence of Compliance**	**Plan of Action/ Measure of Success (if needed)**	**Due Date**
1. Are all quality control test results documented, including internal and external (liquid and electronic)?* **C (EP 1) Ⓜ**				
2. Are test results documented in the clinical record? **C (EP 2) Ⓜ**				
3. Are individual test results associated with quality control and instrument records?† **A (EP 3)**				
4. Are quality control and test result records retained for at least two years? **A (EP 4)**				

* Quality control results may be located in the clinical record.

† A formal log is not required, but a functional audit trail is maintained that allows retrieval of individual test results and their association with quality control and instrument records.

Key: 0 = Insufficient compliance; 1 = Partial compliance; 2 = Satisfactory compliance; NA = Not applicable; **A** indicates scoring category A; **C** indicates scoring category C; ▲ indicates situational decision rules apply; △ indicates direct impact requirements apply; Ⓜ indicates Measure of success is needed; ☆ indicates this standard also applies to organizations seeking Joint Commission's Medicare/Medicaid certification–based long term care accreditation

Medication Management (MM)

Standard MM.1.10	Standard Score: ❑ Compliant ❑ Not Compliant			
Assessment Question	**Level of Compliance**	**Evidence of Compliance**	**Plan of Action/ Measure of Success (if needed)**	**Due Date**
1. Does written policy describe the minimum amount of information about the resident that is to be available to those involved in medication management? **A (EP 1)**				
2. At a minimum, does the information include the following: • The resident's age • The resident's sex • The resident's current medications • The resident's diagnoses, comorbidities, and concurrently occurring conditions • The resident's relevant laboratory values • The resident's allergies and past sensitivities? As appropriate to the resident, does the organization also include information regarding the following: • The resident's height and weight • Pregnancy and lactation status • Any other information required by the organization for safe medication management? **A (EP 2)**				
3. Is the information accessible when needed (except in emergency situations when time does not permit) to licensed independent practitioners, health care professionals, and other staff? **C (EP 3) Ⓜ**				

Standard MM.2.10	Standard Score: ❑ Compliant ❑ Not Compliant			
Assessment Question	**Level of Compliance**	**Evidence of Compliance**	**Plan of Action/ Measure of Success (if needed)**	**Due Date**
1. Do licensed independent practitioners,and health care staff involved in ordering, dispensing, administering, and/or monitoring effects of medications, including the medical director, develop criteria for determining what medications are available for dispensing or administration? **A (EP 1)**				
2. At a minimum, does the criteria include the indication for use, effectiveness, risks, (including propensity for medication errors, abuse potential, and sentinel events), and costs? **A (EP 2)**				

Key: 0 = Insufficient compliance; 1 = Partial compliance; 2 = Satisfactory compliance; NA = Not applicable; **A** indicates scoring category A; **C** indicates scoring category C; ▲ indicates situational decision rules apply; △ indicates direct impact requirements apply; Ⓜ indicates Measure of success is needed; ☆ indicates this standard also applies to organizations seeking Joint Commission's Medicare/Medicaid certification–based long term care accreditation

Standard MM.2.10

Assessment Question	Level of Compliance	Evidence of Compliance	Plan of Action/ Measure of Success (if needed)	Due Date
3. Does the organization maintain a list of medications for dispensing or administration (including strength and dosage) that is maintained and readily available?* **A (EP 3)**				
4. Are processes and mechanisms established to monitor resident responses to a newly added medication before the medication is made available for dispensing or administration within the organization? **A (EP 4)**				
5. Are medications designated as available for dispensing or administration reviewed at least annually based on emerging safety and efficacy information? **A (EP 5)**				
6. Does the organization have processes to approve and procure medications that are not on the organization's medication list? **A (EP 6)**				
7. Does the organization have processes to address medication shortages and outages, including the following: • Communicating with appropriate prescribers and staff who participate in the medication management system • Developing approved substitution protocols • Educating appropriate licensed independent practitioners, and health care staff who participate in medication management systems about these protocols • Obtaining medications in the event of a disaster? **A (EP 7)**				

* **Note:** *Sample medications are not required to be on this list.*

Key: 0 = Insufficient compliance; 1 = Partial compliance; 2 = Satisfactory compliance; NA = Not applicable; **A** indicates scoring category A; **C** indicates scoring category C; ▲(2) indicates situational decision rules apply; △(3) indicates direct impact requirements apply; Ⓜ indicates Measure of success is needed; ☆ indicates this standard also applies to organizations seeking Joint Commission's Medicare/Medicaid certification–based long term care accreditation

Standard MM.2.20★	**Standard Score: ❑ Compliant ❑ Not Compliant**			
Assessment Question	**Level of Compliance**	**Evidence of Compliance**	**Plan of Action/ Measure of Success (if needed)**	**Due Date**
1. Does the organization routinely stock or store only approved medications?*† **A (EP 1)** Ⓜ				
2. Are medications stored under conditions suitable for product stability?† **A (EP 2)** Ⓜ				
3. Is there a written policy addressing the storage of medication between receipt of a medication by an individual health care provider and medication administration and, at a minimum, does the policy address the following:† • Safe storage • Safe handling • Security • Disposition of these medications including return to the medication storage area at the end of the individual's shift? **A (EP 3)**				
4. Is the policy addressing the storage of medication between receipt of a medication by an individual health care provider and medication administration implemented?† **C (EP 4)** Ⓜ				
5. Are unauthorized persons, in accordance with the organization's policy and law or regulation, unable to obtain access to medications?† **A (EP 5)**				
6. Are controlled substances stored to prevent diversion and according to state and federal laws and regulations?† **A (EP 6)**				
7. Are all expired, damaged, and/or contaminated medications segregated until they are removed from the organization?† **A (EP 7)**				

* **Note:** See *Standard MM.2.40 for the exception to this EP: The organization has a process to safely manage medications brought in by the resident or the resident's family.*

† This assessment question is not applicable to organizations seeking Joint Commission's Medicare/Medicaid Certification–based long term care accreditation.

Key: 0 = Insufficient compliance; 1 = Partial compliance; 2 = Satisfactory compliance; NA = Not applicable; **A** indicates scoring category A; **C** indicates scoring category C; ▲ indicates situational decision rules apply; △ indicates direct impact requirements apply; Ⓜ indicates Measure of success is needed; ☆ indicates this standard also applies to organizations seeking Joint Commission's Medicare/Medicaid certification–based long term care accreditation

Standard MM.2.20★

Assessment Question	Level of Compliance	Evidence of Compliance	Plan of Action/ Measure of Success (if needed)	Due Date
8. Does the organization identify and, at a minimum, annually review a list of look-alike/sound-alike drugs used in the organization, and take action to prevent errors involving the interchange of these drugs? (The preceding requirement is not scored here. It is scored at NPSG.03.03.01.) **(EP 8)**				
9. Are those medications and chemicals used to prepare medications accurately labeled with contents, expiration dates, and warnings?* **A (EP 9)**				
10. Are drug concentrations that are available in the organization standardized and limited in number? **A (EP 10)**				
11. Are concentrated electrolytes removed from care units or areas (unless resident safety is at risk if the concentrated electrolyte is not immediately available on a specific care unit or area; in such situations, specific precautions are taken to prevent inadvertent administration)? **A (EP 11)** Ⓜ △3				
12. Are all medication storage areas periodically inspected according to the organization's policy to make sure medications are stored properly?* **C (EP 15)** Ⓜ				

* This assessment question is not applicable to organizations seeking Joint Commission's Medicare/Medicaid certification–based long term care accreditation.

Key: 0 = Insufficient compliance; 1 = Partial compliance; 2 = Satisfactory compliance; NA = Not applicable; **A** indicates scoring category A; **C** indicates scoring category C; ▲2 indicates situational decision rules apply; △3 indicates direct impact requirements apply; Ⓜ indicates Measure of success is needed; ☆ indicates this standard also applies to organizations seeking Joint Commission's Medicare/Medicaid certification–based long term care accreditation

Standard MM.2.30	Standard Score: ❑ Compliant ❑ Not Compliant			
Assessment Question	**Level of Compliance**	**Evidence of Compliance**	**Plan of Action/ Measure of Success (if needed)**	**Due Date**
1. Do organization leaders, in conjunction with licensed independent practitioners and other health care staff whose scope of practice includes the dispensing or administration of emergency medications, decide which emergency medications and/or supplies, if any, will be readily available in care areas? **A (EP 1)**				
2. Are emergency medications available in unit-dose, age-specific, and ready-to-administer forms, whenever possible? **A (EP 3)** ⚠3				
3. Are emergency medications sealed or stored in containers (for example, crash carts, tackle boxes, emergency drug kits, closed bags that are clearly labeled and so forth) in such a way that staff can readily determine that the contents are complete and have not expired? **A (EP 4)** Ⓜ				
4. Are emergency medications stored in sealed or in locked containers; in a locked room; or under constant supervision in accordance with law or regulation? **A (EP 6)** Ⓜ				
5. Are emergency medications and supplies replaced as soon as possible after their use in accordance with the organization's policies and procedures? **A (EP 7)**				

Standard MM.2.40	Standard Score: ❑ Compliant ❑ Not Compliant			
Assessment Question	**Level of Compliance**	**Evidence of Compliance**	**Plan of Action/ Measure of Success (if needed)**	**Due Date**
1. Does the organization address the use of medications brought into the organization by residents or their families, including defining when such medications can be used or administered? **A (EP 1)**				

Key: 0 = Insufficient compliance; 1 = Partial compliance; 2 = Satisfactory compliance; NA = Not applicable; **A** indicates scoring category A; **C** indicates scoring category C; ▲2 indicates situational decision rules apply; ⚠3 indicates direct impact requirements apply; Ⓜ indicates Measure of success is needed; ☆ indicates this standard also applies to organizations seeking Joint Commission's Medicare/Medicaid certification–based long term care accreditation

Standard MM.2.40

Assessment Question	Level of Compliance	Evidence of Compliance	Plan of Action/ Measure of Success (if needed)	Due Date
2. Does the organization address the use of medications brought into the organization by residents or their families, including identifying the medication and visually evaluating its integrity, when medications brought in by the resident or family are allowed? **A (EP 2)**				
3. Does the organization address the use of medications brought into the organization by residents or their families including informing the prescriber and resident if the medications brought into the organization by residents or their families are not permitted? **A (EP 3)**				

Standard MM.3.10

Standard Score: ❑ Compliant ❑ Not Compliant

Assessment Question	Level of Compliance	Evidence of Compliance	Plan of Action/ Measure of Success (if needed)	Due Date
1. Is there a documented diagnosis, condition, or indication for use for each medication ordered? **C (EP 1)** Ⓜ				

Standard MM.3.20

Standard Score: ❑ Compliant ❑ Not Compliant

Assessment Question	Level of Compliance	Evidence of Compliance	Plan of Action/ Measure of Success (if needed)	Due Date
1. Does a written policy(ies) for medication orders address the required elements of a complete medication order? **A (EP 1)**				
2. Does a written policy(ies) for medication orders address when generic or brand names are acceptable or required as part of a medication order? **A (EP 2)**				
3. Does a written policy(ies) for medication orders address whether or when indication for use is required on a medication order? **A (EP 3)**				

Key: 0 = Insufficient compliance; 1 = Partial compliance; 2 = Satisfactory compliance; NA = Not applicable; **A** indicates scoring category A; **C** indicates scoring category C; ▲(2) indicates situational decision rules apply; △(3) indicates direct impact requirements apply; Ⓜ indicates Measure of success is needed; ☆ indicates this standard also applies to organizations seeking Joint Commission's Medicare/Medicaid certification–based long term care accreditation

Standard MM.3.20

Assessment Question	Level of Compliance	Evidence of Compliance	Plan of Action/ Measure of Success (if needed)	Due Date
4. Does a written policy(ies) for medication orders address any special precautions or procedures for ordering drugs with look-alike or sound-alike names? **A (EP 4)**				
5. Does a written policy(ies) for medication orders address actions to take when medication orders are incomplete, illegible, or unclear? **A (EP 5)**				
6. Does the organization specify the required elements of the following types of orders that it deems acceptable for use: • "As needed" (PRN) orders—orders acted upon based on the occurence of a specific indication or symptom • Standing orders—written instruction to administer a medication to a person in circumstances specified in instructions without a prescription • Hold orders—instruction to temporarily suspend (place medication orders on hold) under specified conditions and to alert users at specified times while a medication is on hold • Automatic stop orders—a date or time to discontinue a medication • Resume orders—restart an order which was previously held • Titrating orders—orders in which the dose is either progressively increased or decreased in response to the resident's status • Taper orders—orders in which the dose is decreased by a particular amount with each dosing interval • Range orders—orders in which the dose or dosing interval varies over a prescribed range, depending on the situation or resident's status • Orders for compounded drugs or drug mixtures not commercially available • Orders for medication-related devices (for example, nebulizers and catheters) • Orders for investigational medications • Orders for herbal products • Orders for medications at discharge or transfer? **A (EP 6)**				

Key: 0 = Insufficient compliance; 1 = Partial compliance; 2 = Satisfactory compliance; NA = Not applicable; **A** indicates scoring category A; **C** indicates scoring category C; ▲2 indicates situational decision rules apply; △3 indicates direct impact requirements apply; Ⓜ indicates Measure of success is needed; ☆ indicates this standard also applies to organizations seeking Joint Commission's Medicare/Medicaid certification–based long term care accreditation

Standard MM.3.20

Assessment Question	Level of Compliance	Evidence of Compliance	Plan of Action/ Measure of Success (if needed)	Due Date
7. In addition, does the organization review and update preprinted order sheets as needed to support clarity, accuracy, and safety? **A (EP 8)**				
8. In addition, does the organization specify that blanket reinstatement of previous orders—a summary order to resume all previous orders—for medications are not acceptable? **A (EP 9)**				
9. Are policies and procedures regarding medication orders implemented? **C (EP 13) Ⓜ**				
10. Are influenza and pneumococcal polysaccharide vaccines administered according to a physician order, or, as permitted by law and regulation, according to physician-approved, organization-specific protocol(s)? **A (EP 14)**				

Standard MM.4.10

Standard Score: ❑ Compliant ❑ Not Compliant

Assessment Question	Level of Compliance	Evidence of Compliance	Plan of Action/ Measure of Success (if needed)	Due Date
1. Does a pharmacist review all prescription or medication orders: • Before dispensing • Before removal from stock • Before removal from automated storage and distribution devices • Unless a licensed independent practitioner controls the ordering, preparation, and administration of the medication • Unless there is an urgent situation when the resulting delay would harm the resident, including situations in which the resident experiences a sudden change in clinical status (for example, new onset of nausea)? **C (EP 1) Ⓜ △3**				

Key: 0 = Insufficient compliance; 1 = Partial compliance; 2 = Satisfactory compliance; NA = Not applicable; **A** indicates scoring category A; **C** indicates scoring category C; ▲2 indicates situational decision rules apply; △3 indicates direct impact requirements apply; Ⓜ indicates Measure of success is needed; ☆ indicates this standard also applies to organizations seeking Joint Commission's Medicare/Medicaid certification–based long term care accreditation

Standard MM.4.10

Assessment Question	Level of Compliance	Evidence of Compliance	Plan of Action/ Measure of Success (if needed)	Due Date
2. Does the organization have a process to review all prescriptions for the following: • The appropriateness of the drug, dose, frequency, and route of administration • Therapeutic duplication • Real or potential allergies or sensitivities • Real or potential interactions between the prescription and other medications' current or potential impact as evidenced by laboratory values or food • Other contraindications • Variation from organizational criteria for use • Other relevant medication-related issues or concerns? **A (EP 5)**				
3. Are all concerns, issues, or questions clarified with the individual prescriber before dispensing the medication? **A (EP 6)** △3				

Standard MM.4.20

Standard Score: ❑ Compliant ❑ Not Compliant

Assessment Question	Level of Compliance	Evidence of Compliance	Plan of Action/ Measure of Success (if needed)	Due Date
1. When an on-site licensed pharmacy is available, does only the pharmacy compound or admix all sterile medications, intravenous admixtures, or other drugs except in emergencies or when not feasible (for example, when the product's stability is short)? **A (EP 1)** △3				
2. Does the organization have a written policy that addresses the safety and use of medications acquired by a practitioner from sources other than the organization for use in resident care in that organization and does the policy address the following: • Whether such medications are allowed to be used • If allowed, a process to evaluate the integrity of medications brought in by a practitioner prior to use in resident care? **A (EP 2)**				

Key: 0 = Insufficient compliance; 1 = Partial compliance; 2 = Satisfactory compliance; NA = Not applicable; **A** indicates scoring category A; **C** indicates scoring category C; ▲2 indicates situational decision rules apply; △3 indicates direct impact requirements apply; Ⓜ indicates Measure of success is needed; ☆ indicates this standard also applies to organizations seeking Joint Commission's Medicare/Medicaid certification–based long term care accreditation

Standard MM.4.20

Assessment Question	Level of Compliance	Evidence of Compliance	Plan of Action/ Measure of Success (if needed)	Due Date
3. Is the written policy that addresses the safety and use of medications acquired by a practitioner from sources other than the organization for use in resident care implemented? **A (EP 3)**				
4. Wherever medications are prepared, do staff members use safety materials and equipment while preparing hazardous medications? **C (EP 4)** Ⓜ				
5. Wherever medications are prepared, do staff members use techniques to assure accuracy in medication preparation? **C (EP 5)** Ⓜ △3				
6. Wherever medications are prepared, do staff members use appropriate techniques to avoid contamination during medication preparation, including but not limited to the following: • Using clean or sterile technique as appropriate • Maintaining clean, uncluttered, and functionally separate areas for product preparation to minimize the possibility of contamination • Using a laminar flow hood or other class 100 environment while preparing any intravenous (IV) admixture in the pharmacy, any sterile product made from nonsterile ingredients, or any sterile product that will not be used within 24 hours • Visually inspecting the integrity of the medications? **C (EP 6)** Ⓜ △3				

Standard MM.4.30

Standard Score: ❑ Compliant ❑ Not Compliant

Assessment Question	Level of Compliance	Evidence of Compliance	Plan of Action/ Measure of Success (if needed)	Due Date
1. Are medications labeled in a standardized manner according to law or regulation and standards of practice? **A (EP 1)** △3				

Key: 0 = Insufficient compliance; 1 = Partial compliance; 2 = Satisfactory compliance; NA = Not applicable; **A** indicates scoring category A; **C** indicates scoring category C; ▲2 indicates situational decision rules apply; △3 indicates direct impact requirements apply; Ⓜ indicates Measure of success is needed; ☆ indicates this standard also applies to organizations seeking Joint Commission's Medicare/Medicaid certification–based long term care accreditation

Standard MM.4.30

Assessment Question	Level of Compliance	Evidence of Compliance	Plan of Action/ Measure of Success (if needed)	Due Date
2. Are medication containers* labeled properly any time one or more medications or solutions are prepared but not administered immediately? **A (EP 2)** △3				
3. At a minimum, are all medications prepared in the organization labeled with the following: • Drug name, strength, amount (if not apparent from the container) • Expiration date† when not used within 24 hours • Expiration time when expiration occurs in less than 24 hours • The date prepared and the diluent for all compounded IV admixtures and parenteral nutrition solutions? **A (EP 3)** △3				
4. When preparing individualized medications for multiple residents, when the person preparing the individualized medications is not the same person administering the medication, does the label include the following: • Resident name • Resident location • Directions for use and any applicable cautionary statements either on the label or attached as an accessory label (for example, "requires refrigeration," or "for IM use only")? **A (EP 4)** △3				
5. Do organizations that do not operate a pharmacy validate that all medications coming into the organization are appropriately labeled? **A (EP 5)** △3				
6. If not labeled, is action taken to have the medications correctly labeled? **A (EP 6)** △3				

* A container can be any storage device such as a plastic bag, syringe, bottle, box, medicine cup, or basin.

† Expiration date, also called the "beyond use date," refers to the last date that the product should be used by the resident.

Key: 0 = Insufficient compliance; 1 = Partial compliance; 2 = Satisfactory compliance; NA = Not applicable; **A** indicates scoring category A; **C** indicates scoring category C; ▲2 indicates situational decision rules apply; △3 indicates direct impact requirements apply; Ⓜ indicates Measure of success is needed; ☆ indicates this standard also applies to organizations seeking Joint Commission's Medicare/Medicaid certification–based long term care accreditation

Standard MM.4.40	**Standard Score:** ❑ Compliant ❑ Not Compliant			
Assessment Question	**Level of Compliance**	**Evidence of Compliance**	**Plan of Action/ Measure of Success (if needed)**	**Due Date**
1. Are quantities of medications dispensed which minimize diversion yet are still consistent with the resident's needs? **A (EP 1)**				
2. Does dispensing adhere to law, regulation, licensure, and professional standards of practice, including record keeping? **A (EP 2)**				
3. Are medications dispensed in a timely manner to meet resident needs? **C (EP 3)** Ⓜ				
4. Are medications dispensed in the most ready-to-administer forms available from the manufacturer or, if feasible, in unit-doses that have been repackaged by the pharmacy or licensed repackager? **C (EP 4)** Ⓜ ⚠3				
5. Does the organization consistently use the same dose packaging system, or if a different system is used, provide education about the use of the dose packaging system to the residents impacted by the change? **A (EP 5)**				

Standard MM.4.50	**Standard Score:** ❑ Compliant ❑ Not Compliant			
Assessment Question	**Level of Compliance**	**Evidence of Compliance**	**Plan of Action/ Measure of Success (if needed)**	**Due Date**
1. Does the organization have a process for providing medications to meet resident needs when the pharmacy is closed? **A (EP 1)**				

Standard MM.4.60	**Standard Score:** ❑ Compliant ❑ Not Compliant			
Assessment Question	**Level of Compliance**	**Evidence of Compliance**	**Plan of Action/ Measure of Success (if needed)**	**Due Date**
1. If the organization does not operate a pharmacy, does the organization have a process for obtaining medications from a pharmacy for its residents? **A (EP 1)**				

Key: 0 = Insufficient compliance; 1 = Partial compliance; 2 = Satisfactory compliance; NA = Not applicable; **A** indicates scoring category A; **C** indicates scoring category C; ▲2 indicates situational decision rules apply; ⚠3 indicates direct impact requirements apply; Ⓜ indicates Measure of success is needed; ☆ indicates this standard also applies to organizations seeking Joint Commission's Medicare/Medicaid certification–based long term care accreditation

Standard MM.4.60

Assessment Question	Level of Compliance	Evidence of Compliance	Plan of Action/ Measure of Success (if needed)	Due Date
2. If the organization obtains medications from a pharmacy that is not open 24 hours a day, 7 days a week, does the organization have a process for obtaining medications from another source for urgent or emergent conditions when the pharmacy is closed? **A (EP 2)** △3				

Standard MM.4.70

Standard Score: ❑ Compliant ❑ Not Compliant

Assessment Question	Level of Compliance	Evidence of Compliance	Plan of Action/ Measure of Success (if needed)	Due Date
1. When the organization has been informed of a medication recall or discontinuation by the manufacturer or the Food and Drug Administration (FDA) for safety reasons, are medications within the organization retrieved* and handled per organization policy and law or regulation? **A (EP 1)**				
2. Does the organization notify all those ordering, dispensing, and/or administering active† medication of any manufacturer or FDA recall or discontinuance? **A (EP 2)**				
3. When the organization has been informed of a medication recall or discontinuation by the manufacturer or the FDA for safety reasons, are residents who are actively receiving the medication identified and informed of the recall or discontinuation? **A (EP 3)**				

Standard MM.4.80

Standard Score: ❑ Compliant ❑ Not Compliant

Assessment Question	Level of Compliance	Evidence of Compliance	Plan of Action/ Measure of Success (if needed)	Due Date
1. Does the organization have a process in place that addresses if and when unused, expired, or returned medications will be managed by the pharmacy or by the organization? **A (EP 1)**				

* Although recalls are generally by lot number, an organization may retrieve all lots of a recalled medication instead of recording and identifying medications by their lot number.

† Dispensed medications that have not passed expiration date and prescriptions that can be refilled without an additional physician order.

Key: 0 = Insufficient compliance; 1 = Partial compliance; 2 = Satisfactory compliance; NA = Not applicable; **A** indicates scoring category A; **C** indicates scoring category C; ▲ indicates situational decision rules apply; △3 indicates direct impact requirements apply; Ⓜ indicates Measure of success is needed; ☆ indicates this standard also applies to organizations seeking Joint Commission's Medicare/Medicaid certification–based long term care accreditation

Standard MM.4.80

Assessment Question	Level of Compliance	Evidence of Compliance	Plan of Action/ Measure of Success (if needed)	Due Date
2. Does the organization have a process in place that addresses how medications are returned to the pharmacy's or organization's control, including procedures that address preventing diversion of medications and account for all unused, expired, or returned medications? **A (EP 2)**				
3. Does the organization have a process in place that addresses how outside sources, if any, are used for destruction of medications? **A (EP 3)**				
4. Are these processes for addressing medications returned to the pharmacy or organization implemented? **C (EP 4) Ⓜ**				

Standard MM.5.10

Standard Score: ❑ Compliant ❑ Not Compliant

Assessment Question	Level of Compliance	Evidence of Compliance	Plan of Action/ Measure of Success (if needed)	Due Date
1. Do medication administration policies and procedures address health care staff members who are allowed to administer medications, with or without supervision, consistent with law or regulation and organization policy? **A (EP 1)**				
2. Before administering a medication, does the licensed independent practitioner or qualified individual administering the medication verify that the medication selected for administration is the correct one based on the medication order and product label? **C (EP 2) Ⓜ ⚠3**				
3. Before administering a medication, does the licensed independent practitioner or qualified individual administering the medication verify that the medication is stable based on visual examination for particulates or discoloration and that the medication has not expired? **C (EP 3) Ⓜ ⚠3**				

Key: 0 = Insufficient compliance; 1 = Partial compliance; 2 = Satisfactory compliance; NA = Not applicable; **A** indicates scoring category A; **C** indicates scoring category C; ▲2 indicates situational decision rules apply; ⚠3 indicates direct impact requirements apply; Ⓜ indicates Measure of success is needed; ☆ indicates this standard also applies to organizations seeking Joint Commission's Medicare/Medicaid certification–based long term care accreditation

Standard MM.5.10

Assessment Question	Level of Compliance	Evidence of Compliance	Plan of Action/ Measure of Success (if needed)	Due Date
4. Before administering a medication, does the licensed independent practitioner or qualified individual administering the medication verify that there is no contraindication for administering the medication? **C (EP 4)** Ⓜ △3				
5. Before administering a medication, does the licensed independent practitioner or qualified individual administering the medication verify that the medication is being administered at the proper time, in the prescribed dose, and by the correct route? **C (EP 5)** Ⓜ △3				
6. Before administering a medication, does the licensed independent practitioner or qualified individual administering the medication advise the resident, or if appropriate, the resident's family about any potential clinically significant adverse reaction, or other concerns about administering a new medication? **C (EP 6)** Ⓜ				
7. Before administering a medication, does the licensed independent practitioner or qualified individual administering the medication discuss any unresolved, significant concerns about the medication with the resident's physician, prescriber (if different from the physician), and/or relevant staff involved with the resident's care, treatment, and services? **C (EP 7)** Ⓜ △3				
8. Do policies and procedures address guidelines for prescriber notification in the event of an adverse drug reaction or medication error? **A (EP 8)**				

Key: 0 = Insufficient compliance; 1 = Partial compliance; 2 = Satisfactory compliance; NA = Not applicable; **A** indicates scoring category A; **C** indicates scoring category C; ▲2 indicates situational decision rules apply; △3 indicates direct impact requirements apply; Ⓜ indicates Measure of success is needed; ☆ indicates this standard also applies to organizations seeking Joint Commission's Medicare/Medicaid certification–based long term care accreditation

Standard MM 5.20	**Standard Score:** ❑ Compliant ❑ Not Compliant			
Assessment Question	**Level of Compliance**	**Evidence of Compliance**	**Plan of Action/ Measure of Success (if needed)**	**Due Date**
1. If self-administration* is allowed, do procedures guide the safe and accurate self-administration of medications by a person who is not a staff member and address training, supervision, and administration documentation? **A (EP 1)**				
2. Do persons who administer medications, but are not staff members (for example, the resident), receive information about the following: • The nature of the medication to be administered • How to administer medications, such as the frequency, route of administration, and dose • The expected actions and side effects of the medications to be administered • How to monitor the effects of the medication on the resident? **C (EP 2) Ⓜ**				
3. Are persons who administer medications but are not staff members (including the resident if self-administering) determined to be competent at medication administration before being allowed to administer medications? **C (EP 3) Ⓜ**				

Standard MM.6.10	**Standard Score:** ❑ Compliant ❑ Not Compliant			
Assessment Question	**Level of Compliance**	**Evidence of Compliance**	**Plan of Action/ Measure of Success (if needed)**	**Duo Date**
1. Is each resident's response to his or her medication monitored according to the clinical needs of the resident and does it address the resident's response to the prescribed medication and actual or potential medication-related problems? **C (EP 1) Ⓜ ⚠3**				

* Self-administration includes those instances where a resident independently uses a medication, including medications that may be held by the organization for the independent use by the resident.

Key: 0 = Insufficient compliance; 1 = Partial compliance; 2 = Satisfactory compliance; NA = Not applicable; **A** indicates scoring category A; **C** indicates scoring category C; ▲2 indicates situational decision rules apply; △3 indicates direct impact requirements apply; Ⓜ indicates Measure of success is needed; ☆ indicates this standard also applies to organizations seeking Joint Commission's Medicare/Medicaid certification–based long term care accreditation

Standard MM.6.10

Assessment Question	Level of Compliance	Evidence of Compliance	Plan of Action/ Measure of Success (if needed)	Due Date
2. Does monitoring a medication's effect on a resident include the following: • Gathering the resident's own perception about side effects and, when appropriate, perceived efficacy • Referring to information from the resident's medical record, relevant laboratory results, clinical response, and medication profile? **C (EP 2)** Ⓜ				
3. Does the organization have a process for monitoring the resident's response to the first dose(s) of a medication new to a resident while he or she is under the direct care of the organization? **A (EP 3)**				
4. Does the consultant pharmacist review each resident's medication regimen at least monthly? **C (EP 5)** Ⓜ				
5. Are the findings, conclusions, and recommendations of medication monitoring documented in the clinical record and communicated to the physician, prescriber (if different from the physician), and those involved in the resident's care? **C (EP 6)** Ⓜ				

Standard MM.6.20

Standard Score: ❑ Compliant ❑ Not Compliant

Assessment Question	Level of Compliance	Evidence of Compliance	Plan of Action/ Measure of Success (if needed)	Due Date
1. Does the organization have a process to respond to actual or potential adverse drug events and medication errors? **A (EP 1)**				
2. Is action taken when an actual or potential adverse drug event is identified, depending on the organization's services (this may be limited to calling for outside assistance, for example, community-sponsored 911 service)? **C (EP 2)** Ⓜ △3				

Key: 0 = Insufficient compliance; 1 = Partial compliance; 2 = Satisfactory compliance; NA = Not applicable; **A** indicates scoring category A; **C** indicates scoring category C; ▲2 indicates situational decision rules apply; △3 indicates direct impact requirements apply; Ⓜ indicates Measure of success is needed; ☆ indicates this standard also applies to organizations seeking Joint Commission's Medicare/Medicaid certification–based long term care accreditation

Standard MM.6.20

Assessment Question	Level of Compliance	Evidence of Compliance	Plan of Action/ Measure of Success (if needed)	Due Date
3. Does the organization or responsible individual comply with internal and external reporting requirements for actual or potential adverse drug events (for example, to the United States Pharmacopeia, the FDA, the Institute for Safe Medication Practices)? **C (EP 3)** Ⓜ				

Standard MM.7.10

Standard Score: ❑ Compliant ❑ Not Compliant

Assessment Question	Level of Compliance	Evidence of Compliance	Plan of Action/ Measure of Success (if needed)	Due Date
1. Does the organization identify the high-risk or high-alert medications used within the organization, if any? **A (EP 1)** ⚠3				
2. Based on the services provided does the organization develop processes for procuring, storing, ordering, transcribing, preparing, dispensing, administering, and/or monitoring high-risk or high-alert medications? **A (EP 2)**				
3. Are the processes for managing high-risk or high-alert medications implemented? **C (EP 3)** Ⓜ ⚠3				

Standard MM.7.20

Standard Score: ❑ Compliant ❑ Not Compliant

Assessment Question	Level of Compliance	Evidence of Compliance	Plan of Action/ Measure of Success (if needed)	Due Date
1. Does the organization use an interdisciplinary process that includes the physician, pharmacist, nurse, and other members of the health care team involved in the resident's care to monitor psychotropic medications? **A (EP 1)**				

Key: 0 = Insufficient compliance; 1 = Partial compliance; 2 = Satisfactory compliance; NA = Not applicable; **A** indicates scoring category A; **C** indicates scoring category C; ▲2 indicates situational decision rules apply; ⚠3 indicates direct impact requirements apply; Ⓜ indicates Measure of success is needed; ☆ indicates this standard also applies to organizations seeking Joint Commission's Medicare/Medicaid certification–based long term care accreditation

Standard MM.7.20

Assessment Question	Level of Compliance	Evidence of Compliance	Plan of Action/ Measure of Success (if needed)	Due Date
2. Does the organization specify that psychotropic medications are used only during the following circumstances: • When indicated by assessment and medical necessity • After other nonpharmacological interventions or alternatives have been considered or used • At the lowest effective therapeutic dose? **A (EP 2)**				
3. Is the use of PRN orders for psychotropic medications periodically reviewed to determine the appropriateness and effectiveness of these PRN orders, with the objective of decreasing their use as much as possible? **A (EP 3)**				
4. Is the organization's compliance with its own monitoring process evaluated regularly? **A (EP 4)**				

Standard MM.7.40

Standard Score: ❑ Compliant ❑ Not Compliant

Assessment Question	Level of Compliance	Evidence of Compliance	Plan of Action/ Measure of Success (if needed)	Due Date
1. Do procedures for the use of investigational medications specify a written process for reviewing, approving, supervising, and monitoring investigational medications use? **A (EP 1)**				
2. When the organization operates a pharmacy, do procedures specify that the pharmacy controls the storage, dispensing, labeling, and distribution of the investigational medication? **A (EP 2)**				
3. Do procedures specify that when a patient is involved in an investigational protocol that is independent of the organization, does the organization review and accommodate the resident's continued participation in the protocol? **A (EP 3)**				
4. Are the procedures for the use of investigational medications implemented? **A (EP 4)**				

Key: 0 = Insufficient compliance; 1 = Partial compliance; 2 = Satisfactory compliance; NA = Not applicable; **A** indicates scoring category A; **C** indicates scoring category C; ▲ indicates situational decision rules apply; △ indicates direct impact requirements apply; Ⓜ indicates Measure of success is needed; ☆ indicates this standard also applies to organizations seeking Joint Commission's Medicare/Medicaid certification–based long term care accreditation

Standard MM.8.10	**Standard Score:** ❑ Compliant ❑ Not Compliant			
Assessment Question	**Level of Compliance**	**Evidence of Compliance**	**Plan of Action/ Measure of Success (if needed)**	**Due Date**
1. Does the organization evaluate its medication management system for risk points and identify areas to improve safety? **A (EP 1)**				
2. Does the organization routinely evaluate the literature for new technologies or successful practices that have been demonstrated to enhance safety in other organizations to determine if it can improve its own medication management system? **A (EP 2)**				
3. Does the organization review internally generated reports to identify trends or issues in its medication management system? (*See* Standards PI.2.10 and PI.2.20.) **A (EP 3)**				
4. Does the organization act to implement improvements based on the following: • Evaluation of its medication management system • Review of new technologies • External data • Successful practices that have been demonstrated to enhance safety **A (EP 4)**				
5. Is the performance of new and modified medication management processes measured? **A (EP 5)**				
6. Does the organization use information from data analysis to identify subsequent changes to improve its medication management system? **A (EP 6)**				
7. Do the pharmacy and long term care facility collaborate to determine whether the medication management system is effective? **A (EP 7)**				
8. When the pharmacy is the primary provider of pharmaceutical services to a long term care facility, does the pharmacy collaborate with the long term care facility to implement a medication management system to control all medications? **A (EP 8)**				

Key: 0 = Insufficient compliance; 1 = Partial compliance; 2 = Satisfactory compliance; NA = Not applicable; **A** indicates scoring category A; **C** indicates scoring category C; ▲ indicates situational decision rules apply; △ indicates direct impact requirements apply; Ⓜ indicates Measure of success is needed; ☆ indicates this standard also applies to organizations seeking Joint Commission's Medicare/Medicaid certification–based long term care accreditation

Standard MM.8.10

Assessment Question	Level of Compliance	Evidence of Compliance	Plan of Action/ Measure of Success (if needed)	Due Date
9. When the pharmacy is the primary provider of pharmaceutical services to a long term care facility or consultant pharmacist services are provided, does the pharmacy or pharmacist participate in educating the long term care facility about the following: • The collection and use of performance measures for medication management • Techniques to reduce medication errors and minimize waste of medications? **A (EP 9)**				

Key: 0 = Insufficient compliance; 1 = Partial compliance; 2 = Satisfactory compliance; NA = Not applicable; **A** indicates scoring category A; **C** indicates scoring category C; ▲ indicates situational decision rules apply; △ indicates direct impact requirements apply; Ⓜ indicates Measure of success is needed; ☆ indicates this standard also applies to organizations seeking Joint Commission's Medicare/Medicaid certification–based long term care accreditation

Surveillance, Prevention, and Control of Infection (IC)

Standard IC.1.10	**Standard Score: ❑ Compliant ❑ Not Compliant**			
Assessment Question	**Level of Compliance**	**Evidence of Compliance**	**Plan of Action/ Measure of Success (if needed)**	**Due Date**
1. Is an organizationwide IC program implemented? **A (EP1)**				
2. Are individuals and/or positions with the authority to take steps to prevent or control the acquisition and transmission of infectious agents identified? **A (EP 2)**				
3. Are all applicable organizational components and functions integrated into the IC program? **A (EP 3)**				
4. Are systems in place to communicate with licensed independent practitioners; staff; students/trainees; volunteers; and, as appropriate, visitors, residents, and families about infection prevention and control issues, including their responsibilities in preventing the spread of infection within the organization? **A (EP 4)**				
5. Does the organization have systems for reporting infection surveillance, prevention, and control information to the following: • The appropriate staff within the organization • Federal, state, and local public health authorities in accordance with law and regulation • Accrediting bodies (*see* Sentinel Event Reporting and National Patient Safety Goals in the *Comprehensive Accreditation Manual for Long Term Care*) • The referring or receiving organization when an organization was transferred or referred and the presence of an infection was not known at the time of transfer or referral?* **A (EP 5)**				
6. Are systems for the investigation of outbreaks of infectious diseases in place? **A (EP 6)**				
7. Are applicable policies and procedures in place throughout the organization? **A (EP 7)**				

* When a referring organization becomes aware that a resident it has transferred has an active infection for which treatment should start or change, the referring organization communicates this to the receiving organization. If a receiving organization identifies an infection not identified by the referring organization (such as an infected wound), the receiving organization should communicate the omission to the referring organization. This action will aid the referring organization's improvement efforts.

Key: 0 = Insufficient compliance; 1 = Partial compliance; 2 = Satisfactory compliance; NA = Not applicable; **A** indicates scoring category A; **C** indicates scoring category C; ▲(2) indicates situational decision rules apply; △(3) indicates direct impact requirements apply; Ⓜ indicates Measure of success is needed; ☆ indicates this standard also applies to organizations seeking Joint Commission's Medicare/Medicaid certification–based long term care accreditation

Standard IC.1.10

Assessment Question	Level of Compliance	Evidence of Compliance	Plan of Action/ Measure of Success (if needed)	Due Date
8. Do written policies and procedures include at least the following departments' participation in infection prevention and control activities: clinical services, food services, housekeeping, maintenance, laundry services, hotel service (for example, beauty shops), resident activities, and staff health? **A (EP 8)**				
9. Does the organization have a written IC* plan that includes the following: • A description of prioritized risks • A statement of the goals of the IC program • A description of the organization's strategies to minimize, reduce, or eliminate the prioritized risks • A description of how the strategies will be evaluated? **A (EP 9)**				

Standard IC.2.10

Standard Score: ❑ Compliant ❑ Not Compliant

Assessment Question	Level of Compliance	Evidence of Compliance	Plan of Action/ Measure of Success (if needed)	Due Date
1. Does the organization identify risks for the transmission and acquisition of infectious agents throughout the organization based on the following factors: • The geographic location and community environment of the organization, program/services provided, and the characteristics of the population served • The results of the analysis of the organization's infection prevention and control data • The care, treatment, and services provided? **A (EP 1)**				
2. Is the risk analysis formally reviewed at least annually and whenever significant changes occur in any of the preceding factors? **A (EP 2)**				

* A succinct, useful document, formulated beforehand, that identifies needs, lists strategies to meet those needs, and sets goals and objectives. The format of the "plan" may include narratives, policies and procedures, protocols, practice guidelines, clinical paths, care maps, or a combination of these.

Key: 0 = Insufficient compliance; 1 = Partial compliance; 2 = Satisfactory compliance; NA = Not applicable; **A** indicates scoring category A; **C** indicates scoring category C; ▲(2) indicates situational decision rules apply; △(3) indicates direct impact requirements apply; Ⓜ indicates Measure of success is needed; ☆ indicates this standard also applies to organizations seeking Joint Commission's Medicare/Medicaid certification–based long term care accreditation

Standard IC.2.10

Assessment Question	Level of Compliance	Evidence of Compliance	Plan of Action/ Measure of Success (if needed)	Due Date
3. Are surveillance activities, including data collection and analysis, used to identify infection prevention and control risks pertaining to the following: • Residents • Licensed independent practitioners, staff, volunteers, and student/trainees • Visitors and families, as warranted? **A (EP 3)**				

Standard IC.3.10

Standard Score: ❑ Compliant ❑ Not Compliant

Assessment Question	Level of Compliance	Evidence of Compliance	Plan of Action/ Measure of Success (if needed)	Due Date
1. Are priorities established and goals related to preventing the acquisition and transmission of potentially infectious agents developed based on the risks identified? **A (EP 1)**				
2. Do the goals related to preventing the acquisition and transmission of potentially infectious agents developed based on the risks identified include, but are not limited to, limiting unprotected exposure to pathogens throughout the organization? **A (EP 2)**				
3. Do the goals related to preventing the acquisition and transmission of potentially infectious agents developed based on the risks identified include, but are not limited to, enhancing hand hygiene? **A (EP 3)**				
4. Do the goals related to preventing the acquisition and transmission of potentially infectious agents developed based on the risks identified include, but are not limited to, minimizing the risk of transmitting infections associated with the use of procedures, medical equipment, and medical devices? **A (EP 5)**				

Key: 0 = Insufficient compliance; 1 = Partial compliance; 2 = Satisfactory compliance; NA = Not applicable; **A** indicates scoring category A; **C** indicates scoring category C; ▲ indicates situational decision rules apply; △ indicates direct impact requirements apply; Ⓜ indicates Measure of success is needed; ☆ indicates this standard also applies to organizations seeking Joint Commission's Medicare/Medicaid certification–based long term care accreditation

Standard IC.4.10	**Standard Score:** ❑ Compliant ❑ Not Compliant			
Assessment Question	**Level of Compliance**	**Evidence of Compliance**	**Plan of Action/ Measure of Success (if needed)**	**Due Date**
1. Are interventions designed to incorporate relevant guidelines* for infection prevention and control activities? **A (EP 1)**				
2. Are interventions implemented which include an organizationwide hand hygiene program that complies with current World Health Organization hand hygiene rules and Centers for Disease Control and Prevention (CDC) hand hygiene guidelines?† (The preceding requirement is not scored here. It is scored at NPSG.07.01.01.) **(EP 2)**				
3. Are interventions implemented which include methods to reduce the risks associated with procedures, medical equipment,‡ and medical devices, including the following: • Appropriate storage, cleaning, disinfection, sterilization, and/or disposal of supplies and equipment • Reuse of equipment designated by the manufacturer as disposable in a manner that is consistent with regulatory and professional standards • The appropriate use of personal protective equipment? **A (EP 3)** ⚠3				
4. Is implementation of applicable precautions, as appropriate, based on the following: • The potential for transmission • The mechanism of transmission • The care, treatment, and service setting • The emergence and reemergence of pathogens in the community that could affect the organization? **A (EP 4)** ⚠3				
5. Are interventions implemented which include screening for exposure and/or immunity to infectious diseases that licensed independent practitioners, staff, students/trainees, and volunteers may come in contact with in their work is available as warranted? **C (EP 5)** Ⓜ				

* Examples of guidelines include those offered by the CDC, Healthcare Infection Control Practices Advisory Committee (HICPAC), and National Quality Forum (NQF).

† Organizations are required to comply with all 1A, 1B, 1C CDC or WHO guidelines.

‡ **Medical equipment** Fixed and portable equipment used for the diagnosis, treatment, monitoring, and direct care of individuals.

Key: 0 = Insufficient compliance; 1 = Partial compliance; 2 = Satisfactory compliance; NA = Not applicable; **A** indicates scoring category A; **C** indicates scoring category C; ▲ indicates situational decision rules apply; ⚠ indicates direct impact requirements apply; Ⓜ indicates Measure of success is needed; ☆ indicates this standard also applies to organizations seeking Joint Commission's Medicare/Medicaid certification–based long term care accreditation

Standard IC.4.10

Assessment Question	Level of Compliance	Evidence of Compliance	Plan of Action/ Measure of Success (if needed)	Due Date
6. Are interventions implemented which include referral for assessment, potential testing, immunization and/or prophylaxis/treatment, and counseling as appropriate of licensed independent practitioners, staff, students/trainees, and volunteers who are identified as potentially having an infectious disease or risk of infectious disease that may put the population they serve at risk? **C (EP 6) Ⓜ**				
7. Are interventions implemented which include referral for assessment, potential testing, immunization and/or prophylaxis/treatment, and counseling as appropriate of residents, students/trainees, and volunteers who have been exposed to infectious disease(s) at the organization and licensed independent practitioners or staff who are occupationally exposed? **C (EP 7) Ⓜ**				
8. Are interventions implemented which include the reduction of risks associated with animals brought into the organization (such as, management of animal waste)? **A (EP 8)**				

Standard IC.4.15

Standard Score: ❑ Compliant ❑ Not Compliant

Assessment Question	Level of Compliance	Evidence of Compliance	Plan of Action/ Measure of Success (if needed)	Due Date
1. Does the organization establish an annual influenza vaccination program that includes at least staff and licensed independent practitioners? **A (EP 1)**				
2. Does the organization provide access to influenza vaccination on-site? **A (EP 2)**				
3. Does the organization educate staff and licensed independent practitioners about the following: • Flu vaccination • Nonvaccine control measures (such as the use of appropriate precautions) • The diagnosis, transmission, and potential impact of influenza? **A (EP 3)**				

Key: 0 = Insufficient compliance; 1 = Partial compliance; 2 = Satisfactory compliance; NA = Not applicable; **A** indicates scoring category A; **C** indicates scoring category C; ▲ indicates situational decision rules apply; △ indicates direct impact requirements apply; Ⓜ indicates Measure of success is needed; ☆ indicates this standard also applies to organizations seeking Joint Commission's Medicare/Medicaid certification–based long term care accreditation

Standard IC.4.15

Assessment Question	Level of Compliance	Evidence of Compliance	Plan of Action/ Measure of Success (if needed)	Due Date
4. Does the organization annually evaluate vaccination rates and reasons for nonparticipation in the organization's immunization program? **A (EP 4)**				
5. Does the organization implement enhancements to the program to increase participation? **A (EP 5)**				

Standard IC.5.10

Standard Score: ❑ Compliant ❑ Not Compliant

Assessment Question	Level of Compliance	Evidence of Compliance	Plan of Action/ Measure of Success (if needed)	Due Date
1. Does the organization formally evaluate and revise the IC goals and program (or portions of the program) at least annually and whenever risks significantly change? **A (EP 1)**				
2. Does the evaluation address changes in the scope of the IC program (for example, resulting from the introduction of new services or new sites of care)? **A (EP 2)**				
3. Does the evaluation address changes in the results of the IC program risk analysis? **A (EP 3)**				
4. Does the evaluation address emerging and reemerging problems in the health care community that potentially affect the organization (for example, highly infectious agents)? **A (EP 4)**				
5. Does the evaluation address the assessment of the success or failure of interventions for preventing and controlling infection? **A (EP 5)**				
6. Does the evaluation address responses to concerns raised by leaders and others within the organization? **A (EP 6)**				

Key: 0 = Insufficient compliance; 1 = Partial compliance; 2 = Satisfactory compliance; NA = Not applicable; **A** indicates scoring category A; **C** indicates scoring category C; ▲(2) indicates situational decision rules apply; △(3) indicates direct impact requirements apply; Ⓜ indicates Measure of success is needed; ☆ indicates this standard also applies to organizations seeking Joint Commission's Medicare/Medicaid certification–based long term care accreditation

Standard IC.5.10

Assessment Question	Level of Compliance	Evidence of Compliance	Plan of Action/ Measure of Success (if needed)	Due Date
7. Does the evaluation address the evolution of relevant infection prevention and control guidelines that are based on evidence or, in the absence of evidence, expert consensus? **A (EP 7)**				

Standard IC.6.10

Standard Score: ❑ Compliant ❑ Not Compliant

Assessment Question	Level of Compliance	Evidence of Compliance	Plan of Action/ Measure of Success (if needed)	Due Date
1. Does the organization plan its response to an influx or risk of an influx of infectious residents? **A (EP 1)**				
2. If the organization will continue to accept or treat residents, does the organization have a plan for managing an ongoing influx of potentially infectious residents over an extended period? **A (EP 2)**				
3. Does the organization do the following: • Determine how it will keep abreast of current information about the emergence of epidemics or new infections which may result in the organization activating its response • Determine how it will disseminate critical information to staff and other key practitioners • Identify resources in the community (through local, state, and/or federal public health systems) for obtaining additional information? **A (EP 3)**				

Standard IC.7.10

Standard Score: ❑ Compliant ❑ Not Compliant

Assessment Question	Level of Compliance	Evidence of Compliance	Plan of Action/ Measure of Success (if needed)	Due Date
1. Does the organization assign responsibility for managing IC program activities to one or more individuals whose number, competency, and skill mix are determined by the goals and objectives of the IC activities? **A (EP 1)**				

Key: 0 = Insufficient compliance; 1 = Partial compliance; 2 = Satisfactory compliance; NA = Not applicable; **A** indicates scoring category A; **C** indicates scoring category C; ▲ indicates situational decision rules apply; △ indicates direct impact requirements apply; Ⓜ indicates Measure of success is needed; ☆ indicates this standard also applies to organizations seeking Joint Commission's Medicare/Medicaid certification–based long term care accreditation

Standard IC.7.10

Assessment Question	Level of Compliance	Evidence of Compliance	Plan of Action/ Measure of Success (if needed)	Due Date
2. Are the qualifications* of the individual(s) responsible for managing the IC program determined by the risks entailed in the care, treatment, and services provided, the organization's resident population(s), and the complexity of the activities that will be carried out? **A (EP 2)**				
3. Does this individual(s) coordinate all infection prevention and control activities within the organization? **A (EP 3)**				
4. Does this individual(s) facilitate ongoing monitoring of the effectiveness of prevention and/or control activities and interventions? **A (EP 4)**				

Standard IC.8.10

Standard Score: ❑ Compliant ❑ Not Compliant

Assessment Question	Level of Compliance	Evidence of Compliance	Plan of Action/ Measure of Success (if needed)	Due Date
1. Do organization leaders, with licensed independent practitioners and other direct and indirect resident care staff including, when applicable, administration, building maintenance/engineering, food services, housekeeping, and pharmacy collaborate on an ongoing basis with qualified individual(s) managing the IC program? **A (EP 1)**				
2. Do these representatives participate in the following: • Development of strategies for each component's/function's role in the IC program • Assessment of the adequacy of the human, information, physical, and financial resources allocated to support infection prevention and control activities • Assessment of the overall failure or success of key processes for preventing and controlling infection • The review and revision of the IC program as warranted to improve outcomes? **A (EP 2)**				

* Qualifications may be met through ongoing education, training, experience, and/or certification (such as that offered by the Certification Board for Infection Control [CBIC]) in the prevention and control of infections.)

Key: 0 = Insufficient compliance; 1 = Partial compliance; 2 = Satisfactory compliance; NA = Not applicable; **A** indicates scoring category A; **C** indicates scoring category C; ▲(2) indicates situational decision rules apply; △(3) indicates direct impact requirements apply; Ⓜ indicates Measure of success is needed; ☆ indicates this standard also applies to organizations seeking Joint Commission's Medicare/Medicaid certification–based long term care accreditation

Standard IC.9.10	**Standard Score:** ❑ Compliant ❑ Not Compliant			
Assessment Question	**Level of Compliance**	**Evidence of Compliance**	**Plan of Action/ Measure of Success (if needed)**	**Due Date**
1. Is the effectiveness of the organization's infection prevention and control activities reviewed on an ongoing basis, and are findings reported to the integrated resident safety program at least annually? **A (EP 1)**				
2. Are adequate systems to access information provided to support infection prevention and control activities? **A (EP 2)**				
3. When applicable, is adequate laboratory support provided to support infection prevention and control activities? **A (EP 3)**				
4. Are adequate equipment and supplies provided to support infection prevention and control activities? **A (EP 4)**				

Key: 0 = Insufficient compliance; 1 = Partial compliance; 2 = Satisfactory compliance; NA = Not applicable; **A** indicates scoring category A; **C** indicates scoring category C; ▲(2) indicates situational decision rules apply; △(3) indicates direct impact requirements apply; Ⓜ indicates Measure of success is needed; ☆ indicates this standard also applies to organizations seeking Joint Commission's Medicare/Medicaid certification–based long term care accreditation

Improving Organization Performance (PI)

Standard PI.1.10 ★	**Standard Score: ❑ Compliant ❑ Not Compliant**			
Assessment Question	**Level of Compliance**	**Evidence of Compliance**	**Plan of Action/ Measure of Success (if needed)**	**Due Date**
1. Does the organization collect data for priorities identified by leaders (*see* standard LD.4.50)? **A (EP 1)**				
2. Does the organization consider collecting data in the following areas: • Staff opinions and needs • Staff perceptions of risks to individuals and suggestions for improving resident safety • Staff willingness to report unanticipated adverse events? **A (EP 2)**				
3. Does the organization collect data on the perceptions of care, treatment, and services* of residents about the following: • Their specific needs and expectations • How well the organization meets these needs and expectations • How the organization can improve resident safety • The effectiveness of pain management, when applicable? **A (EP 3)**				
4. Does the organization collect data that measure the performance of medication management, when provided? **A (EP 4)**				
5. Does the organization collect data that measure the performance of blood and blood product use, when provided? **A (EP 5)**				
6. Does the organization collect data that measure the performance of restraint use, when provided? **A (EP 6)**				
7. Does the organization collect data that measure the performance of behavior management and treatment, when provided? **A (EP 8)**				

* The Joint Commission is moving from the phrase *satisfaction with care, treatment, and services* toward the more inclusive phrase *perception of care, treatment, and services* to better measure the performance of organizations meeting the needs, expectations, and concerns of residents. By using this term, the organization will be prompted to assess not only residents' and/or families' satisfaction with care, treatment, or services, but also whether the organization meets their needs and expectations.

Key: 0 = Insufficient compliance; 1 = Partial compliance; 2 = Satisfactory compliance; NA = Not applicable; **A** indicates scoring category A; **C** indicates scoring category C; ▲(2) indicates situational decision rules apply; △(3) indicates direct impact requirements apply; Ⓜ indicates Measure of success is needed; ☆ indicates this standard also applies to organizations seeking Joint Commission's Medicare/Medicaid certification–based long term care accreditation

Standard PI.1.10 ★

Assessment Question	Level of Compliance	Evidence of Compliance	Plan of Action/ Measure of Success (if needed)	Due Date
8. Is relevant information developed from risk management activities integrated into performance improvement initiatives? Does this occur in a way that is consistent with any organization policies or procedures intended to preserve any confidentiality or privilege of information established by applicable law? **A (EP 13)**				
9. Is relevant information developed from utilization management activities integrated into performance improvement initiatives? Does this occur in a way that is consistent with any organization policies or procedures intended to preserve any confidentiality or privilege of information established by applicable law? **A (EP 14)**				
10. Is relevant information developed from quality control activities integrated into performance improvement initiatives? Does this occur in a way that is consistent with any organization policies or procedures intended to preserve any confidentiality or privilege of information established by applicable law? **A (EP 15)**				
11. Is relevant information developed from infection control surveillance and reporting activities integrated into performance improvement initiatives? Does this occur in a way that is consistent with any organization policies or procedures intended to preserve any confidentiality or privilege of information established by applicable law? **A (EP 16)**				
12. Is relevant information developed from research activities (as applicable) integrated into performance improvement initiatives? Does this occur in a way that is consistent with any organization policies or procedures intended to preserve any confidentiality or privilege of information established by applicable law? **A (EP 17)**				

Key: 0 = Insufficient compliance; 1 = Partial compliance; 2 = Satisfactory compliance; NA = Not applicable; **A** indicates scoring category A; **C** indicates scoring category C; ▲ indicates situational decision rules apply; △ indicates direct impact requirements apply; Ⓜ indicates Measure of success is needed; ☆ indicates this standard also applies to organizations seeking Joint Commission's Medicare/Medicaid certification–based long term care accreditation

Standard PI.2.10 ★	Standard Score: ❑ Compliant ❑ Not Compliant			
Assessment Question	**Level of Compliance**	**Evidence of Compliance**	**Plan of Action/ Measure of Success (if needed)**	**Due Date**
1. Are the collected data aggregated and analyzed? **A (EP 1)**				
2. Are data aggregated at the frequency appropriate to the activity or process being studied? **A (EP 2)**				
3. Are statistical tools and techniques used to analyze and display data? **A (EP 3)**				
4. Are data analyzed and compared internally over time and externally* with other sources of information when available? **A (EP 4)**				
5. Are comparative data used to determine if there is excessive variability or unacceptable levels of performance when available? **A (EP 5)**				

Standard PI.2.20 ★	Standard Score: ❑ Compliant ❑ Not Compliant			
Assessment Question	**Level of Compliance**	**Evidence of Compliance**	**Plan of Action/ Measure of Success (if needed)**	**Due Date**
1. Is analysis performed when data comparisons indicate that levels of performance, patterns, or trends vary substantially from those expected? **A (EP 1)**				
2. Does analysis occur for those topics chosen by leaders as performance improvement priorities? **A (EP 2)**				
3. Is analysis performed when undesirable variation occurs which changes priorities? **A (EP 3)**				
4. Is an analysis performed for all confirmed transfusion reactions, if applicable to the organization? **A (EP 4)**				
5. Is an analysis performed for all serious adverse drug events, if applicable and as defined by the organization? **A (EP 5)**				

* External sources of information include recent scientific, clinical, and management literature, including *Sentinel Event Alerts;* well-formulated practice guidelines or parameters; performance measures; reference databases; other organizations with similar processes; and standards that are periodically reviewed and revised.

Key: 0 = Insufficient compliance; 1 = Partial compliance; 2 = Satisfactory compliance; NA = Not applicable; **A** indicates scoring category A; **C** indicates scoring category C; ▲ indicates situational decision rules apply; △ indicates direct impact requirements apply; Ⓜ indicates Measure of success is needed; ☆ indicates this standard also applies to organizations seeking Joint Commission's Medicare/Medicaid certification–based long term care accreditation

Standard PI.2.20 ★

Assessment Question	Level of Compliance	Evidence of Compliance	Plan of Action/ Measure of Success (if needed)	Due Date
6. Is an analysis performed for all significant medication errors, if applicable and as defined by the organization? **A (EP 6)**				
7. Is an analysis performed for hazardous conditions? **A (EP 9)**				
8. Is an analysis performed for staffing effectiveness issues? **A (EP 10)**				

Standard PI.3.10 ★

Standard Score: ❑ Compliant ❑ Not Compliant

Assessment Question	Level of Compliance	Evidence of Compliance	Plan of Action/ Measure of Success (if needed)	Due Date
1. Does the organization use the information from data analysis to identify and implement changes that will improve the quality of care, treatment, and services? **A (EP 1)**				
2. Does the organization identify and implement changes that will reduce the risk of sentinel events? **A (EP 2)**				
3. Does the organization use the information from data analysis to identify changes that will improve resident safety? **A (EP 3)**				
4. Are changes made to improve processes or outcomes evaluated to ensure that they achieve the expected results? **A (EP 4)**				
5. Are appropriate actions undertaken when planned improvements are not achieved or sustained? **A (EP 5)**				

Key: 0 = Insufficient compliance; 1 = Partial compliance; 2 = Satisfactory compliance; NA = Not applicable; **A** indicates scoring category A; **C** indicates scoring category C; ▲ indicates situational decision rules apply; △ indicates direct impact requirements apply; Ⓜ indicates Measure of success is needed; ☆ indicates this standard also applies to organizations seeking Joint Commission's Medicare/Medicaid certification–based long term care accreditation

Leadership (LD)

Standard LD.01.01.01	The organization has a leadership structure.			
Assessment Question	**Level of Compliance**	**Evidence of Compliance**	**Plan of Action/ Measure of Success (if needed)**	**Due Date**
1. Does the organization identify those responsible for governance? **A (EP 1)**				
2. Does the governance identify those responsible for planning, administration, and operational activities? **A (EP 2)**				
3. Does governance identify those responsible for the provision of care, treatment, and services? **A (EP 3)**				

Standard LD.01.03.01 ★	Governance is ultimately accountable for the safety and quality of care, treatment, or services.			
Assessment Question	**Level of Compliance**	**Evidence of Compliance**	**Plan of Action/ Measure of Success (if needed)**	**Due Date**
1. Does governance define in writing its responsibilities? **A (EP 1)**				
2. Does governance provide for organization management and planning? **A (EP 2)**				
3. Does governance approve the organization's written scope of services? **A (EP 3)**				
4. Does the governance select the administrator? **A (EP 4)**				
5. Does governance provide for the resources needed to maintain safe, quality care, treatment, and services? **A (EP 5)** ⚠3				
6. Does governance work with other leaders to annually evaluate the organization's performance in relation to its mission, vision, and goals? **A (EP 6)**				
7. If the organization has an organized medical staff, does the governance approve its bylaws, rules and regulations? **A (EP 11)**				

Key: 0 = Insufficient compliance; 1 = Partial compliance; 2 = Satisfactory compliance; NA = Not applicable; **A** indicates scoring category A; **C** indicates scoring category C; ▲2 indicates situational decision rules apply; ⚠3 indicates direct impact requirements apply; Ⓜ indicates Measure of success is needed; ☆ indicates this standard also applies to organizations seeking Joint Commission's Medicare/Medicaid certification–based long term care accreditation

Standard LD.01.04.01	An administrator manages the organization.			
Assessment Question	**Level of Compliance**	**Evidence of Compliance**	**Plan of Action/ Measure of Success (if needed)**	**Due Date**
1. Does the administrator provide for information and support systems? **A (EP 1)**				
2. Does the administrator provide for recruitment and retention of staff? **A (EP 2)**				
3. Does the administrator provide for physical and financial assets? **A (EP 3)**				
4. Does the administrator identify a registered nurse, qualified by education and experience, to direct nursing services? **A (EP 6)**				
5. When the director of nursing is responsible for more than one organization or specialty program, is an appropriately qualified registered nurse assigned responsibility for the nursing staff activities in each setting? **A (EP 7)**				
6. When the director of nursing is absent, is responsibility for continuity and supervision of nursing care delegated to a registered nurse? **A (EP 8)**				
7. Is the individual with the authority to address administrative issues accessible to the organization on a full-time basis? **A (EP 9)**				
8. When the administrator is absent from the organization, is a qualified individual designated to perform the duties of this position? **A (EP 11)**				

Key: 0 = Insufficient compliance; 1 = Partial compliance; 2 = Satisfactory compliance; NA = Not applicable; **A** indicates scoring category A; **C** indicates scoring category C; ▲ indicates situational decision rules apply; △ indicates direct impact requirements apply; Ⓜ indicates Measure of success is needed; ☆ indicates this standard also applies to organizations seeking Joint Commission's Medicare/Medicaid certification–based long term care accreditation

Standard LD.01.06.01	A medical director oversees the care, treatment, and services provided to residents.			
Assessment Question	**Level of Compliance**	**Evidence of Compliance**	**Plan of Action/ Measure of Success (if needed)**	**Due Date**
1. Is the medical director appointed by the chief executive or designated by the organized medical staff? **A (EP 1)**				
2. Are the responsibilities of the medical director defined in a written agreement with the governing body? **A (EP 2)**				
3. Does the medical director: • Direct and coordinate medical care in the organization • Participate in establishing policies, procedures, and guidelines for comprehensive services • Help develop emergency treatment procedures for residents • Help develop resident transfer procedures • Participate in the resident care management system • Participate in in-service training programs? **A (EP 3)**				
4. Does the medical director advise the administration, the governance, and other professionals on: • Credentialing and privileging recommendations • The development and maintenance of the medical record system • The organization's ability to meet residents' needs • Adequacy and appropriateness of the organization's scope of services, medical equipment, and its professional and support staff • Future resident care programs • Hazards to health and safety identified in environmental incident reports (or summaries of incident reports) • Improving the performance of medical services as an integral part of improving organization performance • Employees' health status and employee health policies • Policies requiring health care professionals to practice within the scope of their licenses? **A (EP 4)**				

Key: 0 = Insufficient compliance; 1 = Partial compliance; 2 = Satisfactory compliance; NA = Not applicable; **A** indicates scoring category A; **C** indicates scoring category C; ▲(2) indicates situational decision rules apply; △(3) indicates direct impact requirements apply; Ⓜ indicates Measure of success is needed; ☆ indicates this standard also applies to organizations seeking Joint Commission's Medicare/Medicaid certification–based long term care accreditation

Standard LD.01.06.01

Assessment Question	Level of Compliance	Evidence of Compliance	Plan of Action/ Measure of Success (if needed)	Due Date
5. Does the medical director serve as a liaison for the organization in the following ways: • Helping to arrange and communicate physician availability and coverage • Communicating medical staff responsibilities and medical care policies, procedures, and guidelines to all licensed independent practitioners providing or ordering care • Serving as a member of the organized medical staff if the organization has one • Collaborating with the administrator and the organized medical staff, if the organization has one, to formulate the bylaws and the rules and regulations • Being responsible, when there is no medical staff, for the written rules and regulations for all licensed independent practitioners who attend residents in the organization • Being familiar with the policies and programs of public health agencies that affect resident care programs • Acting as the organization's medical representative in the community? **Note:** *This standard does not require the creation of a medical staff where one does not exist. That is entirely the decision of the long term care organization.* **A (EP 5)**				

Key: 0 = Insufficient compliance; 1 = Partial compliance; 2 = Satisfactory compliance; NA = Not applicable; **A** indicates scoring category A; **C** indicates scoring category C; ▲ indicates situational decision rules apply; △ indicates direct impact requirements apply; Ⓜ indicates Measure of success is needed; ☆ indicates this standard also applies to organizations seeking Joint Commission's Medicare/Medicaid certification–based long term care accreditation

Standard LD.01.07.01	Individual leaders have the knowledge needed for their roles in the organization, or they seek guidance to fulfill their roles.			
Assessment Question	**Level of Compliance**	**Evidence of Compliance**	**Plan of Action/ Measure of Success (if needed)**	**Due Date**
1. Are leaders oriented to all of the following: • The organization's mission and vision • The organization's safety and quality goals • The organization's structure and the decision-making process • The development of the budget as well as the interpretation of the organization's financial statements • The population(s) served by the organization and any issues related to that population(s) • The individual and interdependent responsibilities and accountabilities of leaders as they relate to supporting the mission of the organization and to providing safe and quality care • Applicable law and regulation? **C (EP 2) Ⓜ**				
2. Does governance provide leaders with access to information and training in areas where they need additional skills or expertise? **A (EP 3)**				
3. If the facility's medical director does not have the expertise to direct specialty programs, is another physician with that expertise identified to direct the medical care provided? Is the relationship between these two positions clearly defined? **A (EP 4)**				

Standard LD.02.01.01 ★	The mission, vision, and goals of the organization support the safety and quality of care, treatment, or services.			
Assessment Question	**Level of Compliance**	**Evidence of Compliance**	**Plan of Action/ Measure of Success (if needed)**	**Due Date**
1. Do leaders work together to create the organization's mission, vision, and goals? **A (EP 1)**				
2. Do the organization's mission, vision, and goals guide the actions of leaders? **A (EP 2)**				
3. Do leaders communicate the mission, vision, and goals to staff and the population(s) the organization serves? **A (EP 3)**				

Key: 0 = Insufficient compliance; 1 = Partial compliance; 2 = Satisfactory compliance; NA = Not applicable; **A** indicates scoring category A; **C** indicates scoring category C; ▲2 indicates situational decision rules apply; △3 indicates direct impact requirements apply; Ⓜ indicates Measure of success is needed; ☆ indicates this standard also applies to organizations seeking Joint Commission's Medicare/Medicaid certification–based long term care accreditation

Standard LD.02.03.01

Leaders regularly communicate with each other on issues of safety and quality.

Assessment Question	Level of Compliance	Evidence of Compliance	Plan of Action/ Measure of Success (if needed)	Due Date
1. Do leaders discuss issues that affect the organization and the population it serves, including the following: • Performance improvement activities • Reported safety and quality issues • Proposed solutions and their impact on the organization's resources • Reports on key quality measures and safety indicators • Safety and quality issues specific to the population(s) served • Input from the population(s) served? **A (EP 1)**				
2. Does the organization establish time frames for the discussion of issues that affect the organization and the population(s) it serves? **A (EP 2)**				

Standard LD.03.01.01 ★

Leaders create and maintain a culture of safety and quality throughout the organization.

Assessment Question	Level of Compliance	Evidence of Compliance	Plan of Action/ Measure of Success (if needed)	Due Date
1. Do leaders regularly evaluate the culture of safety and quality? **A (EP 1)**				
2. Do leaders prioritize and implement changes identified by the evaluation? **A (EP 2)**				
3. Do leaders provide opportunities for all individuals who work in the organization to participate in safety and quality initiatives? **A (EP 3)**				
4. Does the organization have a code of conduct that defines acceptable, disruptive, and inappropriate behaviors? **A (EP 4)**				
5. Do leaders create and implement a process for managing disruptive and inappropriate behaviors? **A (EP 5)** ⚠3				

Key: 0 = Insufficient compliance; 1 = Partial compliance; 2 = Satisfactory compliance; NA = Not applicable; **A** indicates scoring category A; **C** indicates scoring category C; ▲ indicates situational decision rules apply; △3 indicates direct impact requirements apply; Ⓜ indicates Measure of success is needed; ☆ indicates this standard also applies to organizations seeking Joint Commission's Medicare/Medicaid certification–based long term care accreditation

Standard LD.03.01.01 ★

Assessment Question	Level of Compliance	Evidence of Compliance	Plan of Action/ Measure of Success (if needed)	Due Date
6. Do leaders provide education that focuses on safety and quality for all individuals? (*See also* Standard LD.04.04.05, EP 6) **A (EP 6)**				
7. Do leaders establish a team approach among all staff at all levels? **A (EP 7)**				
8. Do all individuals who work in the organization, including staff and licensed independent practitioners, openly discuss issues of safety and quality? **A (EP 8)**				
9. Are literature and advisories relevant to resident safety available to all individuals who work in the organization? **A (EP 9)**				
10. Do leaders define how members of the population(s) served can help identify and manage issues of safety and quality within the organization? **A (EP 10)**				

Standard LD.03.02.01 ★

The organization uses data and information to guide decisions and to understand variation in the performance of processes supporting safety and quality.

Assessment Question	Level of Compliance	Evidence of Compliance	Plan of Action/ Measure of Success (if needed)	Due Date
1. Do leaders set expectations for using data and information to improve the safety and quality of care, treatment, or services? **A (EP 1)**				
2. Are leaders able to describe how data and information are used to create a culture of safety and quality? **A (EP 2)**				
3. Does the organization use processes to support systematic data and information use? **A (EP 3)**				
4. Do leaders provide the resources needed for data and information use, including staff, equipment, and information systems? **A (EP 4)**				

Key: 0 = Insufficient compliance; 1 = Partial compliance; 2 = Satisfactory compliance; NA = Not applicable; **A** indicates scoring category A; **C** indicates scoring category C; ▲ indicates situational decision rules apply; △ indicates direct impact requirements apply; Ⓜ indicates Measure of success is needed; ☆ indicates this standard also applies to organizations seeking Joint Commission's Medicare/Medicaid certification–based long term care accreditation

Standard LD.03.02.01 ★

Assessment Question	Level of Compliance	Evidence of Compliance	Plan of Action/ Measure of Success (if needed)	Due Date
5. Does the organization use data and information in decision making that supports the safety and quality of care, treatment, or services? **A (EP 5)**				
6. Does the organization use data and information to identify and respond to internal and external changes in the environment? **A (EP 6)**				
7. Do leaders evaluate the effectiveness of the use of data and information used throughout the organization? **A (EP 7)**				

Standard LD.03.03.01 ★

Leaders use organizationwide planning to establish structures and processes that focus on safety and quality.

Assessment Question	Level of Compliance	Evidence of Compliance	Plan of Action/ Measure of Success (if needed)	Due Date
1. Do planning activities focus on improving resident safety and health care quality? **A (EP 1)**				
2. Can leaders describe how planning supports a culture of safety and quality? **A (EP 2)**				
3. Is planning systematic, and does it involve designated individuals and information sources? **A (EP 3)**				
4. Do leaders provide the resources needed to support the safety and quality of care, treatment, or services? **A (EP 4)** ⚠3				
5. Is safety and quality planning organizationwide? **A (EP 5)**				
6. Do planning activities adapt to changes in the environment? **A (EP 6)**				
7. Do leaders evaluate the effectiveness of planning activities? **A (EP 7)**				

Key: 0 = Insufficient compliance; 1 = Partial compliance; 2 = Satisfactory compliance; NA = Not applicable; **A** indicates scoring category A; **C** indicates scoring category C; ▲2 indicates situational decision rules apply; ⚠3 indicates direct impact requirements apply; Ⓜ indicates Measure of success is needed; ☆ indicates this standard also applies to organizations seeking Joint Commission's Medicare/Medicaid certification–based long term care accreditation

Standard LD.03.04.01 ★	The organization communicates information related to safety and quality to those who need it, including staff, residents, families, and external interested parties.			
Assessment Question	**Level of Compliance**	**Evidence of Compliance**	**Plan of Action/ Measure of Success (if needed)**	**Due Date**
1. Do communication processes foster the safety of the resident and the quality of care? **A (EP 1)**				
2. Are leaders able to describe how communication supports a culture of safety and quality? **A (EP 2)**				
3. Is communication designed to meet the needs of internal and external users? **A (EP 3)**				
4. Do leaders provide the resources required for communication, based on the needs of residents, staff, and administration? **A (EP 4)**				
5. Does communication support safety and quality throughout the organization? (*See also* Standard LD.04.04.05, EPs 6 and 12) **A (EP 5)**				
6. When changes in the environment occur, does the organization communicate those changes effectively? **A (EP 6)**				
7. Do leaders evaluate the effectiveness of communication methods? **A (EP 7)**				

Standard LD.03.05.01 ★	Leaders implement changes in existing processes to improve the performance of the organization.			
Assessment Question	**Level of Compliance**	**Evidence of Compliance**	**Plan of Action/ Measure of Success (if needed)**	**Due Date**
1. Do structures for managing change and performance improvements exist that foster the safety of the resident and the quality of care, treatment, or services? **A (EP 1)**				
2. Are leaders able to describe how the organization's approach to performance improvement and its capacity for change support a culture of safety and quality? **A (EP 2)**				

Key: 0 = Insufficient compliance; 1 = Partial compliance; 2 = Satisfactory compliance; NA = Not applicable; **A** indicates scoring category A; **C** indicates scoring category C; ▲(2) indicates situational decision rules apply; △(3) indicates direct impact requirements apply; Ⓜ indicates Measure of success is needed; ☆ indicates this standard also applies to organizations seeking Joint Commission's Medicare/Medicaid certification–based long term care accreditation

Standard LD.03.05.01 ★				
Assessment Question	**Level of Compliance**	**Evidence of Compliance**	**Plan of Action/ Measure of Success (if needed)**	**Due Date**
3. Does the organization have a systematic approach to change and performance improvement? **A (EP 3)**				
4. Do leaders provide the resources required for performance improvement and change management, including sufficient staff, access to information, and training? **A (EP 4)**				
5. Does the management of change and performance improvement support both safety and quality throughout the organization? **A (EP 5)**				
6. Can the organization's internal structures adapt to changes in the environment? **A (EP 6)**				
7. Do leaders evaluate the effectiveness of processes for the management of change and performance improvement? **A (EP 7)**				

Standard LD.03.06.01 ★	Those who work in the organization are focused on improving safety and quality.			
Assessment Question	**Level of Compliance**	**Evidence of Compliance**	**Plan of Action/ Measure of Success (if needed)**	**Due Date**
1. Do leaders design work processes to focus individuals on safety and quality issues? **A (EP 1)**				
2. Are leaders able to describe how those who work in the organization support a culture of safety and quality? **A (EP 2)**				
3. Do leaders provide for a sufficient number and mix of individuals to support safe, quality care, treatment, or services? **A (EP 3)** ⚠3				
4. Are those who work in the organization competent to complete their assigned responsibilities? **A (EP 4)** ⚠3				

Key: 0 = Insufficient compliance; 1 = Partial compliance; 2 = Satisfactory compliance; NA = Not applicable; **A** indicates scoring category A; **C** indicates scoring category C; ▲2 indicates situational decision rules apply; ⚠3 indicates direct impact requirements apply; Ⓜ indicates Measure of success is needed; ☆ indicates this standard also applies to organizations seeking Joint Commission's Medicare/Medicaid certification–based long term care accreditation

Standard LD.03.06.01 ★				
Assessment Question	**Level of Compliance**	**Evidence of Compliance**	**Plan of Action/ Measure of Success (if needed)**	**Due Date**
5. Do those who work in the organization adapt to changes in the environment? **A (EP 5)**				
6. Do leaders evaluate the effectiveness of those who work in the organization to promote safety and quality? **A (EP 6)**				

Standard LD.04.01.01 ★	The organization complies with law and regulation.			
Assessment Question	**Level of Compliance**	**Evidence of Compliance**	**Plan of Action/ Measure of Success (if needed)**	**Due Date**
1. Is the organization licensed, certified, or has a permit, in accordance with law and regulation, to provide the care, treatment, or services for which the organization is seeking accreditation from The Joint Commission? **Note:** *Applicable law and regulation include, but are not limited to, individual and facility licensure, certification, Food and Drug Administration regulations, Drug Enforcement Agency regulations, Center for Medicare & Medicaid Services regulations, Occupational Safety and Health Administration regulations, Department of Transportation regulations, Health Insurance Portability and Accountability Act, and other local, state, and federal laws and regulations.* **Note:** *Each service location that performs laboratory testing (waived or non waived) must have a Clinical Laboratory Improvement Amendments of 1988 (CLIA '88) certificate as specified by the federal CLIA regulations (42 CFR 493.55 and 493.3) and applicable state law.** **A (EP 1)** ▲2				
2. Does the organization provide care, treatment, or services in accordance with licensure requirements, laws, and rules and regulations? **A (EP 2)** △3				

* For more information on how to obtain a CLIA certificate, *see* http://www.cms.hhs.gov/CLIA/downloads/HowObtainCLIACertificate.pdf.

Key: 0 = Insufficient compliance; 1 = Partial compliance; 2 = Satisfactory compliance; NA = Not applicable; **A** indicates scoring category A; **C** indicates scoring category C; ▲ indicates situational decision rules apply; △ indicates direct impact requirements apply; Ⓜ indicates Measure of success is needed; ☆ indicates this standard also applies to organizations seeking Joint Commission's Medicare/Medicaid certification–based long term care accreditation

Standard LD.04.01.01 ★

Assessment Question	Level of Compliance	Evidence of Compliance	Plan of Action/ Measure of Success (if needed)	Due Date
3. Do leaders act on or comply with reports or recommendations from external authorized agencies, such as accreditation, certification, or regulatory bodies? **A (EP 3)**				

Standard LD.04.01.03

The organization develops an annual operating budget and, when needed, a long-term capital expenditure plan.

Assessment Question	Level of Compliance	Evidence of Compliance	Plan of Action/ Measure of Success (if needed)	Due Date
1. Do leaders solicit comments from those who work in the organization when developing the operational and capital budgets? **A (EP 1)**				
2. Does the operating budget reflect the organization's goals and objectives? **A (EP 3)**				
3. Does the governance approve an annual operating budget and, when needed, a long-term capital expenditure plan? **A (EP 4)**				
4. Do the leaders monitor the implementation of the budget and long-term capital expenditure plan? **A (EP 5)**				
5. Does an independent public accountant conduct an annual audit of the organization's finances, unless otherwise provided by law? **A (EP 6)**				

Standard LD.04.01.05

The organization effectively manages its programs, services, sites, or departments.

Assessment Question	Level of Compliance	Evidence of Compliance	Plan of Action/ Measure of Success (if needed)	Due Date
1. Do leaders of the program, service, site, or department oversee operations? **A (EP 1)**				

Key: 0 = Insufficient compliance; 1 = Partial compliance; 2 = Satisfactory compliance; NA = Not applicable; **A** indicates scoring category A; **C** indicates scoring category C; ▲(2) indicates situational decision rules apply; △(3) indicates direct impact requirements apply; Ⓜ indicates Measure of success is needed; ☆ indicates this standard also applies to organizations seeking Joint Commission's Medicare/Medicaid certification–based long term care accreditation

Standard LD.04.01.05

Assessment Question	Level of Compliance	Evidence of Compliance	Plan of Action/ Measure of Success (if needed)	Due Date
2. Are programs, services, sites, or departments providing resident care directed by one or more qualified professionals or by a qualified licensed independent practitioner with clinical privileges? **A (EP 2)**				
3. Does the organization define in writing the responsibility of those with administrative and clinical direction of its programs, services, sites, or departments? **A (EP 3)**				
4. Are staff members held accountable for their responsibilities? **A (EP 4)**				
5. Do leaders provide for the coordination of care, treatment, or services among the organization's different programs, services, sites, or departments? **A (EP 5)**				

Standard LD.04.01.07 ★

The organization has policies and procedures that guide and support resident care, treatment, or services.

Assessment Question	Level of Compliance	Evidence of Compliance	Plan of Action/ Measure of Success (if needed)	Due Date
1. Do leaders review and approve policies and procedures that guide and support resident care, treatment, or services? **A (EP 1)**				
2. Does the organization manage the implementation of policies and procedures? **A (EP 2)**				

Standard LD.04.01.11

The organization makes space and equipment available as needed for the provision of care, treatment, or services.

Assessment Question	Level of Compliance	Evidence of Compliance	Plan of Action/ Measure of Success (if needed)	Due Date
1. Does the arrangement and allocation of space support safe, efficient, and effective care, treatment, or services? **A (EP 2)**				

Key: 0 = Insufficient compliance; 1 = Partial compliance; 2 = Satisfactory compliance; NA = Not applicable; **A** indicates scoring category A; **C** indicates scoring category C; ▲ indicates situational decision rules apply; △ indicates direct impact requirements apply; Ⓜ indicates Measure of success is needed; ☆ indicates this standard also applies to organizations seeking Joint Commission's Medicare/Medicaid certification–based long term care accreditation

Standard LD.04.01.11

Assessment Question	Level of Compliance	Evidence of Compliance	Plan of Action/ Measure of Success (if needed)	Due Date
2. Does the interior and exterior space provided for care, treatment, or services meet the needs of residents? **A (EP 3)**				
3. Are the grounds, equipment, and special activity areas safe, maintained, and supervised? **A (EP 4)**				
4 Do the leaders provide for equipment, supplies, and other resources? **A (EP 5)** △3				

Standard LD.04.02.01

The leaders address any conflict of interest involving licensed independent practitioners and/or staff that affects or has the potential to affect the safety or quality of care, treatment, or services.

Assessment Question	Level of Compliance	Evidence of Compliance	Plan of Action/ Measure of Success (if needed)	Due Date
1. Do the leaders define in writing conflict of interest involving licensed independent practitioners or staff? **A (EP 1)**				
2. Do the leaders develop a written policy that defines how the organization will address conflict of interest involving licensed independent practitioners and/or staff? **A (EP 2)**				
3. Are existing or potential conflicts of interest involving licensed independent practitioners and/or staff, as defined by the organization, disclosed? **A (EP 3)**				
4. Does the organization review its relationships with other care providers, educational institutions, manufacturers, and payors to determine whether conflicts of interest exist and whether they are within law and regulation? **A (EP 4)**				

Key: 0 = Insufficient compliance; 1 = Partial compliance; 2 = Satisfactory compliance; NA = Not applicable; **A** indicates scoring category A; **C** indicates scoring category C; ▲2 indicates situational decision rules apply; △3 indicates direct impact requirements apply; Ⓜ indicates Measure of success is needed; ☆ indicates this standard also applies to organizations seeking Joint Commission's Medicare/Medicaid certification–based long term care accreditation

Standard LD.04.02.01

Assessment Question	Level of Compliance	Evidence of Compliance	Plan of Action/ Measure of Success (if needed)	Due Date
5. Are policies, procedures, and information about the relationship between care, treatment, or services and financial incentives available upon request to all residents, and those individuals who work in the organization, including staff and licensed independent practitioners? **A (EP 5)**				

Standard LD.04.02.03 ★

Ethical principles guide the organization's business practices.

Assessment Question	Level of Compliance	Evidence of Compliance	Plan of Action/ Measure of Success (if needed)	Due Date
1. Does the organization have a process that allows staff, residents, and families to address ethical issues or issues prone to conflict? **A (EP 1)**				
2. Does the organization use its process to address ethical issues or issues prone to conflict? **A (EP 2)**				
3. Does the organization follow ethical practices for marketing and billing? **A (EP 3)**				
4. Do marketing materials accurately represent the organization and address the care, treatment, or services that the organization provides either directly or by contractual arrangement? **A (EP 4)**				
5. Are care, treatment, or services based on resident needs, regardless of compensation or financial risk sharing with those who work in the organization, including staff and licensed independent practitioners? **A (EP 5)**				
6. Are care, treatment, or services not negatively affected when leaders excuse a staff member from a job responsibility? **A (EP 6)**				
7. Do residents receive information about charges for which they will be responsible? **A (EP 7)**				

Key: 0 = Insufficient compliance; 1 = Partial compliance; 2 = Satisfactory compliance; NA = Not applicable; **A** indicates scoring category A; **C** indicates scoring category C; ▲2 indicates situational decision rules apply; △3 indicates direct impact requirements apply; Ⓜ indicates Measure of success is needed; ☆ indicates this standard also applies to organizations seeking Joint Commission's Medicare/Medicaid certification–based long term care accreditation

Standard LD.04.02.03 ★

Assessment Question	Level of Compliance	Evidence of Compliance	Plan of Action/ Measure of Success (if needed)	Due Date
8. Are residents informed whenever services, charges, or coverage changes? **A (EP 8)**				
9. When a resident becomes eligible for Medicaid after admission to the organization, does the organization only charge the resident the Medicaid-allowable charge? **C (EP 15)** Ⓜ				

Standard LD.04.02.05 ★

When internal or external review results in the denial of care, treatment, or services or payment, the organization makes decisions regarding the ongoing provision of care, treatment, or services and discharge or transfer, based on the assessed needs of the resident.

Assessment Question	Level of Compliance	Evidence of Compliance	Plan of Action/ Measure of Success (if needed)	Due Date
1. Are decisions regarding the provision of ongoing care, treatment, or services, discharge, or transfer based on the assessed needs of the resident, regardless of the recommendations of any internal or external review? **A (EP 1)**				
2. Do the safety and quality of care, treatment, or services not depend on the resident's ability to pay? **A (EP 2)**				

Standard LD.04.03.01

The organization provides services that meet resident needs.

Assessment Question	Level of Compliance	Evidence of Compliance	Plan of Action/ Measure of Success (if needed)	Due Date
1. Do the needs of the population(s) served guide decisions about which services will be provided directly or through referral, consultation, contractual arrangements, or other agreements? **A (EP 1)**				

Key: 0 = Insufficient compliance; 1 = Partial compliance; 2 = Satisfactory compliance; NA = Not applicable; **A** indicates scoring category A; **C** indicates scoring category C; ▲ indicates situational decision rules apply; △ indicates direct impact requirements apply; Ⓜ indicates Measure of success is needed; ☆ indicates this standard also applies to organizations seeking Joint Commission's Medicare/Medicaid certification–based long term care accreditation

Standard LD.04.03.07	Patients with comparable needs receive the same standard of care, treatment, or services throughout the organization.			
Assessment Question	**Level of Compliance**	**Evidence of Compliance**	**Plan of Action/ Measure of Success (if needed)**	**Due Date**
1. Are outcomes of care, treatment, or services not negatively affected by variance in staff, setting, or payment source? **A (EP 1)**				
2. Is care, treatment, or services consistent with the organization's mission, vision, and goals? **A (EP 2)**				

Standard LD.04.03.09 ★	Care, treatment, or services provided through contractual agreement are provided safely and effectively.			
Assessment Question	**Level of Compliance**	**Evidence of Compliance**	**Plan of Action/ Measure of Success (if needed)**	**Due Date**
1. Do clinical leaders have an opportunity to provide advice about the sources of clinical services to be provided through contractual agreement? **A (EP 1)**				
2. Does the organization describe in writing the nature and scope of services provided through contractual agreements? **A (EP 2)**				
3. Do designated leaders approve contractual agreements? **A (EP 3)**				
4. Do leaders monitor contracted services by establishing expectations for the performance of the contracted services? **Note:** *When the organization contracts with another accredited organization for resident care, treatment, or services to be provided off-site, it can do the following:* • *Verify that all licensed independent practitioners who will be providing resident care, treatment, or services have appropriate privileges by obtaining, for example, a copy of the list of privileges.* • *Specify in the written agreement that the contracted organization will ensure that all contracted services provided by licensed independent practitioners will be within the scope of their privileges.* **A (EP 4)**				

Key: 0 = Insufficient compliance; 1 = Partial compliance; 2 = Satisfactory compliance; NA = Not applicable; **A** indicates scoring category A; **C** indicates scoring category C; ▲(2) indicates situational decision rules apply; △(3) indicates direct impact requirements apply; Ⓜ indicates Measure of success is needed; ☆ indicates this standard also applies to organizations seeking Joint Commission's Medicare/Medicaid certification–based long term care accreditation

Standard LD.04.03.09 ★

Assessment Question	Level of Compliance	Evidence of Compliance	Plan of Action/ Measure of Success (if needed)	Due Date
5. Do leaders monitor contracted services by communicating the expectations in writing to the provider of the contracted services? **Note:** *A written description of the expectations can be provided either as part of the written agreement or in addition to it.* **A (EP 5)**				
6. Do leaders monitor contracted services by evaluating these services in relation to the organization's expectations? **A (EP 6)**				
7. Do the leaders take steps to improve contracted services that do not meet expectations? **Note:** *Examples of improvement efforts to consider include the following:* • *Increase monitoring of the contracted services* • *Provide consultation or training to the contractor* • *Renegotiate the contract terms* • *Apply defined penalties* • *Terminate the contract* **A (EP 7)**				
8. When contractual agreements are renegotiated or terminated, does the organization maintain the continuity of resident care? **A (EP 8)** △3				
9. Do reference and contract lab services meet the federal regulations for clinical laboratories and maintain evidence of the same? **A (EP 10)**				

Standard LD.04.04.01 ★

Leaders establish priorities for performance improvement. (*See also* the "Improving Organization Performance" [PI] chapter.)

Assessment Question	Level of Compliance	Evidence of Compliance	Plan of Action/ Measure of Success (if needed)	Due Date
1. Do leaders set priorities for performance improvement activities and resident health outcomes? **A (EP 1)**				
2. Do leaders give priority to high-volume, high-risk, or problem-prone processes for performance improvement activities? **A (EP 2)**				

Key: 0 = Insufficient compliance; 1 = Partial compliance; 2 = Satisfactory compliance; NA = Not applicable; **A** indicates scoring category A; **C** indicates scoring category C; ▲2 indicates situational decision rules apply; △3 indicates direct impact requirements apply; Ⓜ indicates Measure of success is needed; ☆ indicates this standard also applies to organizations seeking Joint Commission's Medicare/Medicaid certification–based long term care accreditation

Standard LD.04.04.01 ★

Assessment Question	Level of Compliance	Evidence of Compliance	Plan of Action/ Measure of Success (if needed)	Due Date
3. Do leaders reprioritize performance improvement activities in response to changes in the internal or external environment? **A (EP 3)**				
4. Does performance improvement occur organizationwide? **A (EP 4)**				

Standard LD.04.04.03 ★

New or modified services or processes are well designed.

Assessment Question	Level of Compliance	Evidence of Compliance	Plan of Action/ Measure of Success (if needed)	Due Date
1. Does the organization's design of new or modified services or processes incorporate the needs of residents, staff, and others? **A (EP 1)**				
2. Does the organization's design of new or modified services or processes incorporate the results of performance improvement activities? **A (EP 2)**				
3. Does the organization's design of new or modified services or processes incorporate information about potential risks to residents? **A (EP 3)**				
4. Does the organization's design of new or modified services or processes incorporate evidence-based information in the decision-making process? **Note:** *For example, evidence-based information could include practice guidelines, successful practices, information from current literature, and clinical standards.* **A (EP 4)**				
5. Does the organization's design of new or modified services or processes incorporate information about sentinel events? **A (EP 5)**				

Key: 0 = Insufficient compliance; 1 = Partial compliance; 2 = Satisfactory compliance; NA = Not applicable; **A** indicates scoring category A; **C** indicates scoring category C; ▲2 indicates situational decision rules apply; △3 indicates direct impact requirements apply; Ⓜ indicates Measure of success is needed; ☆ indicates this standard also applies to organizations seeking Joint Commission's Medicare/Medicaid certification–based long term care accreditation

Standard LD.04.04.03 ★

Assessment Question	Level of Compliance	Evidence of Compliance	Plan of Action/ Measure of Success (if needed)	Due Date
6. Does the organization test and analyze its design of new or modified services or processes to determine whether the proposed design or modification is an improvement? **A (EP 6)**				
7. Do the leaders involve staff and residents in the design of new or modified services or processes? **A (EP 7)**				

Standard LD.04.04.05 ★

The organization has an organizationwide, integrated resident safety program.

Assessment Question	Level of Compliance	Evidence of Compliance	Plan of Action/ Measure of Success (if needed)	Due Date
1. Does the organization implement an organization-wide resident safety program? **A (EP 1)**				
2. Do one or more qualified individuals or an interdisciplinary group manage the safety program? **A (EP 2)**				
3. Does the scope of the safety program include the full range of safety issues, from potential or no-harm errors (sometimes referred to as near misses, close calls, or good catches) to hazardous conditions and sentinel events? **A (EP 3)**				
4. Do all departments, programs, and services within the organization participate in the safety program? **A (EP 4)**				
5. As part of the safety program, does the organization create procedures for responding to system or process failures? **Note:** *Responses might include continuing to provide care, treatment, or services to those affected, containing the risk to others, and preserving factual information for subsequent analysis.* **A (EP 5)**				

Key: 0 = Insufficient compliance; 1 = Partial compliance; 2 = Satisfactory compliance; NA = Not applicable; **A** indicates scoring category A; **C** indicates scoring category C; ▲ indicates situational decision rules apply; △ indicates direct impact requirements apply; Ⓜ indicates Measure of success is needed; ☆ indicates this standard also applies to organizations seeking Joint Commission's Medicare/Medicaid certification–based long term care accreditation

Standard LD.04.04.05 ★				
Assessment Question	**Level of Compliance**	**Evidence of Compliance**	**Plan of Action/ Measure of Success (if needed)**	**Due Date**
6. Does the organization provide and encourage the use of systems for blame-free internal reporting of a system or process failure, or the results of a proactive risk assessment? (*See also* Standards LD.03.01.01, EP 8; LD.03.04.01, EP 5) **A (EP 6)**				
7. Does the organization define "sentinel event" and communicate this definition throughout the organization? **Note:** *At a minimum, the organization's definition includes those events subject to review under The Joint Commission's Sentinel Event Policy as published in the accreditation manual. The definition may include any process variation that does not affect the outcome or result in an adverse event, but for which a recurrence carries significant chance of a serious adverse outcome or result in an adverse event, often referred to as a "near miss."* **A (EP 7)**				
8. Does the organization conduct thorough and credible root cause analyses in response to sentinel events as described in the sentinel event section of the accreditation manual? **A (EP 8)** ⚠3				
9. Does the organization make support systems available for staff who have been involved in an adverse or sentinel event? **Note:** *Support systems recognize that conscientious health care workers who are involved in sentinel events are themselves victims of the event and require support. Support systems provide staff with additional help and support as well as additional resources through the human resources function or an employee assistance program. Support systems also focus on the process rather than blaming the involved individuals.* **A (EP 9)**				
10. At least every 12 months, does the organization select one high-risk process and conduct a proactive risk assessment?* **A (EP 10)**				

**See* the accreditation manual for suggested components of a proactive risk assessment.

Key: 0 = Insufficient compliance; 1 = Partial compliance; 2 = Satisfactory compliance; NA = Not applicable; **A** indicates scoring category A; **C** indicates scoring category C; ▲2 indicates situational decision rules apply; ⚠3 indicates direct impact requirements apply; Ⓜ indicates Measure of success is needed; ☆ indicates this standard also applies to organizations seeking Joint Commission's Medicare/Medicaid certification–based long term care accreditation

Standard LD.04.04.05 ★

Assessment Question	Level of Compliance	Evidence of Compliance	Plan of Action/ Measure of Success (if needed)	Due Date
11. Does the organization analyze and use information about system or process failures and proactive risk assessments to improve safety? **A (EP 11)**				
12. Does the organization disseminate lessons learned from root cause analyses, system or process failures, and the results of proactive risk assessments to all staff who provide services for the specific situation? (*See also* Standard LD.03.04.01, EP 5) **A (EP 12)**				
13. Does the organization provide governance at least once a year with written reports on the following: • All system or process failures • The number and type of sentinel events • Whether the residents and the families were informed of the event • All actions taken to improve safety, both proactively and in response to actual occurrences? **A (EP 13)**				
14. Does the organization encourage external reporting of significant adverse events, including voluntary reporting programs in addition to mandatory programs? **Note:** *Examples of voluntary programs include The Joint Commission Sentinel Event Database and the Food and Drug Administration (FDA) MedWatch. Mandatory programs are often state initiated.* **A (EP 14)**				

Key: 0 = Insufficient compliance; 1 = Partial compliance; 2 = Satisfactory compliance; NA = Not applicable; **A** indicates scoring category A; **C** indicates scoring category C; ▲ indicates situational decision rules apply; △ indicates direct impact requirements apply; Ⓜ indicates Measure of success is needed; ☆ indicates this standard also applies to organizations seeking Joint Commission's Medicare/Medicaid certification–based long term care accreditation

Management of the Environment of Care (EC)

Standard EC.1.10 ★	Standard Score: ❑ Compliant ❑ Not Compliant			
Assessment Question	**Level of Compliance**	**Evidence of Compliance**	**Plan of Action/ Measure of Success (if needed)**	**Due Date**
1. Does the organization develop and maintain a written management plan describing the processes it implements to effectively manage the environmental safety of residents, staff, and other people coming to the organization's facilities? **A (EP 1)**				
2. Does the organization identify a person(s) as designated by leadership, to coordinate the development, implementation, and monitoring of the safety management activities? **A (EP 2)**				
3. Does the organization identify a person(s) to intervene whenever conditions immediately threaten life or health or threaten damage to equipment or buildings? **A (EP 3)**				
4. Does the organization conduct comprehensive proactive risk assessments that evaluate the potential adverse impact of buildings, grounds, equipment, occupants, and internal physical systems on the safety and health of residents, staff, and other people coming to the organization's facilities? **A (EP 4)**				
5. Does the organization use the risks identified to select and implement procedures and controls to achieve the lowest potential for adverse impact on the safety and health of residents, staff, and other people coming to the organization's facilities? **C (EP 5) Ⓜ**				
6. Does the organization establish safety policies and procedures that are practiced and reviewed as frequently as necessary, but at least every three years? **C (EP 6) Ⓜ**				
7. Does the organization ensure that a process exists for responding to product safety recalls by appropriate organization staff? **A (EP 8)**				
8. Does the organization ensure that all grounds and equipment are maintained appropriately? **A (EP 9)**				

Key: 0 = Insufficient compliance; 1 = Partial compliance; 2 = Satisfactory compliance; NA = Not applicable; **A** indicates scoring category A; **C** indicates scoring category C; ▲ indicates situational decision rules apply; △ indicates direct impact requirements apply; Ⓜ indicates Measure of success is needed; ☆ indicates this standard also applies to organizations seeking Joint Commission's Medicare/Medicaid certification–based long term care accreditation

Standard EC.1.20 ★

Standard Score: ❑ Compliant ❑ Not Compliant

Assessment Question	Level of Compliance	Evidence of Compliance	Plan of Action/ Measure of Success (if needed)	Due Date
1. Does the organization conduct environmental tours to identify environmental deficiencies, hazards, and unsafe practices? **A (EP 1)**				
2. Does the organization conduct environmental tours at least every six months in all areas where residents are served? **C (EP 2) Ⓜ**				
3. Does the organization conduct environmental tours at least annually in areas where residents are not served? **C (EP 3) Ⓜ**				

Standard EC.1.30 ★

Standard Score: ❑ Compliant ❑ Not Compliant

Assessment Question	Level of Compliance	Evidence of Compliance	Plan of Action/ Measure of Success (if needed)	Due Date
1. Does the organization develop a policy regarding smoking in all areas of all building(s) under the organization's control? **A (EP 1)**				
2. Does the organization's policy prohibit smoking in all areas of all building(s) under the organization's control (no medical exceptions allowed) for all children or youth residents? **A (EP 2)**				
3. Is there an organizational policy that permits residents to smoke in the organization's buildings if the resident meets criteria developed and approved by the organization's leaders? **A (EP 3)**				
4. If residents are permitted to smoke in the organization's buildings, do they smoke only under the following circumstances: • In designated locations environmentally separate from care, treatment, or service areas* • After the organization has taken measures to minimize fire risks? **C (EP 4) Ⓜ ⚠3**				

* This does not require that a designated smoking area be a specific distance from care, treatment, or service areas. A physically separate, well-ventilated room (a designated area for authorized smoking by residents that is exhausted to the outside) is acceptable.

Key: 0 = Insufficient compliance; 1 = Partial compliance; 2 = Satisfactory compliance; NA = Not applicable; **A** indicates scoring category A; **C** indicates scoring category C; ▲2 indicates situational decision rules apply; △3 indicates direct impact requirements apply; Ⓜ indicates Measure of success is needed; ☆ indicates this standard also applies to organizations seeking Joint Commission's Medicare/Medicaid certification–based long term care accreditation

Standard EC.1.30 ★

Assessment Question	Level of Compliance	Evidence of Compliance	Plan of Action/ Measure of Success (if needed)	Due Date
5. Are residents who smoke in the organization's buildings provided education, including information about options for smoking cessation? **C (EP 5)** Ⓜ				
6. Does the organization identify and implement a process(es) for monitoring compliance with the policy? **A (EP 6)**				
7. Does the organization develop strategies to eliminate the incidence of policy violations when identified? **A (EP 7)**				

Standard EC.2.10

Standard Score: ❑ Compliant ❑ Not Compliant

Assessment Question	Level of Compliance	Evidence of Compliance	Plan of Action/ Measure of Success (if needed)	Due Date
1. Does the organization develop and maintain a written management plan describing the processes it implements to effectively manage the security of residents, staff, and other people coming to the organization's facilities? **A (EP 1)**				
2. Does the organization identify a person(s), as designated by leadership, to coordinate the development, implementation, and monitoring of the security management activities? **A (EP 2)**				
3. Does the organization conduct proactive risk assessments that evaluate the potential adverse impact of the external environment and the services provided on the security of residents, staff, and other people coming to the organization's facilities?* **A (EP 3)**				
4. Does the organization use the risks identified to select and implement procedures and controls to achieve the lowest potential for adverse impact on security? **C (EP 4)** Ⓜ				

* The potential for workplace violence and for resident elopement or wandering is considered during the risk assessment.

Key: 0 = Insufficient compliance; 1 = Partial compliance; 2 = Satisfactory compliance; NA = Not applicable; **A** indicates scoring category A; **C** indicates scoring category C; ▲2 indicates situational decision rules apply; △3 indicates direct impact requirements apply; Ⓜ indicates Measure of success is needed; ☆ indicates this standard also applies to organizations seeking Joint Commission's Medicare/Medicaid certification–based long term care accreditation

Standard EC.2.10

Assessment Question	Level of Compliance	Evidence of Compliance	Plan of Action/ Measure of Success (if needed)	Due Date
5. Does the organization identify, as appropriate, residents, staff, and other people entering the organization's facilities? **A (EP 5)**				
6. Does the organization control access to and egress from security-sensitive areas, as determined by the organization? **C (EP 6)** Ⓜ △3				
7. Does the organization identify and implement security procedures that address actions taken in the event of a security incident? **A (EP 7)**				
8. Does the organization identify and implement security procedures that address handling of situations involving VIPs or the media? **A (EP 9)**				

Standard EC.3.10 ★

Standard Score: ❑ Compliant ❑ Not Compliant

Assessment Question	Level of Compliance	Evidence of Compliance	Plan of Action/ Measure of Success (if needed)	Due Date
1. Does the organization develop and maintain a written management plan describing the processes it implements to effectively manage hazardous materials and waste? **A (EP 1)**				
2. Does the organization create and maintain an inventory that identifies hazardous materials and waste used, stored, or generated using criteria consistent with applicable law and regulation (for example, the Environmental Protection Agency, the Occupational Safety and Health Administration)? **A (EP 2)**				
3. Does the organization establish and implement processes for selecting, handling, storing, transporting, using, and disposing of hazardous materials and waste from receipt or generation through use and/or final disposal, including managing chemicals? **C (EP 3)** Ⓜ				

Key: 0 = Insufficient compliance; 1 = Partial compliance; 2 = Satisfactory compliance; NA = Not applicable; **A** indicates scoring category A; **C** indicates scoring category C; ▲2 indicates situational decision rules apply; △3 indicates direct impact requirements apply; Ⓜ indicates Measure of success is needed; ☆ indicates this standard also applies to organizations seeking Joint Commission's Medicare/Medicaid certification–based long term care accreditation

Standard EC.3.10 ★

Assessment Question	Level of Compliance	Evidence of Compliance	Plan of Action/ Measure of Success (if needed)	Due Date
4. Does the organization establish and implement processes for selecting, handling, storing, transporting, using, and disposing of hazardous materials and waste from receipt or generation through use and/or final disposal, including managing chemotherapeutic materials? **A (EP 4)** ⚠3				
5. Does the organization establish and implement processes for selecting, handling, storing, transporting, using, and disposing of hazardous materials and waste from receipt or generation through use and/or final disposal, including managing radioactive materials? **A (EP 5)** ⚠3				
6. Does the organization establish and implement processes for selecting, handling, storing, transporting, using, and disposing of hazardous materials and waste from receipt or generation through use and/or final disposal, including managing infectious and regulated medical waste, including sharps? **C (EP 6)** Ⓜ ⚠3				
7. Does the organization provide adequate and appropriate space and equipment for safely handling and storing hazardous materials and waste? **A (EP 7)**				
8. Does the organization identify and implement emergency procedures that include the specific precautions, procedures, and protective equipment used during hazardous materials and waste spills or exposures? **A (EP 9)** ⚠3				
9. Does the organization maintain documentation, including required permits, licenses, and adherence to other regulations? **A (EP 10)**				
10. Does the organization maintain required manifests for handling hazardous materials and waste? **C (EP 11)** Ⓜ				
11. Does the organization properly label hazardous materials and waste? **C (EP 12)** Ⓜ				

Key: 0 = Insufficient compliance; 1 = Partial compliance; 2 = Satisfactory compliance; NA = Not applicable; **A** indicates scoring category A; **C** indicates scoring category C; ▲ indicates situational decision rules apply; ⚠3 indicates direct impact requirements apply; Ⓜ indicates Measure of success is needed; ☆ indicates this standard also applies to organizations seeking Joint Commission's Medicare/Medicaid certification–based long term care accreditation

Standard EC.3.10 ★

Assessment Question	Level of Compliance	Evidence of Compliance	Plan of Action/ Measure of Success (if needed)	Due Date
12. Does the organization effectively separate hazardous materials and waste storage and processing areas from other areas of the facility? **A (EP 13)**				

Standard EC.4.11★

Standard Score: ❑ Compliant ❑ Not Compliant

Assessment Question	Level of Compliance	Evidence of Compliance	Plan of Action/ Measure of Success (if needed)	Due Date
1. Do the organization's leaders, including the administrator, the medical director, the nursing leader, and other clinical leaders, actively participate in emergency management planning? **A (EP 1)**				
2. Does the organization conduct a Hazard Vulnerability Analysis (HVA) to identify events that could affect demand for its services or its ability to provide those services, the likelihood of those events occurring, and the consequences of those events? **Note:** *The HVA is evaluated at least annually as part of EP 11.* **A (EP 2)**				
3. Does the organization prioritize those hazards, threats, and events identified in its HVA? **A (EP 3)**				
4. When developing its emergency operations plan (*see* Standard EC.4.12), does the organization communicate its needs and vulnerabilities to community emergency response agencies and identify the capabilities of its community in meeting their needs? **A (EP 4)**				
5. For each emergency identified in its HVA, does the organization define mitigation activities designed to reduce the risk of and potential damage due to an emergency? **A (EP 5)**				
6. For each emergency identified in its HVA, does the organization define preparedness activities that will organize and mobilize essential resources? **A (EP 6)**				

Key: 0 = Insufficient compliance; 1 = Partial compliance; 2 = Satisfactory compliance; NA = Not applicable; **A** indicates scoring category A; **C** indicates scoring category C; ▲(2) indicates situational decision rules apply; △(3) indicates direct impact requirements apply; Ⓜ indicates Measure of success is needed; ☆ indicates this standard also applies to organizations seeking Joint Commission's Medicare/Medicaid certification–based long term care accreditation

Standard EC.4.11★				
Assessment Question	**Level of Compliance**	**Evidence of Compliance**	**Plan of Action/ Measure of Success (if needed)**	**Due Date**
7. For each emergency identified in its HVA, does the organization define response strategies and actions to be activated during the emergency? **A (EP 7)**				
8. For each emergency identified in its HVA, does the organization define recovery strategies and actions designed to help restore the systems that are critical to resuming normal care, treatment, and services? **A (EP 8)**				
9. Does the organization keep a documented inventory of the assets and resources it has on site, that would be needed during an emergency (at a minimum, personal protective equipment, water, fuel, staffing, medical, and pharmaceuticals resources and assets)? **Note:** *The inventory is evaluated at least annually as part of EP 11.* **A (EP 9)**				
10. Does the organization establish methods for monitoring quantities of assets and resources during an emergency? **A (EP 10)**				
11. Are the objectives, scope, performance, and effectiveness of the organization's emergency management planning efforts evaluated at least annually? **A (EP 11)**				

Standard EC.4.12 ★	Standard Score: ❑ Compliant ❑ Not Compliant			
Assessment Question	**Level of Compliance**	**Evidence of Compliance**	**Plan of Action/ Measure of Success (if needed)**	**Due Date**
1. Does the organization develop and maintain a written emergency operations plan that describes an "all-hazards" command structure for coordinating six critical areas (*see* Standard EC.4.13 through Standard EC.4.18) within the organization during an emergency? **A (EP 1)**				
2. Does the organization's emergency operations plan establish an incident command structure? **A (EP 2)**				

Key: 0 = Insufficient compliance; 1 = Partial compliance; 2 = Satisfactory compliance; NA = Not applicable; **A** indicates scoring category A; **C** indicates scoring category C; ▲ indicates situational decision rules apply; △ indicates direct impact requirements apply; Ⓜ indicates Measure of success is needed; ☆ indicates this standard also applies to organizations seeking Joint Commission's Medicare/Medicaid certification–based long term care accreditation

Standard EC.4.12 ★	**Standard Score: ❑ Compliant ❑ Not Compliant**			
Assessment Question	**Level of Compliance**	**Evidence of Compliance**	**Plan of Action/ Measure of Success (if needed)**	**Due Date**
3. Does the organization's emergency operations plan identify to whom staff members report in the organization's incident command structure? **A (EP 3)**				
4. Does the organization's emergency operations plan describe processes for initiating and terminating the response and recovery phases, including who has the authority to activate the phases? **A (EP 4)**				
5. Does the organization's emergency operations plan describe processes for initiating and terminating the response and recovery phases, including how the phases are to be activated? **A (EP 5)**				
6. Does the organization's emergency operations plan identify the organization's capabilities and establish response efforts when the organization cannot be supported by the local community for at least 96 hours in the six critical areas? **Note:** *Acceptable response efforts could include the following:* • *Conservation of resources* • *Curtailment of services* • *Supplementing of resources from outside the local community* • *Staged evacuation* • *Total evacuation* **A (EP 6)**				
7. Does the organization's emergency operations plan identify alternative sites for care, treatment, or service that meet the needs of its residents during emergencies? **A (EP 7)**				

Standard EC.4.13 ★	**Standard Score: ❑ Compliant ❑ Not Compliant**			
Assessment Question	**Level of Compliance**	**Evidence of Compliance**	**Plan of Action/ Measure of Success (if needed)**	**Due Date**
1. Does the organization plan for notifying the staff when emergency response measures are initiated? **A (EP 1)**				

Key: 0 = Insufficient compliance; 1 = Partial compliance; 2 = Satisfactory compliance; NA = Not applicable; **A** indicates scoring category A; **C** indicates scoring category C; ▲(2) indicates situational decision rules apply; △(3) indicates direct impact requirements apply; Ⓜ indicates Measure of success is needed; ☆ indicates this standard also applies to organizations seeking Joint Commission's Medicare/Medicaid certification–based long term care accreditation

Standard EC.4.13 ★

Assessment Question	Level of Compliance	Evidence of Compliance	Plan of Action/ Measure of Success (if needed)	Due Date
2. Does the organization plan for ongoing communication of information and instructions to its staff once emergency response measures are initiated? **A (EP 2)**				
3. Does the organization define processes for notifying external authorities when emergency response measures are initiated? **A (EP 3)**				
4. Does the organization plan for communicating with external authorities once emergency response measures are initiated? **A (EP 4)**				
5. Does the organization plan for communicating with residents and their families during emergencies, including notification when residents are relocated to alternative care sites? **A (EP 5)**				
6. Does the organization define the circumstances and plan for communicating with the community and/or the media during emergencies? **A (EP 6)**				
7. Does the organization plan for communicating with purveyors of essential supplies, services, and equipment once emergency measures are initiated? **A (EP 7)**				
8. Does the organization plan for communicating in a timely manner with other health care organizations that together provide services to a contiguous geographic area (for example, among health care organizations serving a town or borough) regarding essential elements of their command structures and control centers for emergency response? **A (EP 8)**				
9. Does the organization plan for communicating in a timely manner with other health care organizations that together provide services to a contiguous geographic area (for example, among health care organizations serving a town or borough) regarding names and roles of individuals in their command structures and command center telephone numbers? **A (EP 9)**				

Key: 0 = Insufficient compliance; 1 = Partial compliance; 2 = Satisfactory compliance; NA = Not applicable; **A** indicates scoring category A; **C** indicates scoring category C; ▲ indicates situational decision rules apply; △ indicates direct impact requirements apply; Ⓜ indicates Measure of success is needed; ☆ indicates this standard also applies to organizations seeking Joint Commission's Medicare/Medicaid certification–based long term care accreditation

Standard EC.4.13 ★

Assessment Question	Level of Compliance	Evidence of Compliance	Plan of Action/ Measure of Success (if needed)	Due Date
10. Does the organization plan for communicating in a timely manner with other health care organizations that together provide services to a contiguous geographic area (for example, among health care organizations serving a town or borough) regarding resources and assets that potentially could be shared in an emergency response? **A (EP 10)**				
11. Does the organization plan for communicating in a timely manner with other health care organizations that together provide services to a contiguous geographic area (for example, among health care organizations serving a town or borough) regarding names of residents and deceased individuals brought to their organizations in accordance with applicable law and regulation, when requested? **A (EP 11)**				
12. Does the organization define the circumstances and plans for communicating information about residents to third parties (such as other health care organizations, the state health department, police, FBI, and so on)? **A (EP 12)**				
13. Does the organization plan for communicating with identified alternative care sites? **A (EP 13)**				
14. Does the organization establish backup communication systems and technologies for the activities identified above? **A (EP 14)**				

Key: 0 = Insufficient compliance; 1 = Partial compliance; 2 = Satisfactory compliance; NA = Not applicable; **A** indicates scoring category A; **C** indicates scoring category C; ▲ indicates situational decision rules apply; △ indicates direct impact requirements apply; Ⓜ indicates Measure of success is needed; ☆ indicates this standard also applies to organizations seeking Joint Commission's Medicare/Medicaid certification–based long term care accreditation

Standard EC.4.14 ★	Standard Score: ❑ Compliant ❑ Not Compliant			
Assessment Question	**Level of Compliance**	**Evidence of Compliance**	**Plan of Action/ Measure of Success (if needed)**	**Due Date**
1. Does the organization plan for obtaining supplies that will be required at the onset of emergency response (medical, pharmaceutical, and non-medical)? **A (EP 1)**				
2. Does the organization plan for replenishing medical supplies and equipment that will be required throughout response and recovery, including personal protective equipment where required? **A (EP 2)**				
3. Does the organization plan for replenishing pharmaceutical supplies that will be required throughout response and recovery, including access to and distribution of caches (stockpiled by the organization, its affiliates, or local, state, or federal sources) to which the organization has access? **A (EP 3)**				
4. Does the organization plan for replenishing nonmedical supplies that will be required throughout response and recovery (for example, food, linen, water, fuel for generators and transportation vehicles, and so on)? **A (EP 4)**				
5. Does the organization plan for managing staff support activities (for example, housing, transportation, incident stress debriefing, and so on)? **A (EP 5)**				
6. Does the organization plan for managing staff family support needs (for example, child care, elder care, communication, and so on)? **A (EP 6)**				
7. Does the organization plan for potential sharing of resources and assets (e.g., personnel, beds, transportation, linens, fuel, PPE, medical equipment and supplies, and so on) with other health care organizations within the community that could potentially be shared in an emergency response? **A (EP 7)**				

Key: 0 = Insufficient compliance; 1 = Partial compliance; 2 = Satisfactory compliance; NA = Not applicable; **A** indicates scoring category A; **C** indicates scoring category C; ▲ indicates situational decision rules apply; △ indicates direct impact requirements apply; Ⓜ indicates Measure of success is needed; ☆ indicates this standard also applies to organizations seeking Joint Commission's Medicare/Medicaid certification–based long term care accreditation

Standard EC.4.14 ★

Assessment Question	Level of Compliance	Evidence of Compliance	Plan of Action/ Measure of Success (if needed)	Due Date
8. Does the organization plan for potential sharing of resources and assets with health care organizations outside of the community in the event of a regional or prolonged disaster? **A (EP 8)**				
9. Does the organization plan for evacuating (both horizontally and, when required by circumstances, vertically) when the environment cannot support care, treatment, and services? **A (EP 9)**				
10. Does the organization plan for transporting residents, their medications and equipment, and staff to an alternative care site or sites when the environment cannot support care, treatment, and services? **A (EP 10)**				
11. Does the organization plan for transporting pertinent information, including essential clinical and medication-related information, for residents to an alternative care site or sites when the environment cannot support care, treatment, and services? **A (EP 11)**				

Standard EC.4.15 ★

Standard Score: ❑ Compliant ❑ Not Compliant

Assessment Question	Level of Compliance	Evidence of Compliance	Plan of Action/ Measure of Success (if needed)	Due Date
1. Does the organization establish internal security and safety operations that will be required once emergency measures are initiated? **A (EP 1)**				
2. Does the organization identify the roles of community security agencies (police, sheriff, national guard, etc.) and define how the organization will coordinate security activities with these agencies? **A (EP 2)**				
3. Does the organization identify a process that will be required for managing hazardous materials and waste once emergency measures are initiated? **A (EP 3)**				

Key: 0 = Insufficient compliance; 1 = Partial compliance; 2 = Satisfactory compliance; NA = Not applicable; **A** indicates scoring category A; **C** indicates scoring category C; ▲(2) indicates situational decision rules apply; △(3) indicates direct impact requirements apply; Ⓜ indicates Measure of success is needed; ☆ indicates this standard also applies to organizations seeking Joint Commission's Medicare/Medicaid certification–based long term care accreditation

Standard EC.4.15 ★

Assessment Question	Level of Compliance	Evidence of Compliance	Plan of Action/ Measure of Success (if needed)	Due Date
4. Does the organization identify residents who might be susceptible to wandering once emergency measures are initiated? **A (EP 5)** △3				
5. Does the organization establish processes for controlling entrance into and out of the health care facility during emergencies? **A (EP 6)**				
6. Does the organization establish processes for controlling the movement of individuals within the health care facility during emergencies? **A (EP 7)**				
7. Does the organization establish processes for controlling traffic accessing the health care facility during emergencies? **A (EP 8)**				

Standard EC.4.16 ★

Standard Score: ❑ Compliant ❑ Not Compliant

Assessment Question	Level of Compliance	Evidence of Compliance	Plan of Action/ Measure of Success (if needed)	Due Date
1. Does the organization's emergency operations plan define staff roles and responsibilities for all critical areas (communications, resources and assets, safety and security, utilities, and clinical activities)? **A (EP 1)**				
2. Are the organization's staff members trained for their assigned roles during emergencies? **A (EP 2)**				
3. Does the organization communicate to licensed independent practitioners their roles in emergency response and to whom they report during an emergency? **A (EP 3)**				
4. Does the organization establish a process for identifying care providers and other personnel (such as identification cards, wrist bands, vests, hats, badges, computer printouts, etc.) assigned to particular areas during emergencies? **A (EP 4)**				

Key: 0 = Insufficient compliance; 1 = Partial compliance; 2 = Satisfactory compliance; NA = Not applicable; **A** indicates scoring category A; **C** indicates scoring category C; ▲2 indicates situational decision rules apply; △3 indicates direct impact requirements apply; Ⓜ indicates Measure of success is needed; ☆ indicates this standard also applies to organizations seeking Joint Commission's Medicare/Medicaid certification–based long term care accreditation

Standard EC.4.17 ★

Standard Score: ❑ Compliant ❑ Not Compliant

Assessment Question	Level of Compliance	Evidence of Compliance	Plan of Action/ Measure of Success (if needed)	Due Date
1. Does the organization identify an alternative means of providing electricity in the event that its supply is compromised or disrupted? **A (EP 1)**				
2. Does the organization identify an alternative means of providing water for consumption and essential care activities in the event that its supply is compromised or disrupted? **A (EP 2)**				
3. Does the organization identify an alternative means of providing water needed for equipment and sanitary purposes in the event that its supply is compromised or disrupted? **A (EP 3)**				
4. Does the organization identify an alternative means of providing fuel required for building operations or essential transport activities in the event that its supply is compromised or disrupted? **A (EP 4)**				
5. Does the organization identify an alternative means of providing other essential utility needs (for example, ventilation, etc.) in the event that its supply is compromised or disrupted? **A (EP 5)**				

Standard EC.4.18 ★

Standard Score: ❑ Compliant ❑ Not Compliant

Assessment Question	Level of Compliance	Evidence of Compliance	Plan of Action/ Measure of Success (if needed)	Due Date
1. During an emergency, does the organization plan to manage the clinical activities required as part of resident scheduling, triage, assessment, treatment, admission, transfer, discharge, and evacuation? **A (EP 1)**				
2. During an emergency, does the organization plan to manage clinical services for vulnerable populations served by the organization, including residents who are pediatric, geriatric, disabled, or have serious chronic conditions or addictions? **A (EP 2)**				

Key: 0 = Insufficient compliance; 1 = Partial compliance; 2 = Satisfactory compliance; NA = Not applicable; **A** indicates scoring category A; **C** indicates scoring category C; ▲2 indicates situational decision rules apply; △3 indicates direct impact requirements apply; Ⓜ indicates Measure of success is needed; ☆ indicates this standard also applies to organizations seeking Joint Commission's Medicare/Medicaid certification–based long term care accreditation

Standard EC.4.18 ★

Assessment Question	Level of Compliance	Evidence of Compliance	Plan of Action/ Measure of Success (if needed)	Due Date
3. Does the organization plan to manage personal hygiene and sanitation needs of its residents during emergencies? **A (EP 3)**				
4. Does the organization plan to manage the mental health service needs of its residents during emergencies? **A (EP 4)**				
5. Does the organization plan to manage mortuary services during emergencies? **A (EP 5)**				
6. Does the organization plan for documenting and tracking residents' clinical information? **A (EP 6)**				

Standard EC.4.20

Standard Score: ❑ Compliant ❑ Not Compliant

Assessment Question	Level of Compliance	Evidence of Compliance	Plan of Action/ Measure of Success (if needed)	Due Date
1. Does the organization test its Emergency Operations Plan twice a year, either in response to an actual emergency or in a planned exercise?* **A (EP 1)**				
2. Do organizations that offer emergency services or are community-designated disaster receiving stations conduct at least one exercise a year that includes an influx of actual or simulated residents? **A (EP 2)**				
3. Does the organization perform at least one exercise a year to evaluate how effectively it performs when it cannot be supported by the local community?† **A (EP 3)**				

* Tabletop sessions, though useful, are not acceptable substitutes for exercises.

† **Note:** *Tabletop sessions are acceptable in meeting the community portion of this exercise.*

Key: 0 = Insufficient compliance; 1 = Partial compliance; 2 = Satisfactory compliance; NA = Not applicable; **A** indicates scoring category A; **C** indicates scoring category C; ▲(2) indicates situational decision rules apply; △(3) indicates direct impact requirements apply; Ⓜ indicates Measure of success is needed; ☆ indicates this standard also applies to organizations seeking Joint Commission's Medicare/Medicaid certification–based long term care accreditation

Standard EC.4.20

Assessment Question	Level of Compliance	Evidence of Compliance	Plan of Action/ Measure of Success (if needed)	Due Date
4. Do organizations that have a defined role in the communitywide* emergency management program participate in at least one communitywide exercise a year?† **A (EP 4)**				
5. Are planned exercise scenarios realistic and related to the priority emergencies identified in the organization's hazard vulnerability analysis? **A (EP 6)**				
6. During planned exercises, does an individual whose sole responsibility is to monitor performance and who is knowledgeable in the goals and expectations of the exercise, document opportunities for improvement?‡ **A (EP 8)**				
7. During planned exercises, does the organization monitor, at a minimum, communication including the effectiveness of communication both within the organization as well as with response entities outside of the organization such as local governmental leadership, police, fire, public health, and other health care organizations within the community? **A (EP 9)**				
8. During planned exercises, does the organization monitor, at a minimum, resource mobilization and allocation including responders, equipment, supplies, personal protective equipment, transportation, and security? **A (EP 10)**				
9. During planned exercises, does the organization monitor, at a minimum, safety and security? **A (EP 11)**				
10. During planned exercises, does the organization monitor, at a minimum, staff roles and responsibilities? **A (EP 12)**				

* "Communitywide" may range from a contiguous geographic area served by the same health care providers, to a large borough, town, city, or region. Tabletop sessions are acceptable in meeting the community portion of this exercise.

† Exercises for EPs 2, 3, and 4 may be conducted separately or simultaneously.

‡ This individual may be a staff member of the organization who is not participating in the exercise.

Key: 0 = Insufficient compliance; 1 = Partial compliance; 2 = Satisfactory compliance; NA = Not applicable; **A** indicates scoring category A; **C** indicates scoring category C; ▲(2) indicates situational decision rules apply; △(3) indicates direct impact requirements apply; Ⓜ indicates Measure of success is needed; ☆ indicates this standard also applies to organizations seeking Joint Commission's Medicare/Medicaid certification–based long term care accreditation

Standard EC.4.20

Assessment Question	Level of Compliance	Evidence of Compliance	Plan of Action/ Measure of Success (if needed)	Due Date
11. During planned exercises, does the organization monitor, at a minimum, utility systems? **A (EP 13)**				
12. During planned exercises, does the organization monitor, at a minimum, resident clinical and support care activities? **A (EP 14)**				
13. Are all exercises critiqued to identify deficiencies and opportunities for improvement based on all monitoring activities and observations during the exercise? **A (EP 15)**				
14. Are completed exercises critiqued through a multidisciplinary process that includes administration, clinical, and support staff? **A (EP 16)**				
15. Does the organization modify its emergency management plan in response to critiques of exercise? **A (EP 17)**				
16. Do planned exercises evaluate the effectiveness of improvements that were made in response to critiques of the previous exercise?* **A (EP 18)**				
17. Are the strengths and weaknesses identified during exercises communicated to the multidisciplinary improvement team responsible for monitoring environment of care issues? (*See* Standard EC.9.20) **A (EP 19)**				

* When improvements require substantive resources that cannot be accomplished by the next planned exercise, interim improvements must be put in place until final resolution.

Key: 0 = Insufficient compliance; 1 = Partial compliance; 2 = Satisfactory compliance; NA = Not applicable; **A** indicates scoring category A; **C** indicates scoring category C; ▲2 indicates situational decision rules apply; △3 indicates direct impact requirements apply; Ⓜ indicates Measure of success is needed; ☆ indicates this standard also applies to organizations seeking Joint Commission's Medicare/Medicaid certification–based long term care accreditation

Standard EC.5.10	**Standard Score:** ❑ Compliant ❑ Not Compliant			
Assessment Question	**Level of Compliance**	**Evidence of Compliance**	**Plan of Action/ Measure of Success (if needed)**	**Due Date**
1. Does the organization develop and maintain a written management plan describing the processes it implements to effectively manage fire safety? **A (EP 1)**				
2. Does the organization identify proactive processes for protecting residents, staff, and others coming to the organization's facilities, as well as protecting property from fire, smoke, and other products of combustion? **A (EP 2)**				
3. Does the organization identify processes for regularly inspecting, testing, and maintaining fire protection and fire safety systems, equipment, and components? **A (EP 3)**				
4. Does the organization develop and implement a fire response plan that addresses the following: • Facilitywide fire response • Area-specific needs including fire-evacuation routes • Specific roles and responsibilities of staff, licensed independent practitioners, and volunteers away **at** a fire's point of origin • Specific roles and responsibilities of staff, licensed independent practitioners, and volunteers **away from** a fire's point of origin • Specific roles and responsibilities of staff, licensed independent practitioners, and volunteers in preparing for building evacuation? **A (EP 4)** △3				
5. Does the organization review proposed acquisitions of bedding, window draperies, and other curtains, furnishings, decorations, and other equipment for fire safety? **A (EP 5)**				

Key: 0 = Insufficient compliance; 1 = Partial compliance; 2 = Satisfactory compliance; NA = Not applicable; **A** indicates scoring category A; **C** indicates scoring category C; ▲2 indicates situational decision rules apply; △3 indicates direct impact requirements apply; Ⓜ indicates Measure of success is needed; ☆ indicates this standard also applies to organizations seeking Joint Commission's Medicare/Medicaid certification–based long term care accreditation

Standard EC.5.30	Standard Score: ❑ Compliant ❑ Not Compliant			
Assessment Question	**Level of Compliance**	**Evidence of Compliance**	**Plan of Action/ Measure of Success (if needed)**	**Due Date**
1. Are fire drills conducted quarterly on all shifts in each building defined by the *Life Safety Code* as health care occupancy? **C (EP 1) Ⓜ**				
2. Are at least 50% of the fire drills unannounced? **C (EP 4) Ⓜ**				
3. Are staff in all areas of the building where residents are housed or treated participating in drills to the extent called for in the facility's fire plan?* **A (EP 5)**				
4. Are all fire drills critiqued to identify deficiencies and opportunities for improvement? **A (EP 6)**				
5. Is the effectiveness of the fire response training according to the fire plan evaluated at least annually? **A (EP 7)**				
6. During fire drills, is staff knowledge evaluated for the following? • When and how to sound fire alarms (where such alarms are available) • When and how to transmit for off-site fire responders • Containment of smoke and fire • Transfer of residents to areas of refuge • Fire extinguishment • Specific fire response duties • Preparation for building evacuation? **A (EP 8)**				

* When drills are conducted between 9:00 P.M. and 6:00 A.M., a coded announcement will be permitted to be used instead of audible alarms.

Key: 0 = Insufficient compliance; 1 = Partial compliance; 2 = Satisfactory compliance; NA = Not applicable; **A** indicates scoring category A; **C** indicates scoring category C; ▲ indicates situational decision rules apply; △ indicates direct impact requirements apply; Ⓜ indicates Measure of success is needed; ☆ indicates this standard also applies to organizations seeking Joint Commission's Medicare/Medicaid certification–based long term care accreditation

Standard EC.5.40	**Standard Score:** ❑ Compliant ❑ Not Compliant			
Assessment Question	**Level of Compliance**	**Evidence of Compliance**	**Plan of Action/ Measure of Success (if needed)**	**Due Date**
1. Are initiating devices and fire detection and alarm equipment tested as follows:* • All supervisory signal devices (except valve tamper switches) are tested at least quarterly • All valve tamper switches and water flow devices are tested at least semiannually • All duct detectors, electromechanical releasing devices, heat detectors, manual fire alarm boxes, and smoke detectors are tested at least annually? **C (EP 1)** Ⓜ ⚠3				
2. Are occupant alarm notification devices, including all audible devices, speakers, and visible devices tested at least annually? **C (EP 2)** Ⓜ ⚠3				
3. Is off-premises emergency services notification transmission equipment tested at least quarterly? **A (EP 3)** ⚠3				
4. For water-based automatic fire-extinguishing systems are all fire pumps tested at least weekly under no-flow conditions? **C (EP 4)** Ⓜ ⚠3				
5. For water-based automatic fire-extinguishing systems are all water-storage tank high- and low-water level alarms tested at least semiannually? **C (EP 5)** Ⓜ ⚠3				
6. For water-based automatic fire-extinguishing systems are all water storage tank low-water temperature alarms (during cold weather only) tested at least monthly? **C (EP 6)** Ⓜ ⚠3				
7. For water-based automatic fire-extinguishing systems are main drain tests conducted at least annually at all system risers? **C (EP 7)** Ⓜ ⚠3				
8. For water-based automatic fire-extinguishing systems, are all fire department connections inspected quarterly? **C (EP 8)** Ⓜ ⚠3				

* When drills are conducted between 9:00 P.M. and 6:00 A.M., a coded announcement will be permitted to be used instead of audible alarms.

Key: 0 = Insufficient compliance; 1 = Partial compliance; 2 = Satisfactory compliance; NA = Not applicable; **A** indicates scoring category A; **C** indicates scoring category C; ▲2 indicates situational decision rules apply; ⚠3 indicates direct impact requirements apply; Ⓜ indicates Measure of success is needed; ☆ indicates this standard also applies to organizations seeking Joint Commission's Medicare/Medicaid certification–based long term care accreditation

Standard EC.5.40

Assessment Question	Level of Compliance	Evidence of Compliance	Plan of Action/ Measure of Success (if needed)	Due Date
9. For water-based automatic fire extinguishing systems, are all fire pumps tested at least annually under flow? **A (EP 9)** △3				
10. Are kitchen automatic fire-extinguishing systems inspected for proper operation at least semiannually (actual discharge of the fire-extinguishing system is not required)? **A (EP 10)** △3				
11. Are carbon dioxide and other gaseous automatic fire-extinguishing systems tested for proper operation at least annually (actual discharge of the fire-extinguishing system is not required)? **C (EP 11)** Ⓜ △3				
12. Are all portable fire extinguishers clearly identified, inspected at least monthly, and maintained at least annually? **C (EP 12)** Ⓜ △3				
13. Are standpipe occupant hoses hydrostatically tested five years after installation and at least every three years thereafter, and do systems receive water-flow tests at least every five years? **C (EP 13)** Ⓜ				
14. Are all fire and smoke dampers operated one year after installation and then at least every four years to verify that they fully close? **Note:** *The initial test that must occur one year after installation applies only to dampers installed on and after January 1, 2008.* **C (EP 14)** Ⓜ				
15. Are automatic smoke-detection shutdown devices for air-handling equipment tested at least annually? **A (EP 15)** △3				
16. Are horizontal and vertical sliding and rolling fire doors tested for proper operation and full closure at least annually? **C (EP 16)** Ⓜ △3				

Key: 0 = Insufficient compliance; 1 = Partial compliance; 2 = Satisfactory compliance; NA = Not applicable; **A** indicates scoring category A; **C** indicates scoring category C; ▲2 indicates situational decision rules apply; △3 indicates direct impact requirements apply; Ⓜ indicates Measure of success is needed; ☆ indicates this standard also applies to organizations seeking Joint Commission's Medicare/Medicaid certification–based long term care accreditation

Standard EC.6.10 ★	**Standard Score:** ❑ Compliant ❑ Not Compliant			
Assessment Question	**Level of Compliance**	**Evidence of Compliance**	**Plan of Action/ Measure of Success (if needed)**	**Due Date**
1. Does the organization develop and maintain a written management plan describing the processes it implements to manage the effective, safe, and reliable operation of medical equipment? **A (EP 1)**				
2. Does the organization identify and implement a process(es) for selecting and acquiring medical equipment?* **A (EP 2)**				
3. Does the organization establish and use risk criteria† for identifying, evaluating, and creating an inventory of equipment to be included in the medical management plan before the equipment is used, and do these criteria address the following: • Equipment function (diagnosis, care, treatment, life support, and monitoring) • Physical risks associated with use • Equipment incident history? **A (EP 3)**				
4. Does the organization identify appropriate inspection and maintenance strategies for all equipment on the inventory for achieving effective, safe, and reliable operation of all equipment in the inventory?‡ **A (EP 4)**				
5. Does the organization define intervals for inspecting, testing, and maintaining appropriate equipment on the inventory (that is, those pieces of equipment on the inventory benefiting from scheduled activities to minimize the clinical and physical risks) that are based upon criteria such as manufacturers' recommendations, risk levels, and current organization experience? **A (EP 5)**				
6. Does the organization identify and implement processes for monitoring and acting on equipment hazard notices and recalls? **A (EP 6)**				

* The acquisition process includes initially evaluating the condition and function of the equipment when received and evaluating the training of users before use on residents.

† The organization may choose not to use risk criteria to limit the types of equipment to be included in the medical equipment management plan, but rather include all medical equipment.

‡ Organizations may use different strategies for different items as appropriate. For example, strategies such as predictive maintenance, interval-based inspections, corrective maintenance, or metered maintenance may be selected to ensure reliable performance.

Key: 0 = Insufficient compliance; 1 = Partial compliance; 2 = Satisfactory compliance; NA = Not applicable; **A** indicates scoring category A; **C** indicates scoring category C; ▲(2) indicates situational decision rules apply; △(3) indicates direct impact requirements apply; Ⓜ indicates Measure of success is needed; ☆ indicates this standard also applies to organizations seeking Joint Commission's Medicare/Medicaid certification–based long term care accreditation

Standard EC.6.10 ★				
Assessment Question	**Level of Compliance**	**Evidence of Compliance**	**Plan of Action/ Measure of Success (if needed)**	**Due Date**
7. Does the organization identify and implement processes for monitoring and reporting incidents in which a medical device is suspected or attributed to the death, serious injury, or serious illness of any individual, as required by the Safe Medical Devices Act of 1990? **A (EP 7)**				
8. Does the organization identify and implement processes for emergency procedures that address the following: • What to do in the event of equipment disruption or failure • When and how to perform emergency clinical interventions when medical equipment fails • Availability of back-up equipment • How to obtain repair services? **A (EP 8)**				

Standard EC.6.20 ★	Standard Score: ❑ Compliant ❑ Not Compliant			
Assessment Question	**Level of Compliance**	**Evidence of Compliance**	**Plan of Action/ Measure of Success (if needed)**	**Due Date**
1. Does the organization document a current, accurate, and separate inventory of all equipment identified in the medical equipment management plan, regardless of ownership? **C (EP 1) Ⓜ**				
2. Does the organization document performance and safety testing of all equipment identified in the medical management program before initial use? **A (EP 2)**				
3. Does the organization document inspection and maintenance of equipment used for life support* that is consistent with maintenance strategies to minimize clinical and physical risks identified in the equipment management plan? **A (EP 3)** △3				

* **Life support equipment** Those devices intended to sustain life and whose failure to perform its primary function, when used according to manufacturer's instructions and clinical protocol, is expected to result in imminent death in the absence of immediate intervention (examples include ventilators, anesthesia machines, and heart-lung bypass machines).

Key: 0 = Insufficient compliance; 1 = Partial compliance; 2 = Satisfactory compliance; NA = Not applicable; **A** indicates scoring category A; **C** indicates scoring category C; ▲2 indicates situational decision rules apply; △3 indicates direct impact requirements apply; Ⓜ indicates Measure of success is needed; ☆ indicates this standard also applies to organizations seeking Joint Commission's Medicare/Medicaid certification–based long term care accreditation

Standard EC.6.20 ★

Assessment Question	Level of Compliance	Evidence of Compliance	Plan of Action/ Measure of Success (if needed)	Due Date
4. Does the organization document inspection and maintenance of non–life support equipment on the inventory that is consistent with maintenance strategies to minimize clinical and physical risks identified in the equipment management plan? **C (EP 4) Ⓜ**				
5. Does the organization document chemical and biological testing of water used in renal dialysis and other applicable tests based on regulations, manufacturers' recommendations, and organization experience? **A (EP 6) Ⓜ ⚠3**				

Standard EC.7.10 ★

Standard Score: ❑ Compliant ❑ Not Compliant

Assessment Question	Level of Compliance	Evidence of Compliance	Plan of Action/ Measure of Success (if needed)	Due Date
1. Does the organization develop and maintain a written management plan describing the processes it implements to manage the effective, safe, and reliable operation of utility systems? **A (EP 7)**				
2. Does the organization design and install utility systems that meet the resident care and operational needs of the services in the organization's buildings? **A (EP 8)**				
3. Does the organization establish risk criteria* for identifying, evaluating, and creating an inventory of operating components of systems before the equipment is used and do the criteria address the following: • Life support • Infection control • Support of the environment • Equipment support • Communication? **A (EP 9)**				

* The organization may choose not to use risk criteria to limit the types of utility systems to be included in the utility management plan, but rather include all utility systems.

Key: 0 = Insufficient compliance; 1 = Partial compliance; 2 = Satisfactory compliance; NA = Not applicable; **A** indicates scoring category A; **C** indicates scoring category C; ▲2 indicates situational decision rules apply; ⚠3 indicates direct impact requirements apply; Ⓜ indicates Measure of success is needed; ☆ indicates this standard also applies to organizations seeking Joint Commission's Medicare/Medicaid certification–based long term care accreditation

Standard EC.7.10 ★

Assessment Question	Level of Compliance	Evidence of Compliance	Plan of Action/ Measure of Success (if needed)	Due Date
4. Does the organization develop appropriate strategies for all utility systems equipment on the inventory for ensuring effective, safe, and reliable operation of all equipment in the inventory?* **A (EP 10)**				
5. Does the organization define intervals for inspecting, testing, and maintaining appropriate utility systems equipment on the inventory (that is, those pieces of equipment on the inventory benefiting from scheduled activities to minimize the clinical and physical risks) that are based on criteria such as manufacturers' recommendations, risk levels, or current organization experience? **A (EP 11)**				
6. Does the organization identify and implement emergency procedures for responding to utility system disruptions or failures that address the following: • What to do if utility systems malfunction • Identification of an alternative source of organization-defined essential utilities • Shutting off of the malfunctioning system and notifying staff in affected areas • How and when to perform emergency clinical interventions when utility systems fail • Obtaining repair services? **A (EP 12)** ⚠3				
7. Does the organization map the distribution of utility systems? **A (EP 13)** ⚠3				
8. Does the organization label controls for a partial or complete emergency shutdown? **C (EP 14)** Ⓜ ⚠3				
9. Does the organization identify and implement processes to minimize pathogenic biologic agents in cooling towers, domestic hot/cold water systems, and other aerosolizing water systems? **A (EP 15)** ⚠3				

* Organizations may use different strategies as appropriate. For example, strategies such as predictive maintenance, interval-based inspections, corrective maintenance, or metered maintenance may be selected to ensure reliable performance.

Key: 0 = Insufficient compliance; 1 = Partial compliance; 2 = Satisfactory compliance; NA = Not applicable; **A** indicates scoring category A; **C** indicates scoring category C; ▲2 indicates situational decision rules apply; ⚠3 indicates direct impact requirements apply; Ⓜ indicates Measure of success is needed; ☆ indicates this standard also applies to organizations seeking Joint Commission's Medicare/Medicaid certification–based long term care accreditation

Standard EC.7.10 ★

Assessment Question	Level of Compliance	Evidence of Compliance	Plan of Action/ Measure of Success (if needed)	Due Date
10. Does the organization design, install, and maintain ventilation equipment to provide appropriate pressure relationships, air-exchange rates, and filtration efficiencies for ventilation systems serving areas specially designed* to control air-borne contaminants (such as biological agents, gases, fumes, and dust)? **A (EP 16)** △3				

Standard EC.7.20

Standard Score: ❑ Compliant ❑ Not Compliant

Assessment Question	Level of Compliance	Evidence of Compliance	Plan of Action/ Measure of Success (if needed)	Due Date
1. Does the organization provide a reliable emergency power system, as required by the *Life Safety Code* occupancy requirements, that supplies electricity to alarm systems when normal electricity is interrupted? **A (EP 1)** △3				
2. Does the organization provide a reliable emergency power system, as required by the *Life Safety Code* occupancy requirements, that supplies electricity to exit-route illumination when normal electricity is interrupted? **C (EP 2)** Ⓜ △3				
3. Does the organization provide a reliable emergency power system, as required by the *Life Safety Code* occupancy requirements, that supplies electricity to emergency communication systems when normal electricity is interrupted? **A (EP 3)** △3				
4. Does the organization provide a reliable emergency power system, as required by the *Life Safety Code* occupancy requirements, that supplies illumination of exit signs when normal electricity is interrupted? **C (EP 4)** Ⓜ				
5. Does the organization provide a reliable emergency power system, as required by the services provided and residents served, that supplies electricity to elevators (at least one for nonambulatory clients) when normal electricity is interrupted? **A (EP 8)**				

* **Areas specially designed** include spaces such as rooms for residents diagnosed or suspected of having airborne communicable diseases (for example, pulmonary or laryngeal tuberculosis), residents in "protective isolation" rooms (for example, those receiving bone marrow transplants), laboratories, pharmacies, and sterile supply rooms.

Key: 0 = Insufficient compliance; 1 = Partial compliance; 2 = Satisfactory compliance; NA = Not applicable; **A** indicates scoring category A; **C** indicates scoring category C; ▲2 indicates situational decision rules apply; △3 indicates direct impact requirements apply; Ⓜ indicates Measure of success is needed; ☆ indicates this standard also applies to organizations seeking Joint Commission's Medicare/Medicaid certification–based long term care accreditation

Standard EC.7.20

Assessment Question	Level of Compliance	Evidence of Compliance	Plan of Action/ Measure of Success (if needed)	Due Date
6. Does the organization provide a reliable emergency power system, as required by the services provided and residents served, that supplies electricity to medical air compressors when normal electricity is interrupted? **A (EP 9)** ⚠3				
7. Does the organization provide a reliable emergency power system, as required by the services provided and residents served, that supplies electricity to medical and surgical vacuum systems when normal electricity is interrupted? **A (EP 10)** ⚠3				
8. Does the organization provide a reliable emergency power system, as required by the services provided and residents served, that supplies electricity to areas where electrically powered life-support equipment is used when normal electricity is interrupted? **A (EP 11)** ⚠3				

Standard EC.7.30 ★

Standard Score: ❑ Compliant ❑ Not Compliant

Assessment Question	Level of Compliance	Evidence of Compliance	Plan of Action/ Measure of Success (if needed)	Due Date
1. Does the organization maintain documentation of a current, accurate, and separate inventory of utility components identified in the utility management plan? **C (EP 1)** Ⓜ				
2. Does the organization maintain documentation of performance and safety testing of each critical component identified in the plan before initial use? **A (EP 2)**				
3. Does the organization maintain documentation of maintenance of critical components of life support utility systems/equipment consistent with maintenance strategies identified in the utility management plan? **A (EP 3)**				

Key: 0 = Insufficient compliance; 1 = Partial compliance; 2 = Satisfactory compliance; NA = Not applicable; **A** indicates scoring category A; **C** indicates scoring category C; ▲2 indicates situational decision rules apply; ⚠3 indicates direct impact requirements apply; Ⓜ indicates Measure of success is needed; ☆ indicates this standard also applies to organizations seeking Joint Commission's Medicare/Medicaid certification–based long term care accreditation

Standard EC.7.30 ★

Assessment Question	Level of Compliance	Evidence of Compliance	Plan of Action/ Measure of Success (if needed)	Due Date
4. Does the organization maintain documentation of maintenance of critical components of infection control utility systems/equipment for high-risk residents consistent with maintenance strategies identified in the utility management plan? (*See* Standard EC.7.10) **A (EP 4)**				
5. Does the organization maintain documentation of maintenance of critical components of non–life support utility systems/equipment on the inventory consistent with maintenance strategies identified in the utility management plan? (*See* Standard EC.7.10) **C (EP 5) Ⓜ**				

Standard EC.7.40*

Standard Score: ❑ Compliant ❑ Not Compliant

Assessment Question	Level of Compliance	Evidence of Compliance	Plan of Action/ Measure of Success (if needed)	Due Date
1. Does the organization test each generator 12 times a year with testing intervals not less than 20 days and not more than 40 days apart, and are the tests conducted for at least 30 continuous minutes under a dynamic load that is at least 30% of the nameplate rating of the generator? **C (EP 1) Ⓜ ⚠3**				
2. Does the organization test all automatic transfer switches 12 times a year with testing intervals not less than 20 days and not more than 40 days apart? **C (EP 2) Ⓜ ⚠3**				
3. Does the organization test all battery-powered lights required for egress and include the following: • Functional test at 30-day intervals for a minimum of 30 seconds • Annual test of a duration of 1.5 hours? **C (EP 3) Ⓜ**				

* **Note:** *This standard does not require organizations to have the types of emergency power systems discussed in the EPs. However, if an organization has these types of systems, then the following maintenance, testing, and inspection requirements apply.*

Key: 0 = Insufficient compliance; 1 = Partial compliance; 2 = Satisfactory compliance; NA = Not applicable; **A** indicates scoring category A; **C** indicates scoring category C; ▲2 indicates situational decision rules apply; ⚠3 indicates direct impact requirements apply; Ⓜ indicates Measure of success is needed; ☆ indicates this standard also applies to organizations seeking Joint Commission's Medicare/Medicaid certification–based long term care accreditation

Standard EC.7.40

Assessment Question	Level of Compliance	Evidence of Compliance	Plan of Action/ Measure of Success (if needed)	Due Date
4. Does the organization test Stored Emergency Power Supply Systems (SEPSS) whose malfunction may severely jeopardize the residents' life and safety* and include the following: • Quarterly functional test for 5 minutes or as specified for its class,† whichever is less • Annual test at full load for 60% of the full duration of its class? **C (EP 4)** Ⓜ ⚠3				
5. For facilities that have a generator providing emergency power for the services listed in EPs 8–11 of Standard EC.7.20: Does the organization test each emergency generator at least once every 36 months for a minimum of four continuous hours? And is this test conducted under a load (dynamic or static) that is at least 30% of the nameplate rating of the generator?‡ **A (EP 5)** ⚠3				
6. If a test(s) required by Standard EC.7.40 fails, does the organization implement interim measures to compensate for the risk to patients, visitors, and staff until necessary repairs or corrections are completed? **A (EP 6)** ⚠3				
7. If a test(s) required by Standard EC.7.40 fails, does the organization perform a retest after making the necessary repairs or corrections? **A (EP 7)** ⚠3				

* **Stored Emergency Power Supply Systems (SEPSS)** Are intended to automatically supply illumination or power to critical areas and equipment essential for safety to human life. Included are systems that supply emergency power for such functions as illumination for safe exiting, ventilation where it is essential to maintain life, fire detection and alarm systems, public safety communications systems, and processes where the current interruption would produce serious life safety or health hazards to residents, the public, or staff. **Note:** *Other non–SEPSS battery backup emergency power systems that an organization has determined to be critical for operations during a power failure (for example, laboratory equipment, electronic medical records) should be properly tested and maintained in accordance with manufacturer's recommendations.*

† **Class** Defines the minimum time for which the SEPSS is designed to operate at its rated load without being recharged.

‡ This test may satisfy one of the tests required by EP 1. After the test, the fuel supply should be replenished. Any problems identified during the test shall be resolved promptly. For additional guidance, see NFPA 110 (2005 edition) Standard for Emergency & Standby Power Systems.

Key: 0 = Insufficient compliance; 1 = Partial compliance; 2 = Satisfactory compliance; NA = Not applicable; **A** indicates scoring category A; **C** indicates scoring category C; ▲2 indicates situational decision rules apply; ⚠3 indicates direct impact requirements apply; Ⓜ indicates Measure of success is needed; ☆ indicates this standard also applies to organizations seeking Joint Commission's Medicare/Medicaid certification–based long term care accreditation

Standard EC.7.50 ★	Standard Score: ❑ Compliant ❑ Not Compliant			
Assessment Question	**Level of Compliance**	**Evidence of Compliance**	**Plan of Action/ Measure of Success (if needed)**	**Due Date**
1. Does the organization inspect, test, and maintain critical components of piped medical gas systems including master signal panels, area alarms, automatic pressure switches, shutoff valves, flexible connectors, and outlets? **A (EP 1)** ⚠3				
2. Does the organization test piped medical gas and vacuum systems when the systems are installed, modified, or repaired including cross-connection testing, piping purity testing, and pressure testing? **A (EP 2)** ⚠3				
3. Does the organization maintain the main supply valve and area shut-off valves of piped medical gas and vacuum systems to be accessible and clearly labeled? **A (EP 3)** ⚠3				

Standard EC.8.10	Standard Score: ❑ Compliant ❑ Not Compliant			
Assessment Question	**Level of Compliance**	**Evidence of Compliance**	**Plan of Action/ Measure of Success (if needed)**	**Due Date**
1. Does the physical environment have interior spaces that have the following characteristics: • Are appropriate to the care, treatment, and services provided and the needs of the residents related to age and other characteristics • Include closet and drawer space provided for storing personal property and other items for use by residents; lockers, drawers, or closet space is provided for residents who are in charge of their own personal grooming and who wear street clothes • Allow for good recreational interchange, consider personal preferences when feasible, and accommodate equipment, such as wheelchairs, that are necessary for activities of daily living • Have equipment for rehabilitation and activities adequate to accomplish goals without compromising the environment's safety? **A (EP 1)**				

Key: 0 = Insufficient compliance; 1 = Partial compliance; 2 = Satisfactory compliance; NA = Not applicable; **A** indicates scoring category A; **C** indicates scoring category C; ▲2 indicates situational decision rules apply; ⚠3 indicates direct impact requirements apply; Ⓜ indicates Measure of success is needed; ☆ indicates this standard also applies to organizations seeking Joint Commission's Medicare/Medicaid certification–based long term care accreditation

Standard EC.8.10

Assessment Question	Level of Compliance	Evidence of Compliance	Plan of Action/ Measure of Success (if needed)	Due Date
2. Do furnishings and equipment have the following characteristics: • Maintained to be safe and in good repair • Reflect the resident's level of ability and needs? **A (EP 2)**				
3. Does the physical environment have outside areas that have the following characteristics: • Are appropriate and safe considering the care, treatment, or services provided and the needs of the residents related to age and other characteristics • Used during appropriate seasons? **A (EP 3)**				
4. Are the areas used by residents safe, clean, functional, and comfortable? **C (EP 4)** Ⓜ				
5. Is lighting suitable for care, treatment, or services and the specific activities being conducted? **A (EP 5)** ⚠3				
6. Does ventilation provide for acceptable levels of temperature and humidity and eliminate odors? **A (EP 7)** ⚠3				
7. Are door locks and other structural restraints used, consistent with the needs of the residents, program policy, law, and regulation? **A (EP 11)**				
8. Is emergency access provision provided to all locked and occupied spaces? **A (EP 12)** ⚠3				
9. Are spaces available for safe wandering and exploring? **A (EP 15)**				
10. Does the organization have a sufficient number of electrical outlets with sufficient capacities present to accommodate medically complex services offered to residents? **A (EP 16)**				

Key: 0 = Insufficient compliance; 1 = Partial compliance; 2 = Satisfactory compliance; NA = Not applicable; **A** indicates scoring category A; **C** indicates scoring category C; ▲2 indicates situational decision rules apply; ⚠3 indicates direct impact requirements apply; Ⓜ indicates Measure of success is needed; ☆ indicates this standard also applies to organizations seeking Joint Commission's Medicare/Medicaid certification–based long term care accreditation

Standard EC.8.20	**Standard Score:** ❑ Compliant ❑ Not Compliant			
Assessment Question	**Level of Compliance**	**Evidence of Compliance**	**Plan of Action/ Measure of Success (if needed)**	**Due Date**
1. Does the dining environment encourage eating and socialization, for instance, by minimizing distractions and providing small group settings? **C (EP 1)** Ⓜ				
2. Are dining areas free from loud and distracting noises according to the residents' needs? **C (EP 2)** Ⓜ				
3. Do the dining areas have adequate space for residents with equipment such as ventilators and cardiac monitors? **C (EP 6)** Ⓜ				
4. Do the dining areas have the following characteristics: • Offer residents a selection of seating • Include tables with height(s) to facilitate independent eating • Have staff that help residents sit in a regular dining chair, when possible? **C (EP 7)** Ⓜ				

Standard EC.8.30	**Standard Score:** ❑ Compliant ❑ Not Compliant			
Assessment Question	**Level of Compliance**	**Evidence of Compliance**	**Plan of Action/ Measure of Success (if needed)**	**Due Date**
1. When planning for the size, configuration, and equipping of the space renovated, altered, or new construction, does the organization use one of the following: • Applicable state rules and regulations • *Guidelines for Design and Construction of Hospitals and Healthcare Facilities*, 2001 edition, published by the American Institute of Architects or • Standards or guidelines that provide design criteria? **A (EP 1)**				

Key: 0 = Insufficient compliance; 1 = Partial compliance; 2 = Satisfactory compliance; NA = Not applicable; **A** indicates scoring category A; **C** indicates scoring category C; ▲ indicates situational decision rules apply; △ indicates direct impact requirements apply; Ⓜ indicates Measure of success is needed; ☆ indicates this standard also applies to organizations seeking Joint Commission's Medicare/Medicaid certification–based long term care accreditation

Standard EC.8.30

Assessment Question	Level of Compliance	Evidence of Compliance	Plan of Action/ Measure of Success (if needed)	Due Date
2. When planning demolition, construction, or renovation, does the organization conduct a proactive risk assessment using risk criteria to identify hazards that could potentially compromise care, treatment, and services in occupied areas of the organization's buildings, and does the scope and nature of the activities determine the extent of risk assessment? **A (EP 2)**				
3. When planning demolition, construction, or renovation, does the organization use risk criteria that address the impact of demolition, renovation, or new construction on air quality requirements, infection control, utility requirements, noise, vibration, and emergency procedures? **A (EP 3)**				
4. When planning demolition, construction, or renovation, does the organization select and implement proper controls, as required, to reduce risk and minimize impact of these activities? **A (EP 4)**				

Standard EC.9.10 ★

Standard Score: ❑ Compliant ❑ Not Compliant

Assessment Question	Level of Compliance	Evidence of Compliance	Plan of Action/ Measure of Success (if needed)	Due Date
1. Does the organization establish and implement process(es) for reporting and investigating the following:* • Injuries to residents or others coming to the organization's facilities as well as incidents of property damage • Occupational illnesses and injuries to staff • Security incidents involving residents, staff, or others coming to the organization's facilities or property • Hazardous materials and waste spills, exposures, and other related incidents • Fire-safety management problems, deficiencies, and failures • Equipment-management problems, failures, and user errors • Utility systems management problems, failures, or user errors? **A (EP 1)**				

* Organizations have the flexibility to develop a single reporting method that addresses one or more of the items listed.

Key: 0 = Insufficient compliance; 1 = Partial compliance; 2 = Satisfactory compliance; NA = Not applicable; **A** indicates scoring category A; **C** indicates scoring category C; ▲ indicates situational decision rules apply; △ indicates direct impact requirements apply; Ⓜ indicates Measure of success is needed; ☆ indicates this standard also applies to organizations seeking Joint Commission's Medicare/Medicaid certification–based long term care accreditation

Standard EC.9.10 ★

Assessment Question	Level of Compliance	Evidence of Compliance	Plan of Action/ Measure of Success (if needed)	Due Date
2. Do the organization's leaders assign a person(s) (hereafter referred to as the "assigned person[s]") to monitor and respond to conditions in the organization's environment, and does the assigned person perform the following tasks: • Coordinate the ongoing, organizationwide collection of information about deficiencies and opportunities for improvement in the environment of care • Coordinate the ongoing collection and dissemination of other sources of information, such as published hazard notices or recall reports • Coordinate the preparation of summaries of deficiencies, problems, failures, and user errors related to managing the environment of care* • Coordinate the preparation of summaries on findings, recommendations, actions taken, and results of performance improvement (PI) activities • Participate in hazard surveillance and incident reporting • Participate in developing safety policies and procedures? **A (EP 2)**				
3. Does the organization establish and implement a process(es) for ongoing monitoring of performance regarding actual or potential risk(s) in each of the environment of care management plans?† **A (EP 3)**				
4. Are each of the environment of care management plans evaluated at least annually? **A (EP 4)**				
5. Are the objectives, scope, performance, and effectiveness of each of the environment of care management plans evaluated at least annually? **A (EP 5)**				
6. Are environmental safety monitoring and response activities communicated to the resident safety program as required in the "Leadership" chapter of the *CAMLTC*? **A (EP 10)**				

* Incidents involving residents may be reported to appropriate staff such as staff in quality assessment, improvement, or other functions. However, at least a summary of incidents is shared with the person designated to coordinate safety management activities. Review of incident reports often requires that various legal processes be followed to preserve confidentiality. Opportunities to improve care, treatment, or services or to prevent future similar incidents are not lost as a result of the legal process followed.

† The environment of care plans are for managing safety, security, hazardous materials and waste, emergency management, fire safety, medical equipment, and utilities.

Key: 0 = Insufficient compliance; 1 = Partial compliance; 2 = Satisfactory compliance; NA = Not applicable; **A** indicates scoring category A; **C** indicates scoring category C; ▲(2) indicates situational decision rules apply; △(3) indicates direct impact requirements apply; Ⓜ indicates Measure of success is needed; ☆ indicates this standard also applies to organizations seeking Joint Commission's Medicare/Medicaid certification–based long term care accreditation

Standard EC.9.20 ★	**Standard Score: ❑ Compliant ❑ Not Compliant**			
Assessment Question	**Level of Compliance**	**Evidence of Compliance**	**Plan of Action/ Measure of Success (if needed)**	**Due Date**
1. Does the organization establish an ongoing process for resolving environment of care issues that involves representatives from clinical, administrative, and support services? **A (EP 1)**				
2. Does a multidisciplinary improvement team meet at least bimonthly to address environment of care issues?* **C (EP 2) Ⓜ**				
3. Does the organization analyze environment of care issues in a timely manner? **A (EP 3)**				
4. Are recommendations developed and approved as appropriate? **A (EP 4)**				
5. Do appropriate staff members establish measurement guidelines? **A (EP 5)**				
6. Are environment of care issues communicated to the organization's leaders and person(s) responsible for performance improvement activities? **A (EP 6)**				
7. Is a recommendation for one or more performance improvement activities communicated at least annually to the organization's leaders based on the ongoing performance monitoring of the environment of care management plans? **A (EP 8)**				
8. Are recommendations for resolving environmental safety issues communicated, when appropriate, to those responsible for managing the resident safety program as required in the "Leadership" chapter of the *CAMLTC*? **A (EP 9)**				

* Meetings held less frequently than bimonthly are acceptable when supported by current organization experience and the multidisciplinary improvement team's approval. Ongoing justification of meeting frequency depends on a satisfactory annual evaluation of performance as required by Standard EC.9.10.

Key: 0 = Insufficient compliance; 1 = Partial compliance; 2 = Satisfactory compliance; NA = Not applicable; **A** indicates scoring category A; **C** indicates scoring category C; ▲(2) indicates situational decision rules apply; △(3) indicates direct impact requirements apply; Ⓜ indicates Measure of success is needed; ☆ indicates this standard also applies to organizations seeking Joint Commission's Medicare/Medicaid certification–based long term care accreditation

Standard EC.9.30 ★	**Standard Score: ❑ Compliant ❑ Not Compliant**			
Assessment Question	**Level of Compliance**	**Evidence of Compliance**	**Plan of Action/ Measure of Success (if needed)**	**Due Date**
1. Do appropriate staff members participate in implementing recommendations to improve the environment? **A (EP 1)**				
2. Do appropriate staff members monitor the effectiveness of the recommendations' implementation? **A (EP 2)**				
3. Are monitoring results reported through appropriate channels, including the organization's leaders? **A (EP 3)**				
4. Are monitoring results reported to the multidisciplinary improvement team responsible for resolving environment of care issues? **A (EP 4)**				
5. Are results of monitoring reported (when appropriate) to those responsible for managing the resident safety program required in the "Leadership" chapter of the *CAMLTC*? **A (EP 5)**				

Key: 0 = Insufficient compliance; 1 = Partial compliance; 2 = Satisfactory compliance; NA = Not applicable; **A** indicates scoring category A; **C** indicates scoring category C; ▲(2) indicates situational decision rules apply; △(3) indicates direct impact requirements apply; Ⓜ indicates Measure of success is needed; ☆ indicates this standard also applies to organizations seeking Joint Commission's Medicare/Medicaid certification–based long term care accreditation

Life Safety (LS)

The standards statements are not included with these chapter questions due to the excessive length of the statements. Please refer to your accreditation manual for those standard statements.

Standard LS.01.01.01

Assessment Question	Level of Compliance	Evidence of Compliance	Plan of Action/ Measure of Success (if needed)	Due Date
1. Does the organization assign an individual(s) to assess compliance with the *Life Safety Code*, complete the electronic Statement of Conditions, and manage the resolution of deficiencies? **A (EP 1)**				
2. Does the organization maintain a current electronic Statement of Conditions (e-SOC)? **Note:** *The e-SOC is available through The Joint Commission Connect™ extranet site.* **A (EP 2)**				
3. When the organization plans to resolve a deficiency through a Plan for Improvement (PFI), does the organization meet the time frames identified in the PFI accepted by The Joint Commission? (*See also* Standard LS.01.02.01, EPs 1–14) **A (EP 3)** ▲2				

Standard LS.01.02.01

Assessment Question	Level of Compliance	Evidence of Compliance	Plan of Action/ Measure of Success (if needed)	Due Date
1. Does the organization notify the fire department (or other emergency response group) and initiate a fire watch when a fire alarm or sprinkler system is out of service more than four hours in a 24-hour period in an occupied building? Are the notification and fire watch times documented? (*See also* Standard LS.01.01.01, EP 3) (For full text and any exceptions, refer to NFPA 101-2000: 9.6.1.8 and 9.7.6.1) **A (EP 1)** △3				
2. Does the organization post signage identifying the location of alternate exits to everyone affected? (*See also* Standard LS.01.01.01, EP 3) **A (EP 2)** △3				

Key: 0 = Insufficient compliance; 1 = Partial compliance; 2 = Satisfactory compliance; NA = Not applicable; **A** indicates scoring category A; **C** indicates scoring category C; ▲2 indicates situational decision rules apply; △3 indicates direct impact requirements apply; Ⓜ indicates Measure of success is needed; ☆ indicates this standard also applies to organizations seeking Joint Commission's Medicare/Medicaid certification–based long term care accreditation

Standard LS.01.02.01

Assessment Question	Level of Compliance	Evidence of Compliance	Plan of Action/ Measure of Success (if needed)	Due Date
3. Does the organization have a written interim life safety measure (ILSM) policy that covers situations when *Life Safety Code* deficiencies cannot be immediately corrected or during periods of construction? Do the policy criteria include evaluating when and to what extent the organization follows special measures to compensate for increased life safety risk? (*See also* Standard LS.01.01.01, EP 3) **A (EP 3)** ▲2				
4. When the organization identifies *Life Safety Code* deficiencies that cannot be immediately corrected or during periods of construction, does the organization inspect exits in affected areas on a daily basis? Does the organization determine when these inspections are needed? (*See also* Standard LS.01.01.01, EP 3) **C (EP 4)** Ⓜ △3				
5. When the organization identifies *Life Safety Code* deficiencies that cannot be immediately corrected or during periods of construction, does the organization provide temporary but equivalent fire alarm and detection systems for use when a fire system is impaired? Does the organization determine when these systems are needed? (*See also* Standard LS.01.01.01, EP 3) **A (EP 5)** △3				
6. When the organization identifies *Life Safety Code* deficiencies that cannot be immediately corrected or during periods of construction, does the organization provide additional fire-fighting equipment? Does the organization determine when to provide this equipment? (*See also* Standard LS.01.01.01, EP 3) **A (EP 6)** △3				

Key: 0 = Insufficient compliance; 1 = Partial compliance; 2 = Satisfactory compliance; NA = Not applicable; **A** indicates scoring category A; **C** indicates scoring category C; ▲ indicates situational decision rules apply; △ indicates direct impact requirements apply; Ⓜ indicates Measure of success is needed; ☆ indicates this standard also applies to organizations seeking Joint Commission's Medicare/Medicaid certification–based long term care accreditation

Standard LS.01.02.01

Assessment Question	Level of Compliance	Evidence of Compliance	Plan of Action/ Measure of Success (if needed)	Due Date
7. When the organization identifies *Life Safety Code* deficiencies that cannot be immediately corrected or during periods of construction, does the organization use temporary construction partitions that are smoke-tight, or made of noncombustible material, or made of limited-combustible material that will not contribute to the development or spread of fire? Does the organization determine when to use these partitions? (*See also* Standard LS.01.01.01, EP 3) **A (EP 7)**				
8. When the organization identifies *Life Safety Code* deficiencies that cannot be immediately corrected or during periods of construction, does the organization increase surveillance of buildings, grounds, and equipment, giving special attention to construction areas and storage, excavation, and field offices? Does the organization determine when to increase surveillance? (*See also* Standard LS.01.01.01, EP 3) **C (EP 8) Ⓜ**				
9. When the organization identifies *Life Safety Code* deficiencies that cannot be immediately corrected or during periods of construction, does the organization enforce storage, housekeeping, and debris-removal practices that reduce the building's flammable and combustible fire load to the lowest feasible level? Does the organization determine when these practices are needed? (*See also* Standard LS.01.01.01, EP 3) **C (EP 9) Ⓜ**				
10. When the organization identifies *Life Safety Code* deficiencies that cannot be immediately corrected or during periods of construction, does the organization provide additional training to those who work in the organization on the use of fire-fighting equipment? Does the organization determine when to provide additional training? (*See also* Standard LS.01.01.01, EP 3) **A (EP 10)**				

Key: 0 = Insufficient compliance; 1 = Partial compliance; 2 = Satisfactory compliance; NA = Not applicable; **A** indicates scoring category A; **C** indicates scoring category C; ▲ indicates situational decision rules apply; △ indicates direct impact requirements apply; Ⓜ indicates Measure of success is needed; ☆ indicates this standard also applies to organizations seeking Joint Commission's Medicare/Medicaid certification–based long term care accreditation

Standard LS.01.02.01

Assessment Question	Level of Compliance	Evidence of Compliance	Plan of Action/ Measure of Success (if needed)	Due Date
11. When the organization identifies *Life Safety Code* deficiencies that cannot be immediately corrected or during periods of construction, does the organization conduct one additional fire drill per shift per quarter? Does the organization determine when these additional fire drills are needed? (*See also* Standards EC.5.30, EP 1; LS.01.01.01, EP 3) **A (EP 11)**				
12. When the organization identifies *Life Safety Code* deficiencies that cannot be immediately corrected or during periods of construction, does the organization inspect and test temporary systems monthly? Does the organization determine when these inspections and tests are needed? (*See also* Standard LS.01.01.01, EP 3) **C (EP 12) Ⓜ**				
13. Does the organization conduct education to promote awareness of building deficiencies, construction hazards, and temporary measures implemented to maintain fire safety? Does the organization determine when this education is needed? (*See also* Standard LS.01.01.01, EP 3) **A (EP 13)** △3				
14. Does the organization train those who work in the organization to compensate for impaired structural or compartmental fire safety features? (*See also* Standard LS.01.01.01, EP 3) **Note:** *Compartmentalization is the concept of using various building components (fire-rated walls and doors, smoke barriers, fire-rated floor slabs) to prevent the spread of fire and the products of combustion, and to provide a safe means of egress to an approved exit. The presence of these features varies depending on the building occupancy classification.* **C (EP 14) Ⓜ** △3				

Key: 0 = Insufficient compliance; 1 = Partial compliance; 2 = Satisfactory compliance; NA = Not applicable; **A** indicates scoring category A; **C** indicates scoring category C; ▲2 indicates situational decision rules apply; △3 indicates direct impact requirements apply; Ⓜ indicates Measure of success is needed; ☆ indicates this standard also applies to organizations seeking Joint Commission's Medicare/Medicaid certification–based long term care accreditation

Standard LS.02.01.10

Assessment Question	Level of Compliance	Evidence of Compliance	Plan of Action/ Measure of Success (if needed)	Due Date
1. Do buildings meet requirements for height and construction type in accordance with NFPA 101-2000 18/19.1.6.2? **A (EP 1)** △3				
2. Do new buildings contain approved automatic sprinkler systems? Do existing buildings contain approved automatic sprinkler systems as required by the construction type? (For full text and any exceptions, refer to NFPA 101-2000: 18.3.5.1. and 19.1.6.2) **A (EP 2)** △3				
3. Do walls that are fire-rated for two hours (such as common walls between buildings and occupancy separation walls within buildings) extend from the floor slab to the floor or roof slab above, and from exterior wall to exterior wall? (For full text and any exceptions, refer to NFPA 101-2000: 8.2.2.2) **A (EP 3)**				
4. Are openings in two-hour fire-rated walls fire-rated for 1 ½ hours? (*See also* Standards LS.02.01.20, EP 3 and LS.02.01.34, EP 2) (For full text and any exceptions, refer to NFPA 101-2000: 8.2.3.2.3.1) **A (EP 4)**				
5. Do doors required to be fire-rated have functioning hardware, including positive latching devices, self-closing, or automatic-closing devices? Are gaps between meeting edges of door pairs no more than 1/8 inch wide, and are undercuts no larger than 3/4 inch? (*See also* Standard LS.02.01.30, EP 2) (For full text and any exceptions, refer to NFPA 101-2000: 8.2.3.2.3.1, 8.2.3.2.1 and NFPA 80-1999: 2-4.4.3, 2-3.1.7, and 1-11.4) **C (EP 5)**				
6. Do doors that are fire-rated have approved protective plates that are no higher than 16 inches above the bottom of the door? (For full text and any exceptions, refer to NFPA 80-1999: 2-4.5; NFPA 101-2000:19.3.2.1) **Note:** *Doors for hazardous rooms may have non-rated protective plates that are placed no higher than 48 inches from the bottom of the door.* **C (EP 6)**				

Key: 0 = Insufficient compliance; 1 = Partial compliance; 2 = Satisfactory compliance; NA = Not applicable; **A** indicates scoring category A; **C** indicates scoring category C; ▲ indicates situational decision rules apply; △3 indicates direct impact requirements apply; Ⓜ indicates Measure of success is needed; ☆ indicates this standard also applies to organizations seeking Joint Commission's Medicare/Medicaid certification–based long term care accreditation

Standard LS.02.01.10

Assessment Question	Level of Compliance	Evidence of Compliance	Plan of Action/ Measure of Success (if needed)	Due Date
7. Are doors requiring a fire rating of 3/4 hour or longer free of coverings, decorations, or other objects applied to the door face, with the exception of informational signs? (For full text and any exceptions, refer to NFPA 80-1999: 1-3.5) **C (EP 7)**				
8. When ducts penetrate a two-hour fire-rated separation, are they protected by dampers that are fire-rated for 1½ hours? (For full text and any exceptions, refer to NFPA 101-2000: 8.2.3.2.4.1 and NFPA 90A-1999: 3-3.1) **A (EP 8)**				
9. When pipes, conduits, bus ducts, cables/wires, air ducts or pneumatic tubes penetrate fire-rated walls and floors, are the spaces around the penetration protected with an approved fire-rated material? (For full text and any exceptions, refer to NFPA 101-2000: 8.2.3.2.4.2) **Note:** *Polyurethane expanding foam is not an accepted fire-rated material for this purpose.* **C (EP 9)**				
10. Does the organization meet all other *Life Safety Code* requirements related to NFPA 101-2000: 18/19.1? **C (EP 10)**				

Standard LS.02.01.20

Assessment Question	Level of Compliance	Evidence of Compliance	Plan of Action/ Measure of Success (if needed)	Due Date
1. Are doors in a means of egress unlocked in the direction of egress? (For full text and any exceptions, refer to NFPA 101-2000: 18/19.2.2.2.4) **A (EP 1)** △3				
2. Do doors in a means of egress swing in the direction of egress in organizations whose occupancy is 50 or more? (For full text and any exceptions, refer to NFPA 101-2000: 7.2.1.4.2) **C (EP 2)**				

Key: 0 = Insufficient compliance; 1 = Partial compliance; 2 = Satisfactory compliance; NA = Not applicable; **A** indicates scoring category A; **C** indicates scoring category C; ▲2 indicates situational decision rules apply; △3 indicates direct impact requirements apply; Ⓜ indicates Measure of success is needed; ☆ indicates this standard also applies to organizations seeking Joint Commission's Medicare/Medicaid certification–based long term care accreditation

Standard LS.02.01.20

Assessment Question	Level of Compliance	Evidence of Compliance	Plan of Action/ Measure of Success (if needed)	Due Date
3. Are walls containing horizontal exits fire-rated for two or more hours, extending from the lowest floor slab to the floor or roof slab above, and continuously from exterior wall to exterior wall? (*See also* Standard LS.02.01.10 EP 4) (For full text and any exceptions, refer to NFPA 101-2000: 7.2.4.3.1 and 8.2.2.2) **C (EP 3)**				
4. Are outside exit stairs separated from the interior of the building by walls with the same fire rating required for enclosed stairs? Does the wall extend vertically from the ground to a point 10 feet or more above the top landing of the stairs or roofline (whichever is lower) and extend 10 feet or more horizontally? (For full text and any exceptions, refer to NFPA 101-2000: 7.2.2.6.3) **C (EP 4)**				
5. Do doors in new buildings that are a part of horizontal exits have approved vision panels and are installed without a center mullion? (For full text and any exceptions, refer to NFPA 101-2000: 18.2.2.5.6) **C (EP 5)**				
6. When horizontal exit walls in new buildings terminate at outside walls at an angle of less than 180 degrees, are the outside walls fire-rated for one hour for a distance of 10 or more feet? And are openings in the walls in the 10-foot span fire rated for 3/4 hour? (For full text and any exceptions, refer to NFPA 101-2000: 7.2.4.3.2) **C (EP 6)**				
7. Do stairs and ramps serving as a required means of egress have handrails and guards on both sides in new buildings and at least on one side in existing buildings? (For full text and any exceptions, refer to NFPA 101-2000: 7.2.2.4.2) **C (EP 7)**				
8. Do exits discharge to the outside at grade level or through an approved exit passageway that is continuous and terminates at a public way or at an exterior exit discharge? (For full text and any exceptions, refer to NFPA 101-2000: 7.7) **C (EP 8)**				

Key: 0 = Insufficient compliance; 1 = Partial compliance; 2 = Satisfactory compliance; NA = Not applicable; **A** indicates scoring category A; **C** indicates scoring category C; ▲ indicates situational decision rules apply; △ indicates direct impact requirements apply; Ⓜ indicates Measure of success is needed; ☆ indicates this standard also applies to organizations seeking Joint Commission's Medicare/Medicaid certification–based long term care accreditation

Standard LS.02.01.20

Assessment Question	Level of Compliance	Evidence of Compliance	Plan of Action/ Measure of Success (if needed)	Due Date
9. When stair doors are held open and the sprinkler or fire alarm system activates the release of one door in a stairway, do all doors serving that stairway close? (For full text and any exceptions, refer to NFPA 101-2000: 18/19.2.2.2.7) **C (EP 9)**				
10. Are doors to new boiler rooms, new heater rooms, and new mechanical equipment rooms located in a means of egress not held open by an automatic release device? (For full text and any exceptions, refer to NFPA 101-2000: 18.2.2.2.6) **C (EP 10)**				
11. In new buildings, are exit corridors at least 8 feet wide? And in existing buildings, are exit corridors at least 4 feet wide? If modifying existing buildings with exit corridors that exceed 8 feet, are the exit corridors not reduced to less then 8 feet? (For full text and any exceptions, refer to NFPA 101-2000: 18/19.2.3.3) **C (EP 11)**				
12. Is the corridor width not obstructed by wall projections? (For full text and any exceptions, refer to NFPA 101-2000: 18/19.2.3.3) **Note:** *When corridors are 6 feet wide or more, The Joint Commission permits certain objects to project into the corridor, such as hand rub dispensers or computer desks that are retractable. They must be no more than 36 inches wide and cannot project more than 6 inches into the corridor. These items must be installed at least 48 inches apart and above the handrail height.* **C (EP 12)**				
13. Are exits, exit accesses, and exit discharges clear of obstructions or impediments to the public way, such as clutter (for example, equipment, carts, furniture), construction material, and snow and ice? (For full text and any exceptions, refer to NFPA 101-2000: 7.1.10.1) **C (EP 13)**				

Key: 0 = Insufficient compliance; 1 = Partial compliance; 2 = Satisfactory compliance; NA = Not applicable; **A** indicates scoring category A; **C** indicates scoring category C; ▲ indicates situational decision rules apply; △ indicates direct impact requirements apply; Ⓜ indicates Measure of success is needed; ☆ indicates this standard also applies to organizations seeking Joint Commission's Medicare/Medicaid certification–based long term care accreditation

Standard LS.02.01.20

Assessment Question	Level of Compliance	Evidence of Compliance	Plan of Action/ Measure of Success (if needed)	Due Date
14. Are exit access doors and exit doors free of mirrors, hangings, or draperies that might conceal, obscure, or confuse the direction of exit? (For full text and any exceptions, refer to NFPA 101-2000: 7.5.2.2) **C (EP 14)**				
15. Do floors or compartments in a building have two or more approved exits arranged and constructed to be remotely located from each other? (For full text and any exceptions, refer to NFPA 101-2000: 18/19.2.4.1) **C (EP 15)**				
16. Are resident sleeping rooms or suites that are larger than 1,000 square feet provided with at least two exit access doors located remotely from each other? (For full text and any exceptions, refer to NFPA 101-2000: 18/19.2.5.2) **C (EP 16)**				
17. Do rooms or suites larger than 2,500 square feet (not used as resident sleeping rooms) have at least two exit access doors located remotely from each other? (For full text and any exceptions, refer to NFPA 101-2000: 18/19.2.5.3) **C (EP 17)**				
18. Are suites of sleeping rooms limited to 5,000 square feet and suites used for other purposes limited to 10,000 square feet? Are the suites arranged so that no intervening rooms are hazardous areas? (*See also* Standard LS.02.01.30, EP 2) (For full text and any exceptions, refer to NFPA 101-2000: 18/19.2.5.5-7) **C (EP 18)**				
19. In suites of resident sleeping rooms, is the travel distance to an exit access door 100 feet or less from any point in the suite? (For full text and any exceptions, refer to NFPA 101-2000: 18/19.2.5.8) **C (EP 19)**				

Key: 0 = Insufficient compliance; 1 = Partial compliance; 2 = Satisfactory compliance; NA = Not applicable; **A** indicates scoring category A; **C** indicates scoring category C; ▲ indicates situational decision rules apply; △ indicates direct impact requirements apply; Ⓜ indicates Measure of success is needed; ☆ indicates this standard also applies to organizations seeking Joint Commission's Medicare/Medicaid certification–based long term care accreditation

Standard LS.02.01.20

Assessment Question	Level of Compliance	Evidence of Compliance	Plan of Action/ Measure of Success (if needed)	Due Date
20. In suites not used as resident sleeping rooms that have up to one intervening room, is the travel distance to an exit access door 100 feet or less from any point in the suite and 50 feet or less from any point in a suite containing two intervening rooms? (For full text and any exceptions, refer to NFPA 101-2000: 18/19.2.5.8) **C (EP 20)**				
21. Do resident sleeping rooms open directly onto an exit access corridor? (For full text and any exceptions, refer to NFPA 101-2000: 18/19.2.5.1) **C (EP 21)**				
22. Are resident sleeping room doors not locked? (For full text and any exceptions, refer to NFPA 101-2000: 18/19.2.2.2.2) **C (EP 22)** ⚠3				
23. Is the travel distance to a room door from any point in a resident sleeping room 50 feet or less? (For full text and any exceptions, refer to NFPA 101-2000: 18/19.2.6.2.3) **C (EP 23)**				
24. In existing buildings, is the travel distance between any room door and an exit 100 feet or less (or 150 feet or less when equipped with an approved automatic sprinkler system)? In new buildings, is the travel distance between any room door and an exit 150 feet or less? (For full text and any exceptions, refer to NFPA 101-2000: 18/19.2.6.2.1) **C (EP 24)**				
25. In existing buildings, is the travel distance between any point in a room and an exit 150 feet or less (or 200 feet or less when equipped with an approved automatic sprinkler system)? In new buildings, is the travel distance between any point in a room and an exit 200 feet or less? (For full text and any exceptions, refer to NFPA 101-2000: 18/19.2.6.2.2) **C (EP 25)**				

Key: 0 = Insufficient compliance; 1 = Partial compliance; 2 = Satisfactory compliance; NA = Not applicable; **A** indicates scoring category A; **C** indicates scoring category C; ▲2 indicates situational decision rules apply; ⚠3 indicates direct impact requirements apply; Ⓜ indicates Measure of success is needed; ☆ indicates this standard also applies to organizations seeking Joint Commission's Medicare/Medicaid certification–based long term care accreditation

Standard LS.02.01.20

Assessment Question	Level of Compliance	Evidence of Compliance	Plan of Action/ Measure of Success (if needed)	Due Date
26. In new buildings, is no dead-end corridor longer than 30 feet? (For full text and any exceptions, refer to NFPA 101-2000: 18.2.5.10) **C (EP 26)**				
27. Are means of egress adequately illuminated at all points, including angles and intersections of corridors and passageways, stairways, stairway landings, exit doors, and exit discharge? (For full text and any exceptions, refer to NFPA 101-2000: 18/19.2.8) **C (EP 27)**				
28. Is illumination in the means of egress, including exit discharge, arranged so that failure of any single light fixture or bulb will not leave the area in darkness? (For full text and any exceptions, refer to NFPA 101-2000: 7.8.1.4) **C (EP 28)**				
29. Do stairs serving five or more stories have signs on each floor landing in the stairwell that identify the story, the stairwell, the top and bottom, and the direction to and story of exit discharge? Are the signs placed 5 feet above the floor landing in a position that is easily visible when the door is open or closed? (For full text and any exceptions, refer to NFPA 101-2000: 7.2.2.5.4) **C (EP 29)**				
30. Are signs reading "No Exit" posted on any door, passage, or stairway that is neither an exit, nor an access to an exit, nor may be mistaken for an exit? (For full text and any exceptions, refer to NFPA 101-2000: 7.10.8.1) **C (EP 30)**				
31. Are exit signs visible when the path to the exit is not readily apparent? Are signs adequately lit and have letters that are 4 or more inches high (or 6 inches high if externally lit)? (For full text and any exceptions, refer to NFPA 101-2000: 7.10.1.2, 7.10.5, 7.10.6.1 and 7.10.7.1) **C (EP 31)**				

Key: 0 = Insufficient compliance; 1 = Partial compliance; 2 = Satisfactory compliance; NA = Not applicable; **A** indicates scoring category A; **C** indicates scoring category C; ▲ indicates situational decision rules apply; △ indicates direct impact requirements apply; Ⓜ indicates Measure of success is needed; ☆ indicates this standard also applies to organizations seeking Joint Commission's Medicare/Medicaid certification–based long term care accreditation

Standard LS.02.01.20

Assessment Question	Level of Compliance	Evidence of Compliance	Plan of Action/ Measure of Success (if needed)	Due Date
32. Does the organization meet all other *Life Safety Code* means of egress requirements related to NFPA 101-2000: 18/19.2? **C (EP 32)**				

Standard LS.02.01.30

Assessment Question	Level of Compliance	Evidence of Compliance	Plan of Action/ Measure of Success (if needed)	Due Date
1. Are existing vertical openings (other than exit stairs) enclosed with one-hour fire-rated construction? For new construction, are vertical openings (other than exit stairs) enclosed by one-hour fire-rated walls when connecting three or fewer floors and two-hour fire-rated walls when connecting four or more floors? (*See also* Standard LS.02.01.10 EP 4) **Note:** *These vertical openings include, but are not limited to, communicating stairs, ramps, elevator shafts, ventilation shafts, light shafts, trash chutes, linen chutes, and utility chases.* (For full text and any exceptions, refer to NFPA 101-2000: 18/19.3.1.1) **C (EP 1)**				
2. Are all hazardous areas protected by walls and doors in accordance with NFPA 101-2000: 18/19.3.2.1? (*See also* Standards LS.02.01.10, EP 5 and LS.02.01.20, EP 18) Hazardous areas include, but are not limited to: Boiler/fuel fired heater rooms: • Existing boiler/fuel-fired heater rooms have sprinkler systems, resist the passage of smoke, and have doors with self-closing or automatic-closing devices; or the rooms have one-hour fire-rated walls and doors fire-rated for 3/4 hour. • New boiler/fuel fired heater rooms have sprinkler systems and have one-hour fire-rated walls and doors fire-rated for 3/4 hour.				

Key: 0 = Insufficient compliance; 1 = Partial compliance; 2 = Satisfactory compliance; NA = Not applicable; **A** indicates scoring category A; **C** indicates scoring category C; ▲2 indicates situational decision rules apply; △3 indicates direct impact requirements apply; Ⓜ indicates Measure of success is needed; ☆ indicates this standard also applies to organizations seeking Joint Commission's Medicare/Medicaid certification–based long term care accreditation

Standard LS.02.01.30

Assessment Question	Level of Compliance	Evidence of Compliance	Plan of Action/ Measure of Success (if needed)	Due Date
Central/bulk laundries larger than 100 square feet: • Existing central/bulk laundries larger than 100 square feet have sprinkler systems, resist the passage of smoke, and have doors with self-closing or automatic-closing devices; or the laundries have one-hour fire-rated walls and doors fire-rated for 3/4 hour. • New central/bulk laundries larger than 100 square feet have sprinkler systems and have one-hour fire-rated walls and doors fire-rated for 3/4 hour. Flammable liquid storage rooms (NFPA 30-1996:4-4.2, 4-4.4.2): • Existing flammable liquid storage rooms have two-hour fire-rated walls with doors fire-rated for 1½ hours. • New flammable liquid storage rooms have sprinkler systems and have two-hour fire-rated walls with doors fire-rated for 1½ hours. Laboratories (*See* NFPA 45-1996 to determine if a laboratory is a "severe hazard" area): • Existing laboratories that are not severe hazard areas have sprinkler systems, resist the passage of smoke, and have doors with self-closing or automatic-closing devices; or the laboratories have walls fire-rated for one hour with doors fire-rated for 3/4 hour. • New laboratories that are not severe hazard areas have sprinkler systems, resist the passage of smoke, and have doors with self-closing or automatic-closing devices. • Existing laboratories that are severe hazard areas (NFPA 99-1999: 10-3.1.1) have two-hour fire-rated walls with doors fire-rated for 1½ hours. When there is a sprinkler system, the walls are fire-rated for 1 hour with doors fire-rated for 3/4 hour. • New laboratories that are severe hazard areas (NFPA 99-1999: 10-3.1.1) have sprinkler systems and have one-hour fire-rated walls with doors fire-rated for 3/4 hour. Maintenance repair shops: • Existing maintenance repair shops have sprinkler systems, resist the passage of smoke, and have doors with self-closing or automatic-closing devices; or the shop has one-hour fire-rated walls with at least 3/4-hour fire-rated doors.				

Key: 0 = Insufficient compliance; 1 = Partial compliance; 2 = Satisfactory compliance; NA = Not applicable; **A** indicates scoring category A; **C** indicates scoring category C; ▲ indicates situational decision rules apply; △ indicates direct impact requirements apply; Ⓜ indicates Measure of success is needed; ☆ indicates this standard also applies to organizations seeking Joint Commission's Medicare/Medicaid certification–based long term care accreditation

Standard LS.02.01.30

Assessment Question	Level of Compliance	Evidence of Compliance	Plan of Action/ Measure of Success (if needed)	Due Date
• New maintenance repair shops have sprinkler systems and have one-hour fire-rated walls with doors fire-rated for 3/4 hour. Piped oxygen tank supply rooms (NFPA 99-1999: 4-3.1.1.2): • Existing piped oxygen tank supply rooms have one-hour fire-rated walls with doors fire-rated for 3/4 hour. • New piped oxygen tank supply rooms have sprinkler systems and have one-hour fire-rated walls with doors fire-rated for 3/4 hour. Paint shops that are not severe hazard areas: • Existing paint shops that are not severe hazard areas have sprinkler systems, resist the passage of smoke, and have doors with self-closing or automatic-closing devices; or the shops have one-hour fire-rated walls with doors fire-rated for 3/4 hour. • New paint shops that are not severe hazard areas have sprinkler systems and have one-hour fire-rated walls with doors fire-rated for 3/4 hour. Soiled linen rooms: • Existing soiled linen rooms have sprinkler systems, resist the passage of smoke, and have doors with self-closing or automatic-closing devices; or the rooms have one-hour fire-rated walls with doors fire-rated for 3/4 hour. • New soiled linen rooms have sprinkler systems and have one-hour fire-rated walls with doors fire-rated for 3/4 hour. Storage rooms: • Existing storage rooms for combustible materials larger than 50 square feet have sprinkler systems, resist the passage of smoke, and have doors with self-closing or automatic-closing devices; or the rooms have one-hour fire-rated walls with doors fire-rated for more than 3/4 hour. • New storage rooms for combustible materials 50 to 100 square feet are sprinkled, resist the passage of smoke and have doors with self-closing or automatic-closing devices. • New storage rooms for combustible materials larger than 100 square feet are sprinkled, and have one-hour fire-rated walls with doors fire-rated for more than 3/4 hour.				

Key: 0 = Insufficient compliance; 1 = Partial compliance; 2 = Satisfactory compliance; NA = Not applicable; **A** indicates scoring category A; **C** indicates scoring category C; ▲ indicates situational decision rules apply; △ indicates direct impact requirements apply; Ⓜ indicates Measure of success is needed; ☆ indicates this standard also applies to organizations seeking Joint Commission's Medicare/Medicaid certification–based long term care accreditation

Standard LS.02.01.30

Assessment Question	Level of Compliance	Evidence of Compliance	Plan of Action/ Measure of Success (if needed)	Due Date
Trash collection rooms: • Existing trash collection rooms have sprinkler systems, resist the passage of smoke, and have doors with self-closing or automatic-closing devices; or the rooms have one-hour fire-rated walls with doors fire-rated for 3/4 hour. • New trash collection rooms are sprinkled, and have 1-hour fire-rated walls with doors fire-rated for 3/4 hour. **C (EP 2)**				
3. Are gift shops storing or displaying combustibles in quantities considered hazardous separated by walls fire rated for one hour and doors fire rated for 3/4 hour? In existing buildings, are a combination of walls and doors used to limit the passage of smoke and an approved automatic sprinkler system used for gift shops storing or displaying combustibles in quantities considered hazardous? (For full text and any exceptions, refer to NFPA 101-2000: 18/19.3.2.5) **C (EP 3)**				
4. Are existing wall and ceiling interior finishes rated Class A or B for limiting smoke development and the spread of flames? Are newly installed wall and ceiling interior finishes rated Class A? (For full text and any exceptions, refer to NFPA 101-2000: 18/19.3.3.2) **C (EP 4)**				
5. Do newly installed interior floor finishes in corridors of smoke compartments without sprinkler systems have a Class I radiant flux rating? (For full text and any exceptions, refer to NFPA 101-2000: 19.3.3.3) **C (EP 5)**				

Key: 0 = Insufficient compliance; 1 = Partial compliance; 2 = Satisfactory compliance; NA = Not applicable; **A** indicates scoring category A; **C** indicates scoring category C; ▲ indicates situational decision rules apply; △ indicates direct impact requirements apply; Ⓜ indicates Measure of success is needed; ☆ indicates this standard also applies to organizations seeking Joint Commission's Medicare/Medicaid certification–based long term care accreditation

Standard LS.02.01.30

Assessment Question	Level of Compliance	Evidence of Compliance	Plan of Action/ Measure of Success (if needed)	Due Date
6. Are existing corridor partitions fire-rated for 1/2 hour, continuous from the floor slab to the floor or roof slab above, and through any concealed spaces (such as those above suspended ceilings and interstitial spaces), properly sealed, and constructed to limit the transfer of smoke? **Note:** *Unsealed spaces 1/8-inch or less in width around pipes, conduits, ducts, and wires above the ceiling are permitted.* **Note:** *In smoke compartments protected throughout with an approved supervised sprinkler system, corridor walls are allowed to terminate at the ceiling if the ceiling is constructed to limit the passage of smoke. The passage of smoke can be limited by an exposed, suspended-grid acoustical tile ceiling. The following ceiling features also limit the passage of smoke:* • *Sprinkler piping and sprinklers that penetrate the ceiling* • *Ducted heating, ventilating, and air conditioning (HVAC) supply and return-air diffusers* • *Speakers* • *Recessed lighting fixtures* **C (EP 6)**				
7. Are corridor walls in new buildings constructed to limit the transfer of smoke? (For full text and any exceptions, refer to: NFPA 101-2000: 18.3.6.2) **C (EP 7)**				
8. In smoke compartments without sprinkler systems, are fixed fire windows in corridor walls 25% or less of the size of the corridor walls in which they are installed? (For full text and any exceptions, refer to NFPA 101-2000: 19.3.6.3.8. and 8.2.3.2.2(2)) **Note:** *Existing window installations that conform to previously accepted* Life Safety Code *criteria (such as 1,296 square inches or less, fixed wired glass, or fire-rated glazing set in approved metal frames) are permitted.* **C (EP 8)**				

Key: 0 = Insufficient compliance; 1 = Partial compliance; 2 = Satisfactory compliance; NA = Not applicable; **A** indicates scoring category A; **C** indicates scoring category C; ▲(2) indicates situational decision rules apply; △(3) indicates direct impact requirements apply; Ⓜ indicates Measure of success is needed; ☆ indicates this standard also applies to organizations seeking Joint Commission's Medicare/Medicaid certification–based long term care accreditation

Standard LS.02.01.30

Assessment Question	Level of Compliance	Evidence of Compliance	Plan of Action/ Measure of Success (if needed)	Due Date
9. In existing buildings, are all corridor doors constructed of 1 3/4 inch or thicker solid bonded wood core or equivalent material and do not have ventilating louvers or transfer grills (with the exception of bathrooms, toilets, and sink closets that do not contain flammable or combustible materials)? (For full text and any exceptions, refer to NFPA 101-2000: 19.3.6.3.1 and 19.3.6.4) **C (EP 9)**				
10. Are corridor doors free from non-rated protective plates placed higher than 48 inches above the bottom of the door? (For full text and any exceptions, refer to NFPA 101-2000: 18/19.3.6.3.5) **C (EP 10)**				
11. Are corridor doors fitted with positive latching hardware, arranged to restrict the movement of smoke, and hinged so that they swing? Are gaps between meeting edges of door pairs no more than 1/8 inch wide, and undercuts no larger than 1 inch? **Note:** *For existing doors, it is acceptable to use a device that keeps the door closed when a force of 5 foot pounds is applied to the edge of the door.* (For full text and any exceptions, refer to NFPA 101-2000: 18/19.3.6.3.2, 18/19.3.6.3.1, and 7.2.1.4.1) **C (EP 11)**				
12. Are openings in vision panels or doors in corridor walls (other than in smoke compartments containing patient sleeping rooms) installed at or below one half the distance from the floor to the ceiling? Are these openings not larger than 80 square inches in new buildings or larger than 20 square inches in existing buildings? **Note:** *Openings may include, but are not limited to, mail slots and pass-through windows in areas such as laboratories, pharmacies, and cashier stations.* (For full text and any exceptions, refer to NFPA 101-2000: 18/19.3.6.5) **C (EP 12)**				

Key: 0 = Insufficient compliance; 1 = Partial compliance; 2 = Satisfactory compliance; NA = Not applicable; **A** indicates scoring category A; **C** indicates scoring category C; ▲ indicates situational decision rules apply; △ indicates direct impact requirements apply; Ⓜ indicates Measure of success is needed; ☆ indicates this standard also applies to organizations seeking Joint Commission's Medicare/Medicaid certification–based long term care accreditation

Standard LS.02.01.30

Assessment Question	Level of Compliance	Evidence of Compliance	Plan of Action/ Measure of Success (if needed)	Due Date
13. Are corridors serving adjoining areas not used for a portion of an air supply, air return, or exhaust air plenum? **Note:** *The Joint Commission interprets the NFPA code to allow incidental air movement between rooms and corridors (such as isolation rooms) because of the need for pressure differentials in health care organizations. In such cases, the direction of airflow is not the focus for this element of performance. For the purpose of fire protection, air transfer should be limited to the amount necessary to maintain positive or negative pressure differentials.* (For full text and any exceptions, refer to NFPA 90A-1999: 2-3.11.1) **C (EP 13)**				
14. Are at least two smoke compartments provided in existing buildings for every story that has more than 30 residents in sleeping rooms? (For full text and any exceptions, refer to NFPA 101-2000: 19.3.7.1) **A (EP 14)**				
15. Are at least two smoke compartments provided for every story in new buildings with resident sleeping or treatment rooms, and for nonsleeping stories that have an occupant capacity of 50 or more people, and on usable but unoccupied stories? (For full text and any exceptions, refer to NFPA 101-2000: 18.3.7.1 and 18.3.7.2) **A (EP 15)**				
16. Do smoke barriers limit the maximum size of each smoke compartment to 22,500 square feet? Is the travel distance from any point within the compartment to a smoke barrier door no more than 200 feet? (For full text and any exceptions, refer to NFPA 101-2000: 18/19.3.7.1) **C (EP 16)**				
17. Are smoke compartments sized to meet the requirements of NFPA 101-2000: 18/19.3.7.4? **C (EP 17)**				

Key: 0 = Insufficient compliance; 1 = Partial compliance; 2 = Satisfactory compliance; NA = Not applicable; **A** indicates scoring category A; **C** indicates scoring category C; ▲ indicates situational decision rules apply; △ indicates direct impact requirements apply; Ⓜ indicates Measure of success is needed; ☆ indicates this standard also applies to organizations seeking Joint Commission's Medicare/Medicaid certification–based long term care accreditation

Standard LS.02.01.30

Assessment Question	Level of Compliance	Evidence of Compliance	Plan of Action/ Measure of Success (if needed)	Due Date
18. Do smoke barriers extend from the floor slab to the floor or roof slab above, through any concealed spaces (such as those above suspended ceilings and interstitial spaces), and continuously from exterior wall to exterior wall? Are all penetrations properly sealed? (For full text and any exceptions, refer to NFPA 101-2000: 18/19.3.7.3) **C (EP 18)**				
19. In existing buildings, are smoke barriers fire-rated for more than 1/2 hour? In new buildings, are materials fire-rated for one hour? (For full text and any exceptions, refer to NFPA 101-2000: 18/19.3.7.3) **C (EP 19)**				
20. In existing buildings, when ducts penetrate smoke barriers, are they protected by approved smoke dampers that close when a smoke detector is activated? Is the detector located either within the duct system or in the area serving the smoke compartment? **Note:** *In existing buildings with two adjacent compartments with approved automatic sprinkler systems, dampers in common smoke barriers are not required.* (For full text and any exceptions, refer to NFPA 101-2000: 18/19.3.7.3 and 8.3.5.2) **C (EP 20)**				
21. Are air transfer openings through smoke barriers in ceiling spaces used as an unducted common plenum for either supply or return air protected by approved smoke dampers? (For full text and any exceptions, refer to NFPA 101-2000: 8.3.5.1) **C (EP 21)**				
22. Are fixed fire window assemblies in smoke barrier walls or doors fire-rated for 20 minutes and 25% or less of the size of the fire barrier in which they are installed? **Note:** *Existing window installations that have fixed wire glass or have fire-rated glazing, that are 1,296 square inches in size or smaller, and that are set in approved metal frames are acceptable.* (For full text and any exceptions, refer to NFPA 101-2000: 18.3.7.7, 19.3.7.5. and 8.2.3.2.2) **C (EP 22)**				

Key: 0 = Insufficient compliance; 1 = Partial compliance; 2 = Satisfactory compliance; NA = Not applicable; **A** indicates scoring category A; **C** indicates scoring category C; ▲ indicates situational decision rules apply; △ indicates direct impact requirements apply; Ⓜ indicates Measure of success is needed; ☆ indicates this standard also applies to organizations seeking Joint Commission's Medicare/Medicaid certification–based long term care accreditation

Standard LS.02.01.30

Assessment Question	Level of Compliance	Evidence of Compliance	Plan of Action/ Measure of Success (if needed)	Due Date
23. Are doors in smoke barriers self-closing or automatic-closing, constructed of 1-3/4 inch or thicker solid bonded wood core or equivalent, and fitted to resist the passage of smoke? Are gaps between meeting edges of door pairs no more than 1/8 inch wide, and undercuts no larger than 3/4 inch? Non-rated protective plates more than 48 inches above the bottom of the door are not compliant. (For full text and any exceptions, refer to NFPA 101-2000: 18/19.3.7.5, 18/19.3.7.6 and 8.3.4.1) **C (EP 23)**				
24. Does the organization meet all other *Life Safety Code* fire and smoke protection requirements related to NFPA 101-2000 18/19.3? **Note:** *For The Joint Commission's accepted amount of alcohol-based hand rub permitted within a single smoke compartment,* see *http://www.jointcommission.org/lsc.* **C (EP 24)**				

Standard LS.02.01.34

Assessment Question	Level of Compliance	Evidence of Compliance	Plan of Action/ Measure of Success (if needed)	Due Date
1. Does the fire alarm signal automatically transmit to one of the following: • An auxiliary fire alarm system with direct connection to the servicing fire department as described in NFPA 72-1999:6-16 • Central station service as described in NFPA 72-1999:5-2 • A proprietary supervising station system as described in NFPA 72-1999:5-3; or The Joint Commission policy for a manual transmission system • A remote supervising station fire alarm system as described in NFPA 72-1999: 5-4? **A (EP 1)** ⚠3				

Key: 0 = Insufficient compliance; 1 = Partial compliance; 2 = Satisfactory compliance; NA = Not applicable; **A** indicates scoring category A; **C** indicates scoring category C; ▲2 indicates situational decision rules apply; △3 indicates direct impact requirements apply; Ⓜ indicates Measure of success is needed; ☆ indicates this standard also applies to organizations seeking Joint Commission's Medicare/Medicaid certification–based long term care accreditation

Standard LS.02.01.34

Assessment Question	Level of Compliance	Evidence of Compliance	Plan of Action/ Measure of Success (if needed)	Due Date
2. Is the master fire alarm control panel located in a protected environment (an area enclosed with one-hour fire-rated walls and 3/4-hour fire-rated doors) that is continuously occupied or in an area with a smoke detector? (*See also* Standard LS.02.01.10, EP 5) (For full text and any exception, refer to NFPA 101-2000: 9.6.4; NFPA 72-1999:1-5.6 and 3-8.41) **A (EP 2)** ⚠3				
3. Is the remote ancillary annunciator panel in a location approved by the local fire department or its equivalent? (For full text and any exceptions, refer to NFPA 101-2000: 9.6.4) **C (EP 3)**				
4. Does the organization meet all other *Life Safety Code* fire alarm requirements related to NFPA 101-2000: 18.3.4/19.3.4? **C (EP 4)**				

Standard LS.02.01.35

Assessment Question	Level of Compliance	Evidence of Compliance	Plan of Action/ Measure of Success (if needed)	Due Date
1. Does the fire alarm system monitor approved automatic sprinkler system components? (For full text and any exceptions, refer to NFPA 101-2000: 18/19.3.5.2 and 9.7.2.2) **A (EP 1)** ⚠3				
2. Is the fire alarm system connected to water flow alarms? (For full text and any exceptions, refer to NFPA 101-2000: 9.7.2.2) **A (EP 2)** ⚠3				
3. Are piping supports for approved automatic sprinkler systems not damaged or loose? (For full text and any exceptions, refer to NFPA 25-1998: 2-2.2) **C (EP 3)**				
4. Is piping for approved automatic sprinkler systems not used to support any other item? (For full text and any exceptions, refer to NFPA 25-1998: 2-2.3) **C (EP 4)**				

Key: 0 = Insufficient compliance; 1 = Partial compliance; 2 = Satisfactory compliance; NA = Not applicable; **A** indicates scoring category A; **C** indicates scoring category C; ▲2 indicates situational decision rules apply; ⚠3 indicates direct impact requirements apply; Ⓜ indicates Measure of success is needed; ☆ indicates this standard also applies to organizations seeking Joint Commission's Medicare/Medicaid certification–based long term care accreditation

Standard LS.02.01.35

Assessment Question	Level of Compliance	Evidence of Compliance	Plan of Action/ Measure of Success (if needed)	Due Date
5. Are sprinkler heads undamaged and free from corrosion, foreign materials, and paint? (For full text and any exceptions, refer to NFPA 25-1998: 2-2.1.1) **C (EP 5)**				
6. Are 18 inches or more of open space maintained below the sprinkler deflector to the top of storage? (For full text and any exceptions, refer to NFPA 13-1999: 5-8.5.2.1) **Note:** *Perimeter wall and stack shelving may extend up to the ceiling when not located directly below a sprinkler head.* **C (EP 6)** ⚠3				
7. Do limited area sprinkler systems protecting isolated, hazardous areas connected to the domestic water system have a shut-off valve and are limited to six or fewer sprinkler heads? In new installations where two or more sprinkler heads serve one area, is water flow detection provided? (For full text and any exceptions, refer to NFPA 101-2000: 9.7.1.2) **A (EP 7)** ⚠3				
8. Is the travel distance from any point to the nearest fire extinguisher 75 feet or less? (For full text and any exceptions, refer to NFPA 101-2000: 18/19.3.5.6; NFPA 10-1998, 3-1.1) **C (EP 8)**				
9. Are Class K-type portable fire extinguishers located within 30 feet of grease-producing cooking devices such as deep fat fryers, ranges, griddles, or boilers? (For full text and any exceptions, refer to NFPA 101-2000: 18/19.3.5.6; NFPA 10-1998, 2-3.2) **C (EP 9)**				
10. Do grease-producing cooking devices such as deep fat fryers, ranges, griddles, or broilers have an exhaust hood, an exhaust duct system, and grease removal devices without mesh filters? (For full text and any exceptions, refer to NFPA 101-2000: 18/19.3.2.6; NFPA 96-1998:1-3.1) **C (EP 10)**				

Key: 0 = Insufficient compliance; 1 = Partial compliance; 2 = Satisfactory compliance; NA = Not applicable; **A** indicates scoring category A; **C** indicates scoring category C; ▲2 indicates situational decision rules apply; ⚠3 indicates direct impact requirements apply; Ⓜ indicates Measure of success is needed; ☆ indicates this standard also applies to organizations seeking Joint Commission's Medicare/Medicaid certification–based long term care accreditation

Standard LS.02.01.35

Assessment Question	Level of Compliance	Evidence of Compliance	Plan of Action/ Measure of Success (if needed)	Due Date
11. Does the automatic fire extinguishing system for grease-producing cooking devices activate the building fire alarm system? (For full text and any exceptions, refer to NFPA 101-2000: 18/19.3.2.6; NFPA 96-1998:7-1.1 and 7-6.2) **A (EP 11)** △3				
12. Does the automatic fire extinguishing system for grease-producing cooking devices deactivate the fuel source? (For full text and any exceptions, refer to NFPA 101-2000: 18/19.3.2.6; NFPA 96-1998:7-1.1 and 7-4.1) **A (EP 12)** △3				
13. Does the automatic fire extinguishing system for grease-producing cooking devices control the exhaust fans as designed? (For full text and any exceptions, refer to NFPA 101-2000: 18/19.3.2.6; NFPA 96-1998:7-1.1 and 8-1.5) **C (EP 13)**				
14. Does the organization meet all other *Life Safety Code* automatic extinguishing requirements related to NFPA 101-2000: 18/19.3.5? **C (EP 14)**				

Standard LS.02.01.40

Assessment Question	Level of Compliance	Evidence of Compliance	Plan of Action/ Measure of Success (if needed)	Due Date
1. Do windowless buildings or portions of windowless buildings meet the requirements of NFPA 101-2000: 18/19.4.1? (For full text and any exceptions, refer to NFPA 101-2000: 11.7) **C (EP 1)**				
2. Do new high-rise buildings have an approved automatic sprinkler system that meets the requirements of NFPA 101-2000: 18.4.2? (For full text and any exceptions, refer to NFPA 101-2000: 11.8) **A (EP 2)** △3				

Key: 0 = Insufficient compliance; 1 = Partial compliance; 2 = Satisfactory compliance; NA = Not applicable; **A** indicates scoring category A; **C** indicates scoring category C; ▲2 indicates situational decision rules apply; △3 indicates direct impact requirements apply; Ⓜ indicates Measure of success is needed; ☆ indicates this standard also applies to organizations seeking Joint Commission's Medicare/Medicaid certification–based long term care accreditation

Standard LS.02.01.50

Assessment Question	Level of Compliance	Evidence of Compliance	Plan of Action/ Measure of Success (if needed)	Due Date
1. Are fireplaces not permitted in resident sleeping areas? Where allowed, are they separated from resident sleeping spaces by construction fire rated for one hour or more? (For full text and any exceptions, refer to NFPA 101-2000: 18/19.5.2.2) **C (EP 1)**				
2. Are fireplaces equipped with a fireplace enclosure guaranteed against breakage up to a temperature of 650°F and constructed of heat-tempered glass or other approved material? (For full text and any exceptions, refer to NFPA 101-2000: 18/19.5.2.2) **C (EP 2)**				
3. Do newly installed fireplaces have a hearth that is raised at least 4 inches above the floor? (For full text and any exceptions, refer to NFPA 101-2000: 18.5.2.2) **C (EP 3)**				
4. Are new elevators equipped with firefighters service key recall and smoke detector automatic recall, firefighters service emergency in-car key operation, machine room smoke detectors, and elevator lobby smoke detectors? Do existing elevators that have a travel distance of 25 feet or more above or below the level that best serves the needs of firefighters also meet these requirements? (For full text and any exceptions, refer to NFPA 101-2000: 18/19.5.3 and 9.4.3) **C (EP 4)**				
5. Do trash chutes discharge into collection rooms that are not used for any other purpose? (For full text and any exceptions, refer to NFPA 101-2000: 18/19.5.4.3) **C (EP 5)**				
6. In new buildings, are linen and waste chutes vented through the roof and open to the atmosphere? (For full text and any exceptions, refer to NFPA 101-2000: 18.5.4.1; NFPA 82-1999:3-2.2.4) **C (EP 6)**				

Key: 0 = Insufficient compliance; 1 = Partial compliance; 2 = Satisfactory compliance; NA = Not applicable; **A** indicates scoring category A; **C** indicates scoring category C; ▲ indicates situational decision rules apply; △ indicates direct impact requirements apply; Ⓜ indicates Measure of success is needed; ☆ indicates this standard also applies to organizations seeking Joint Commission's Medicare/Medicaid certification–based long term care accreditation

Standard LS.02.01.50

Assessment Question	Level of Compliance	Evidence of Compliance	Plan of Action/ Measure of Success (if needed)	Due Date
7. Is an approved automatic sprinkler system located above the top of the linen and waste chute service openings on the lowest service levels and above the service door opening on alternate floor levels in buildings more than two stories high? (For full text and any exceptions, refer to NFPA 101-2000: 18/19.5.4.2; NFPA 82-1999:3-2.5.1) **C (EP 7)**				
8. In existing buildings, are linen and waste chute service inlet door assemblies fire rated for 3/4 hour (or for one hour when opening into a corridor)? In new buildings, are the inlet door assemblies fire rated for one hour (or for 1½ hours in chutes of four stories or more)? (For full text and any exceptions, refer to NFPA 101-2000: 18/19.5.4.1) **C (EP 8)**				
9. Do all linen and waste chute service doors, both inlet and discharge, have self-closing devices and positive latching? (For full text and any exceptions, refer to NFPA 101-2000: 18/19.5.4.1 and 8.2.3.2.3.1; NFPA 82-1999; 3-2.2.9) **Note:** *Discharge doors may be held open with a fusible link or electrical hold-open devices.* **C (EP 9)**				
10. Are linen and trash chute discharge door assemblies fire rated for one hour? (For full text and any exceptions, refer to NFPA 101-2000: 18/19.5.4.1 and 8.2.3.2.3.1) **C (EP 10)**				
11. Do linen and waste chutes discharge into a collection room separated from the corridor by walls fire rated for one hour? (For full text and any exceptions, refer to NFPA 101-2000: 18/19.5.4.1 and 18/19.3.2.1; NFPA 82-1999; 3-2.6.1) **C (EP 11)**				
12. Does the organization meet all other *Life Safety Code* building service requirements related to NFPA 101-2000: 18/19.5? **C (EP 12)**				

Key: 0 = Insufficient compliance; 1 = Partial compliance; 2 = Satisfactory compliance; NA = Not applicable; **A** indicates scoring category A; **C** indicates scoring category C; ▲2 indicates situational decision rules apply; △3 indicates direct impact requirements apply; Ⓜ indicates Measure of success is needed; ☆ indicates this standard also applies to organizations seeking Joint Commission's Medicare/Medicaid certification–based long term care accreditation

Standard LS.02.01.70

Assessment Question	Level of Compliance	Evidence of Compliance	Plan of Action/ Measure of Success (if needed)	Due Date
1. Does the organization prohibit all combustible decorations that are not flame retardant? (For full text and any exceptions, refer to NFPA 101-2000: 18/19.7.5.4) **C (EP 1)**				
2. Are soiled linen and trash receptacles (including recycling containers) larger than 32 gallons located in a room protected as a hazardous area? (For full text and any exceptions, refer to NFPA 101-2000: 18/19.7.5.5) **C (EP 2)**				
3. Does the organization prohibit portable space heaters within smoke compartments containing sleeping areas and resident treatment areas? (For full text and any exceptions, refer to NFPA 101-2000: 18/19.7.8) **C (EP 3)**				
4. Does the organization meet all other *Life Safety Code* operating feature requirements related to NFPA 101-2000: 18.7/19.7? (*See also* Standard EC.5.30, EP 1) **C (EP 4)**				

Key: 0 = Insufficient compliance; 1 = Partial compliance; 2 = Satisfactory compliance; NA = Not applicable; **A** indicates scoring category A; **C** indicates scoring category C; ▲ indicates situational decision rules apply; △ indicates direct impact requirements apply; Ⓜ indicates Measure of success is needed; ☆ indicates this standard also applies to organizations seeking Joint Commission's Medicare/Medicaid certification–based long term care accreditation

Management of Human Resources (HR)

Standard HR.1.10	**Standard Score:** ❑ Compliant ❑ Not Compliant			
Assessment Question	**Level of Compliance**	**Evidence of Compliance**	**Plan of Action/ Measure of Success (if needed)**	**Due Date**
1. Are nursing care and services provided 24 hours a day, 7 days a week, including relief personnel during vacation periods, sick leaves, emergencies, and holidays? **A (EP 2)** △3				
2. Except when waived by the state, does a registered nurse supervise nursing care at least 8 consecutive hours a day, 7 days a week? **A (EP 3)** △3				
3. If any resident(s) requires a registered nurse's services, is there at least one registered nurse, who is currently licensed by the state in which he or she practices, on duty* on each shift, 7 days a week?† **A (EP 4)** △3				

Standard HR.1.20 ★	**Standard Score:** ❑ Compliant ❑ Not Compliant			
Assessment Question	**Level of Compliance**	**Evidence of Compliance**	**Plan of Action/ Measure of Success (if needed)**	**Due Date**
1. Does the organization define the required competence and qualifications of staff in each program(s) or service(s)?‡ **A (EP 1)**				
2. When the organization requires current licensure, certification, or registration, but these credentials are not required by law or regulation, does the organization verify these credentials at the time of hire and upon expiration of the credentials?‡ **C (EP 2)** Ⓜ				

* The use of a registered nurse "on call" instead of "on duty" should be the exception and must not adversely affect resident care.

† If none of the residents requires a registered nurse's services, registered nurse coverage on each shift is optional; however, a licensed practical (vocational) nurse, who is currently licensed by the state in which he or she practices, is assigned to each shift seven days a week. Supervision is provided on all shifts.

‡ This assessment question is not applicable to organizations seeking Joint Commission's Medicare/Medicaid certification–based long term care accreditation.

Key: 0 = Insufficient compliance; 1 = Partial compliance; 2 = Satisfactory compliance; NA = Not applicable; **A** indicates scoring category A; **C** indicates scoring category C; ▲2 indicates situational decision rules apply; △3 indicates direct impact requirements apply; Ⓜ indicates Measure of success is needed; ☆ indicates this standard also applies to organizations seeking Joint Commission's Medicare/Medicaid certification–based long term care accreditation

Standard HR.1.20 ★

Assessment Question	Level of Compliance	Evidence of Compliance	Plan of Action/ Measure of Success (if needed)	Due Date
3. When current licensure, certification, or registration are required by law or regulation to practice a profession,* does the organization verify these credentials with the primary source at the time of hire and upon expiration of the credentials?† **A (EP 3)**				
4. Does the organization also verify the education, experience, and competence appropriate for assigned responsibilities?‡ **C (EP 4)** Ⓜ				
5. Does the organization also verify information on criminal background if required by law and regulation or organization policy?‡ **C (EP 5)** Ⓜ				
6. Does the organization also verify compliance with applicable health screening requirements if required by law and regulation or established by the organization?‡ **C (EP 6)** Ⓜ				
7. Is the information obtained from EPs 2–6 used in making decisions regarding staff job responsibilities?‡ **A (EP 7)** Ⓜ				
8. Do all staff that provide resident care, treatment, and services possess a license, certification, or registration as required by law and regulation? **A (EP 8)** ▲2				

* **Profession** is a specialized work function within society, generally performed by a professional. It often refers specifically to fields that require extensive study and mastery of specialized knowledge and skills.

† It is acceptable to verify current licensure, certification, or registration with the primary source via a secure electronic communication or by telephone, if this verification is documented. For additional information, *see* "primary source verification" in the *CAMLTC* Glossary. A primary source of information may designate another agency to communicate credentials information. The designated agency then can be used as a primary source. An external organization (for example, a credentials verification organization [CVO]) may be used to collect credentials information. A CVO must meet the CVO guidelines listed in the *CAMLTC* Glossary. This assessment question is not applicable to organizations seeking Joint Commission's Medicare/Medicaid certification–based long term care accreditation.

‡ This assessment question is not applicable to organizations seeking Joint Commission's Medicare/Medicaid certification–based long term care accreditation.

Key: 0 = Insufficient compliance; 1 = Partial compliance; 2 = Satisfactory compliance; NA = Not applicable; **A** indicates scoring category A; **C** indicates scoring category C; ▲2 indicates situational decision rules apply; △3 indicates direct impact requirements apply; Ⓜ indicates Measure of success is needed; ☆ indicates this standard also applies to organizations seeking Joint Commission's Medicare/Medicaid certification–based long term care accreditation

Standard HR.1.20 ★

Assessment Question	Level of Compliance	Evidence of Compliance	Plan of Action/ Measure of Success (if needed)	Due Date
9. Prior to the provision of care, treatment or services, are the qualifications and competence of a non-employee individual, brought into the organization by a licensed independent practitioner to provide care, treatment or services within the scope of the organization's services assessed by the organization and determined to be commensurate with the qualifications and competence required if the individual were to be employed by the organization to perform the same or similar services?* **C (EP 11)** Ⓜ ⚠3				
10. Does the organization review the qualifications, performance, and competence of each non-employee individual brought into the organization by a licensed independent practitioner to provide care, treatment, or services at the same frequency as individuals employed by the organization? **C (EP 12)** Ⓜ				
11. Does the staff supervise students when they provide resident care, treatment, and services as part of their training?† **A (EP 14)**				

Standard HR.1.25 ★

Standard Score: ❑ Compliant ❑ Not Compliant

Assessment Question	Level of Compliance	Evidence of Compliance	Plan of Action/ Measure of Success (if needed)	Due Date
1. Are disaster responsibilities assigned only when the following two conditions are present: the emergency management plan has been activated, and the organization is unable to meet immediate resident needs? **A (EP 1)**				
2. Does the organization identify in writing the individual(s) responsible for assigning disaster responsibilities? **A (EP 2)**				

* When the service to be provided by the individual is not currently performed by anyone employed by the organization, it is leadership's responsibility to consult the appropriate professional organization guidelines with respect to expectations for credentials and competence.

† This assessment question is not applicable to organizations seeking Joint Commission's Medicare/Medicaid certification–based long term care accreditation.

Key: 0 = Insufficient compliance; 1 = Partial compliance; 2 = Satisfactory compliance; NA = Not applicable; **A** indicates scoring category A; **C** indicates scoring category C; ▲2 indicates situational decision rules apply; ⚠3 indicates direct impact requirements apply; Ⓜ indicates Measure of success is needed; ☆ indicates this standard also applies to organizations seeking Joint Commission's Medicare/Medicaid certification–based long term care accreditation

Standard HR.1.25 ★

Assessment Question	Level of Compliance	Evidence of Compliance	Plan of Action/ Measure of Success (if needed)	Due Date
3. Does the organization describe in writing a mechanism (for example, direct observation, mentoring, and clinical record review) to oversee the professional performance of volunteer practitioners who are assigned disaster responsibilities? **A (EP 3)**				
4. Does the organization have a mechanism to identify volunteer practitioners that have been assigned disaster responsibilities? **A (EP 4)**				
5. For volunteer practitioners to be assigned disaster responsibilities, does the organization obtain for each volunteer practitioner at a minimum, a valid government-issued photo identification issued by a state or federal agency (e.g., driver's license or passport) and at least one of the following: • A current health care organization (such as a long term care, ambulatory care, laboratory, or hospital) picture identification card that clearly identifies professional designation • A current license, certification, or registration • Primary source verification of licensure, certification, or registration (if required by law and regulation to practice a profession) • Identification indicating that the individual is a member of a Disaster Medical Assistance Team (DMAT*), or MRC, ESAR-VHP, or other recognized state or federal organizations or groups • Identification indicating that the individual has been granted authority to render resident care, treatment, and services in disaster circumstances (such authority having been granted by a federal, state, or municipal entity) • Identification by current organization member(s) who possesses personal knowledge regarding the volunteer practitioner's qualifications? **A (EP 5)**				

* **DMAT** A group of medical and support personnel designed to provide emergency medical care during a disaster or other unusual event. The DMAT is a component of the National Disaster Medical System (NDMS). The Department of Health and Human Services in partnership with other Federal Agencies such as Department of Defense, Department of Veterans Affairs, and the Federal Emergency Management Agency administer the program.

Key: 0 = Insufficient compliance; 1 = Partial compliance; 2 = Satisfactory compliance; NA = Not applicable; **A** indicates scoring category A; **C** indicates scoring category C; ▲ indicates situational decision rules apply; △ indicates direct impact requirements apply; Ⓜ indicates Measure of success is needed; ☆ indicates this standard also applies to organizations seeking Joint Commission's Medicare/Medicaid certification–based long term care accreditation

Standard HR.1.25 ★				
Assessment Question	**Level of Compliance**	**Evidence of Compliance**	**Plan of Action/ Measure of Success (if needed)**	**Due Date**
6. Does primary source verification of licensure, certification, or registration (if required by law and regulation to practice a profession) begin as soon as the immediate situation is under control, and is completed within 72 hours from the time the volunteer practitioner presents to the organization?* **A (EP 6)**				
7. Does the organization oversee the professional practice of volunteer practitioners? **A (EP 7)**				
8. Does the organization make a decision (based on information obtained regarding the professional practice of the volunteer practitioner) within 72 hours related to the continuation of the disaster responsibilities initially assigned? **A (EP 8)**				

Standard HR.1.30 ★	Standard Score: ❑ Compliant ❑ Not Compliant			
Assessment Question	**Level of Compliance**	**Evidence of Compliance**	**Plan of Action/ Measure of Success (if needed)**	**Due Date**
1. Does the organization identify no fewer than two inpatient populations/settings for which data on staffing effectiveness are to be collected?† **A (EP 1)**				

* In the extraordinary circumstance that primary source verification of licensure, certification, or registration (if required by law and regulation to practice a profession) cannot be completed in 72 hours (for example, no means of communication or a lack of resources), it is expected that it be done as soon as possible. In this extraordinary circumstance, there must be documentation of the following: why primary source verification could not be performed in the required time frame; evidence of a demonstrated ability to continue to provide adequate care, treatment, and services; and an attempt to rectify the situation as soon as possible. Primary source verification of licensure, certification, or registration (if required by law and regulation to practice a profession) would not be required if the volunteer practitioner has not provided care, treatment, and services under the disaster responsibilities.

† If the organization has only one population/setting, the organization may collect data for that single population/setting.

Key: 0 = Insufficient compliance; 1 = Partial compliance; 2 = Satisfactory compliance; NA = Not applicable; **A** indicates scoring category A; **C** indicates scoring category C; ▲(2) indicates situational decision rules apply; △(3) indicates direct impact requirements apply; Ⓜ indicates Measure of success is needed; ☆ indicates this standard also applies to organizations seeking Joint Commission's Medicare/Medicaid certification–based long term care accreditation

Standard HR.1.30 ★

Assessment Question	Level of Compliance	Evidence of Compliance	Plan of Action/ Measure of Success (if needed)	Due Date
2. Does the organization identify the populations/settings (no less than two) based on assessment of relevant information or risk, including the following: • Knowledge about staffing issues likely to impact resident safety or quality of care • Resident population served • Type of setting • Review of existing data (for example, incident logs, sentinel event data, performance improvement reports) • Input from clinical staff who provide resident care? **Note:** *If the organization has only one population/setting, the organization need not apply these criteria.* **A (EP 2)**				
3. Are a minimum set of four indicators selected for each of the identified inpatient populations/settings?* **A (EP 3)**				
4. Does the organization determine the indicators for each population/setting based on assessment of relevant information or risk, including the following: • Knowledge about staffing issues likely to impact resident safety or quality of care • Resident population served • Type of setting • Review of existing data (for example, incident logs, sentinel event data, performance improvement reports) • Input from clinical staff who provide resident care? **A (EP 4)**				
5. Of the four indicators required for each population/setting, are two clinical/service indicators and two human resource indicators? **A (EP 5)**				
6. Is one of the human resource indicators and one of the clinical/service indicators selected from The Joint Commission's list of approved indicators?† **A (EP 6)**				

* Organizations are free to choose the same set, the same set in part or completely different measure sets for each identified population/setting.

† The Joint Commission's list of approved screening indicators consists of National Quality Forum (NQF)–endorsed voluntary consensus standards for nursing home care and Joint Commission consensus measures.

Key: 0 = Insufficient compliance; 1 = Partial compliance; 2 = Satisfactory compliance; NA = Not applicable; **A** indicates scoring category A; **C** indicates scoring category C; ▲ indicates situational decision rules apply; △ indicates direct impact requirements apply; Ⓜ indicates Measure of success is needed; ☆ indicates this standard also applies to organizations seeking Joint Commission's Medicare/Medicaid certification–based long term care accreditation

Standard HR.1.30 ★

Assessment Question	Level of Compliance	Evidence of Compliance	Plan of Action/ Measure of Success (if needed)	Due Date
7. Do the human resource indicators for all identified populations/settings include all nursing staff (including registered nurses, licensed practical nurses, and nursing assistants or aides)?* **A (EP 7)**				
8. When the organization chooses to include other practitioner groups (in addition to nursing staff in the human resource indicators for the identified populations/settings), is this decision based on the impact the absence of such care/service providers would be expected to have on resident outcomes? **A (EP 8)**				
9. Does the organization do the following: • Define the numerator and denominator for indicators chosen • Standardize the data element definitions for each indicator, including those indicators applied in more than one setting • Determine acceptable ranges/parameters/trigger levels† for the indicators? **A (EP 9)**				
10. Does the organization do the following for each population/setting selected: • Collect data for all indicators • Analyze data for all indicators • Review all indicator data together when analyzing variation from desired performance for additional information that may assist in identifying any potential causes of variation • Investigate to identify any staffing effectiveness issues when indicator data varies from expected • Take appropriate action in response to analyzed data? **A (EP 10)**				
11. Does the organization report at least annually to the leaders on the results of data analyses related to staffing effectiveness (*see* Standards PI.1.10 and PI.2.20) and any actions taken to resolve identified problems? **A (EP 11)**				

* Decisions regarding stratification of data by discipline are left to the organization.

† Acceptable ranges/parameters/trigger levels may be reflective of past performance, expert opinion, expert literature, or a combination of these. The ranges/parameters/trigger levels should be reasonable goals that are possible to attain. When desired ranges/parameters/trigger levels are not met, an investigation into the cause(s) is needed.

Key: 0 = Insufficient compliance; 1 = Partial compliance; 2 = Satisfactory compliance; NA = Not applicable; **A** indicates scoring category A; **C** indicates scoring category C; ▲ indicates situational decision rules apply; △ indicates direct impact requirements apply; Ⓜ indicates Measure of success is needed; ☆ indicates this standard also applies to organizations seeking Joint Commission's Medicare/Medicaid certification–based long term care accreditation

Standard HR.2.10 ★	**Standard Score: ❑ Compliant ❑ Not Compliant**			
Assessment Question	**Level of Compliance**	**Evidence of Compliance**	**Plan of Action/ Measure of Success (if needed)**	**Due Date**
1. Does the organization determine what key elements of orientation should occur before the staff and licensed independent practitioners provide care, treatment, and services? **A (EP 1)**				
2. Does the organization orient the staff and licensed independent practitioners to the identified key elements prior to the provision of care, treatment, and services? **C (EP 2) Ⓜ**				
3. As appropriate, does staff and licensed independent practitioner orientation address the organization's mission and goals? **C (EP 3) Ⓜ**				
4. As appropriate, does staff and licensed independent practitioner orientation address organizationwide policies and procedures (including safety and infection control) and relevant unit, setting, or program-specific policies and procedures? **C (EP 4) Ⓜ**				
5. As appropriate, does staff and licensed independent practitioner orientation address specific job duties and responsibilities and service, setting, or program-specific job duties and responsibilities related to safety and infection control? **C (EP 5) Ⓜ**				
6. As appropriate, does staff and licensed independent practitioner orientation address cultural diversity and sensitivity? **C (EP 7) Ⓜ**				
7. Does staff orientation include education about the rights of residents and ethical aspects of care, treatment, and services and the process used to address ethical issues? **C (EP 8) Ⓜ**				
8. Does staff orientation include education about the effects of psychotropic medications as appropriate? **C (EP 9) Ⓜ**				

Key: 0 = Insufficient compliance; 1 = Partial compliance; 2 = Satisfactory compliance; NA = Not applicable; **A** indicates scoring category A; **C** indicates scoring category C; ▲ indicates situational decision rules apply; △ indicates direct impact requirements apply; Ⓜ indicates Measure of success is needed; ☆ indicates this standard also applies to organizations seeking Joint Commission's Medicare/Medicaid certification–based long term care accreditation

Standard HR.2.20 ★	Standard Score: ❑ Compliant ❑ Not Compliant			
Assessment Question	**Level of Compliance**	**Evidence of Compliance**	**Plan of Action/ Measure of Success (if needed)**	**Due Date**
1. Can the staff and licensed independent practitioners, as appropriate, describe or demonstrate risks within the organization's environment? **C (EP 1)** Ⓜ				
2. Can the staff and licensed independent practitioners, as appropriate, describe or demonstrate actions to eliminate, minimize, or report risks? **C (EP 2)** Ⓜ				
3. Can the staff and licensed independent practitioners, as appropriate, describe or demonstrate procedures to follow in the event of an incident? **C (EP 3)** Ⓜ				
4. Can the staff and licensed independent practitioners, as appropriate, describe or demonstrate reporting processes for common problems, failures, and user errors? **C (EP 4)** Ⓜ				

Standard HR.2.30 ★	Standard Score: ❑ Compliant ❑ Not Compliant			
Assessment Question	**Level of Compliance**	**Evidence of Compliance**	**Plan of Action/ Measure of Success (if needed)**	**Due Date**
1. Does staff training occur when job responsibilities or duties change? **A (EP 1)**				
2. Do staff members participate in ongoing in-services, training, or other activities to increase knowledge of work-related issues? **C (EP 2)** Ⓜ				
3. Are ongoing in-services and other education and training of the staff appropriate to the needs of the population(s) served and do they comply with law and regulation? **C (EP 3)** Ⓜ				
4. Do ongoing in-services, training, or other staff activities emphasize specific job-related aspects of safety and infection prevention and control? **C (EP 4)** Ⓜ				

Key: 0 = Insufficient compliance; 1 = Partial compliance; 2 = Satisfactory compliance; NA = Not applicable; **A** indicates scoring category A; **C** indicates scoring category C; ▲2 indicates situational decision rules apply; △3 indicates direct impact requirements apply; Ⓜ indicates Measure of success is needed; ☆ indicates this standard also applies to organizations seeking Joint Commission's Medicare/Medicaid certification–based long term care accreditation

Standard HR.2.30 ★

Assessment Question	Level of Compliance	Evidence of Compliance	Plan of Action/ Measure of Success (if needed)	Due Date
5. Do ongoing in-services, training, or other staff education incorporate methods of team training, when appropriate? **C (EP 5) Ⓜ**				
6. Do ongoing in-services, training, or other staff education reinforce the need and ways to report unanticipated adverse events? **C (EP 6) Ⓜ**				
7. Are ongoing in-services or other staff education offered in response to learning needs identified through performance improvement findings and other data analysis (that is, data from staff surveys, performance evaluations, or other needs assessments)? **C (EP 7) Ⓜ**				
8. Is ongoing staff education documented? **C (EP 8) Ⓜ**				
9. Are staff members educated, as appropriate to their responsibilities, about psychotropic medications including the following: • The need for a medication in relation to the resident's documented diagnosis and condition • The potential for drug-drug and drug-food interactions • Adverse reactions to psychotropic medications • The use of a medication for an appropriate duration • The optimal dose • Frequent monitoring of the medication's effectiveness • Nonmedication interventions and alternatives developed through the interdisciplinary team assessment • Reduction and discontinuation of a medication? **A (EP 10)**				

Key: 0 = Insufficient compliance; 1 = Partial compliance; 2 = Satisfactory compliance; NA = Not applicable; **A** indicates scoring category A; **C** indicates scoring category C; ▲2 indicates situational decision rules apply; △3 indicates direct impact requirements apply; Ⓜ indicates Measure of success is needed; ☆ indicates this standard also applies to organizations seeking Joint Commission's Medicare/Medicaid certification–based long term care accreditation

Standard HR.3.10 ★	Standard Score: ❑ Compliant ❑ Not Compliant			
Assessment Question	**Level of Compliance**	**Evidence of Compliance**	**Plan of Action/ Measure of Success (if needed)**	**Due Date**
1. Is the competence assessment for the staff based on the population(s) served? **A (EP 1)**				
2. Is the competence assessment process for the staff based on the defined competencies to be required? **A (EP 2)**				
3. Is the competence assessment process for staff based on the defined competencies to be assessed during orientation? **A (EP 3)**				
4. Is the competence assessment process for staff based on the defined competencies that need to be assessed and reassessed on an ongoing basis, based on techniques, procedures, technology, equipment, or skills needed to provide care, treatment, and services? **A (EP 4)**				
5. Is the competence assessment process for staff based on a defined time frame for how often competency assessments are performed for each person, minimally, once in the three year accreditation cycle and in accordance with law and regulation? **A (EP 5)**				
6. Is the competence assessment process for staff based on the assessment methods (appropriate to determine the skill being assessed)? **A (EP 6)**				
7. Is the competence assessment process for staff based on the use of qualified individuals to assess competence?* **A (EP 7)**				
8. Does the organization assess and document staff's ability to carry out assigned responsibilities safely, competently, and in a timely manner upon completion of orientation? **C (EP 8) Ⓜ**				

* When there is no qualified individual in the organization that performs comparable care, treatment, and services, the organization may utilize qualified staff from other organizations to assist with the assessment of competence, or consult the appropriate professional organization guidelines with respect to expectations for competence and use these guidelines to assess competence.

Key: 0 = Insufficient compliance; 1 = Partial compliance; 2 = Satisfactory compliance; NA = Not applicable; **A** indicates scoring category A; **C** indicates scoring category C; ▲ indicates situational decision rules apply; △ indicates direct impact requirements apply; Ⓜ indicates Measure of success is needed; ☆ indicates this standard also applies to organizations seeking Joint Commission's Medicare/Medicaid certification–based long term care accreditation

Standard HR.3.10 ★

Assessment Question	Level of Compliance	Evidence of Compliance	Plan of Action/ Measure of Success (if needed)	Due Date
9. Does the organization assess staff according to its competence assessment process? **C (EP 9) Ⓜ**				
10. When improvement activities lead to a determination that a person with performance problems is unable or unwilling to improve, does the organization take appropriate action (which may include modifying the person's job assignments)? **A (EP 10)**				

Standard HR.3.20

Standard Score: ❑ Compliant ❑ Not Compliant

Assessment Question	Level of Compliance	Evidence of Compliance	Plan of Action/ Measure of Success (if needed)	Due Date
1. Does the organization conduct performance evaluations periodically at time frames identified by the organization (at a minimum, at least once in the three-year accreditation cycle)? **C (EP 1) Ⓜ**				
2. Is performance evaluated based on the performance expectations described in job descriptions or through the privileging process? **C (EP 2) Ⓜ**				
3. Are performance evaluations documented? **C (EP 4) Ⓜ**				

Standard HR.4.10 ★

Standard Score: ❑ Compliant ❑ Not Compliant

Assessment Question	Level of Compliance	Evidence of Compliance	Plan of Action/ Measure of Success (if needed)	Due Date
1. Does the organization have a defined process approved by the leaders for appointing and reappointing licensed independent practitioners? **A (EP 5)**				

Key: 0 = Insufficient compliance; 1 = Partial compliance; 2 = Satisfactory compliance; NA = Not applicable; **A** indicates scoring category A; **C** indicates scoring category C; ▲ indicates situational decision rules apply; △ indicates direct impact requirements apply; Ⓜ indicates Measure of success is needed; ☆ indicates this standard also applies to organizations seeking Joint Commission's Medicare/Medicaid certification–based long term care accreditation

Standard HR.4.10 ★

Assessment Question	Level of Compliance	Evidence of Compliance	Plan of Action/ Measure of Success (if needed)	Due Date
2. At the time of initial granting of privileges, does the organization verify, by viewing a valid government-issued photo identification issued by a state or federal agency (e.g., drivers license or passport), that the individual being granted (clinical privileges) is the same individual identified in the credentialing documents?* **A (EP 6)**				
3. As required by the credentialing process, does the organization do the following: • Verifies in writing current licensure, from the primary source at time of initial granting, renewal and revision of clinical privileges, and prior to licensure expiration • Verifies in writing training (required by the organization to perform the clinical privileges) from the primary source at the time of initial granting and renewal and revision of clinical privileges • Verifies in writing current competence from the primary source at time of initial granting of clinical privileges • Obtains a statement from the applicant at the time of initial granting, renewal, or revision of clinical privileges that no health problems exist that could effect his or her ability to perform the privileges requested?†‡ **A (EP 7)**				
4. Do all licensed independent practitioners that provide resident care possess a license, certification, or registration as required by law and regulation? **A (EP 8)** ▲2				

* Any licensed independent practitioner whose only role is to cover for another licensed independent practitioner(s) is exempt from this requirement.

† Verification of current licensure with the primary source through a secure electronic communication or by telephone is acceptable, if this verification is documented. For additional information, *see* "primary source verification" in the *CAMLTC* Glossary. An external organization (for example, a credentials verification organization [CVO] or a Joint Commission–accredited health care organization functioning as a CVO) may be used to collect credentialing information. Both of these organizations must meet the CVO guidelines listed in the Glossary. A primary source of verified information may designate to an agency the role of communicating credentials information. The delegated agency then becomes acceptable to be used as a primary source.

‡ Organizations should consider the applicability of the Americans with Disabilities Act (ADA) to their credentialing and privileging activities, and, if applicable, review their policies and procedures. Federal entities are required to comply with the Rehabilitation Act of 1974.

Key: 0 = Insufficient compliance; 1 = Partial compliance; 2 = Satisfactory compliance; NA = Not applicable; **A** indicates scoring category A; **C** indicates scoring category C; ▲2 indicates situational decision rules apply; △3 indicates direct impact requirements apply; Ⓜ indicates Measure of success is needed; ☆ indicates this standard also applies to organizations seeking Joint Commission's Medicare/Medicaid certification–based long term care accreditation

Standard HR.4.10 ★

Assessment Question	Level of Compliance	Evidence of Compliance	Plan of Action/ Measure of Success (if needed)	Due Date
5. Does the governing body* do the following: • Review recommendations made by the medical director • Review documentation on which recommendations are based • Review records of any hearings or appeals addressing adverse decisions • Grant appropriate clinical privileges? **A (EP 11)**				
6. When the attending licensed independent practitioner designates a licensed independent practitioner (who is not privileged in the organization) to cover in his/her absence for a period of no more than 72 consecutive hours, are the following requirements met: The medical director and the attending licensed independent practitioner determine that the covering licensed independent practitioner can perform those types of care, treatment, and services that are required? **A (EP 22)**				
7. When the attending licensed independent practitioner designates a licensed independent practitioner (who is not privileged in the organization) to cover in his/her absence for a period of no more than 72 consecutive hours, are the following requirements met: The organization verifies the current licensure of the covering licensed independent practitioner from the primary source prior to his or her provision of care, treatment and services?† **A (EP 23)**				
8. When the attending licensed independent practitioner designates a licensed independent practitioner (who is not privileged in the organization) to cover in his/her absence for a period of no more than 72 consecutive hours, are the following requirements met: A documented review of orders issued by the covering licensed independent practitioner is conducted by the attending licensed independent practitioner upon return in the time frame defined by the organization? **C (EP 24)** Ⓜ				

* The organization administrator or a committee of two or more governing body members may substitute for a governing body.

† It may be more efficient to obtain a list of possible covering licensed independent practitioners ahead of time and verify licensure from the primary source in advance of the licensed independent practitioner actually covering for the attending.

Key: 0 = Insufficient compliance; 1 = Partial compliance; 2 = Satisfactory compliance; NA = Not applicable; **A** indicates scoring category A; **C** indicates scoring category C; ▲ indicates situational decision rules apply; △ indicates direct impact requirements apply; Ⓜ indicates Measure of success is needed; ☆ indicates this standard also applies to organizations seeking Joint Commission's Medicare/Medicaid certification–based long term care accreditation

Standard HR.4.10 ★

Assessment Question	Level of Compliance	Evidence of Compliance	Plan of Action/ Measure of Success (if needed)	Due Date
9. When the attending licensed independent practitioner designates a licensed independent practitioner (who is not privileged in the organization) to cover in his/her absence for a period of no more than 72 consecutive hours, are the following requirements met: The modified process for credentialing and privileging can only be utilized for a covering licensed independent practitioner for up to 12 days* per calendar year but no more than 72 consecutive hours?† **A (EP 25)**				

Standard HR.4.20 ★

Standard Score: ❑ Compliant ❑ Not Compliant

Assessment Question	Level of Compliance	Evidence of Compliance	Plan of Action/ Measure of Success (if needed)	Due Date
1. Based on the scope of services provided, does the organization establish criteria for each privilege and do these criteria include the following: • Current licensure and/or certification as appropriate, verified with the primary source • Successful completion of training specific to each requested privilege, verified with the primary source • Peer‡ and or faculty recommendation • Evidence of the ability to perform the requested privilege? **A (EP 1)**				

* A day is considered as any portion of the day (whether it is 1 hour or 24 hours).

† If a licensed independent practitioner will be covering for more than 12 days per calendar year or more than 72 consecutive hours, this individual must undergo the full process for credentialing and privileging by the organization.

‡ *See* the Glossary in the *CAMLTC* for definition of peer recommendation.

Key: 0 = Insufficient compliance; 1 = Partial compliance; 2 = Satisfactory compliance; NA = Not applicable; **A** indicates scoring category A; **C** indicates scoring category C; ▲ indicates situational decision rules apply; △ indicates direct impact requirements apply; Ⓜ indicates Measure of success is needed; ☆ indicates this standard also applies to organizations seeking Joint Commission's Medicare/Medicaid certification–based long term care accreditation

Standard HR.4.20 ★

Assessment Question	Level of Compliance	Evidence of Compliance	Plan of Action/ Measure of Success (if needed)	Due Date
2. Before granting, renewing, or revising privileges, does the medical director evaluate the following: • Challenges to any licensure or registration • Voluntary and involuntary relinquishment of any license or registration • Voluntary and involuntary termination of medical staff membership at another organization • Voluntary and involuntary limitation, reduction, or loss of clinical privileges • Any evidence of an unusual pattern or an excessive number of professional liability actions resulting in a final judgment against the applicant • Documentation as to the applicant's health status? **A (EP 2)**				
3. Does the organization query the National Practitioner Data Bank (NPDB) at the time of initial granting of privileges, as well as at least every two years thereafter for information on physicians and dentists granted clinical privileges? **A (EP 3)**				
4. Are clinical privileges for licensed independent practitioners delineated according to organization policy and based on the licensed independent practitioner's current credentials and competence, as well as the population(s) served and the types of care, treatment, and services provided in the organization? **C (EP 4) Ⓜ**				
5. Is the decision by leaders to appoint licensed independent practitioners based on the credentials information obtained? **A (EP 5)**				
6. Is the licensed independent practitioner notified in writing of the governing body's decision? **C (EP 6) Ⓜ**				
7. Do individuals with clinical privileges practice within the scope of their privileges? **A (EP 7) △3**				

Key: 0 = Insufficient compliance; 1 = Partial compliance; 2 = Satisfactory compliance; NA = Not applicable; **A** indicates scoring category A; **C** indicates scoring category C; ▲ indicates situational decision rules apply; △ indicates direct impact requirements apply; Ⓜ indicates Measure of success is needed; ☆ indicates this standard also applies to organizations seeking Joint Commission's Medicare/Medicaid certification–based long term care accreditation

Standard HR.4.30 ★	**Standard Score: ❑ Compliant ❑ Not Compliant**			
Assessment Question	**Level of Compliance**	**Evidence of Compliance**	**Plan of Action/ Measure of Success (if needed)**	**Due Date**
1. Do policies and procedures, rules, or regulations describe the process for granting temporary privileges for meeting the important needs of residents or for new applicants? **A (EP 1)**				
2. To grant temporary privileges to meet the important needs of residents, is there verification (which can be done by telephone) of current licensure and current competence? **A (EP 2)**				
3. To grant temporary privileges for new applicants, is there verification (which may be done by telephone) of the following: • Current licensure • Relevant education, training, or experience • Current competence • Ability to perform the privileges requested • A query and evaluation of the NPDB? **A (EP 3)**				
4. To grant temporary privileges for new applicants, does the applicant have the following: • A complete application • No current or previously successful challenge to licensure or registration • Not been subject to involuntary termination of professional or medical staff membership at another organization, when applicable to the discipline • Not been subject to involuntary limitation, reduction, denial, or loss of privileges, when applicable to the discipline? **A (EP 4)**				
5. Does the administrator or designee grant temporary privileges for meeting important resident needs and for new applicants upon recommendation of clinical leadership or the medical director? **A (EP 5)**				
6. Are temporary privileges for new applicants granted for no more than 120 days? **A (EP 6)**				

Key: 0 = Insufficient compliance; 1 = Partial compliance; 2 = Satisfactory compliance; NA = Not applicable; **A** indicates scoring category A; **C** indicates scoring category C; ▲ indicates situational decision rules apply; △ indicates direct impact requirements apply; Ⓜ indicates Measure of success is needed; ☆ indicates this standard also applies to organizations seeking Joint Commission's Medicare/Medicaid certification–based long term care accreditation

Standard HR.4.35 ★	**Standard Score:** ❑ Compliant ❑ Not Compliant			
Assessment Question	**Level of Compliance**	**Evidence of Compliance**	**Plan of Action/ Measure of Success (if needed)**	**Due Date**
1. Are disaster privileges granted only when the following two conditions are present: the emergency management plan has been activated, and the organization is unable to meet immediate resident needs? **A (EP 1)**				
2. Does the organization identify in writing the individual(s) responsible for granting disaster privileges? **A (EP 2)**				
3. Does the organization describe in writing a mechanism (for example, direct observation, mentoring, and clinical record review) to oversee the professional performance of volunteer practitioners who receive disaster privileges? **A (EP 3)**				
4. Does the organization have a mechanism to identify the volunteer practitioners who have been granted disaster privileges? **A (EP 4)**				

Key: 0 = Insufficient compliance; 1 = Partial compliance; 2 = Satisfactory compliance; NA = Not applicable; **A** indicates scoring category A; **C** indicates scoring category C; ▲ indicates situational decision rules apply; △ indicates direct impact requirements apply; Ⓜ indicates Measure of success is needed; ☆ indicates this standard also applies to organizations seeking Joint Commission's Medicare/Medicaid certification–based long term care accreditation

Standard HR.4.35 ★

Assessment Question	Level of Compliance	Evidence of Compliance	Plan of Action/ Measure of Success (if needed)	Due Date
5. In order for volunteers to be considered eligible to act as licensed independent practitioners, does the organization obtain for each volunteer practitioner at a minimum, a valid government-issued photo identification issued by a state or federal agency (e.g., driver's license or passport) and at least one of the following: • A current health care organization (such as a long term care, ambulatory care, or hospital) picture identification card that clearly identifies professional designation • A current license to practice • Primary source verification of the license • Identification indicating that the individual is a member of a Disaster Medical Assistance Team (DMAT*), or MRC, ESAR-VHP, or other recognized state or federal organizations or groups • Identification indicating that the individual has been granted authority to render resident care, treatment, and services in disaster circumstances (such authority having been granted by a federal, state, or municipal entity) • Identification by current organization member(s) who possesses personal knowledge regarding the volunteer's ability to act as a licensed independent practitioner during a disaster? **A (EP 5)**				
6. Does primary source verification of licensure begin as soon as the immediate situation is under control, and is completed within 72 hours from the time the volunteer practitioner presents to the organization?† **A (EP 6)**				
7. Does the organization oversee the professional practice of volunteer licensed independent practitioners? **A (EP 7)**				

* **DMAT** A group of medical and support personnel designed to provide emergency medical care during a disaster or other unusual event. The DMAT is a component of the National Disaster Medical System (NDMS). The Department of Health and Human Services in partnership with other federal agencies such as Department of Defense, Department of Veterans Affairs, and the Federal Emergency Management Agency administer the program.

† In the extraordinary circumstance that primary source verification cannot be completed in 72 hours (for example, no means of communication or a lack of resources), it is expected that it be done as soon as possible. In this extraordinary circumstance, there must be documentation of the following: why primary source verification could not be performed in the required time frame; evidence of a demonstrated ability to continue to provide adequate care, treatment, and services; and an attempt to rectify the situation as soon as possible. Primary source verification of licensure would not be required if the volunteer practitioner has not provided care, treatment, and services under the disaster privileges.

Key: 0 = Insufficient compliance; 1 = Partial compliance; 2 = Satisfactory compliance; NA = Not applicable; **A** indicates scoring category A; **C** indicates scoring category C; ▲ indicates situational decision rules apply; △ indicates direct impact requirements apply; Ⓜ indicates Measure of success is needed; ☆ indicates this standard also applies to organizations seeking Joint Commission's Medicare/Medicaid certification–based long term care accreditation

Standard HR.4.35 ★

Assessment Question	Level of Compliance	Evidence of Compliance	Plan of Action/ Measure of Success (if needed)	Due Date
8. Does the organization make a decision (based on information obtained regarding the professional practice of the volunteer) within 72 hours related to the continuation of the disaster privileges initially granted? **A (EP 8)**				

Standard HR.4.40 ★

Standard Score: ❑ Compliant ❑ Not Compliant

Assessment Question	Level of Compliance	Evidence of Compliance	Plan of Action/ Measure of Success (if needed)	Due Date
1. Does the organization develop a fair hearing and appeals process that is designed to provide a uniform and fair process? **A (EP 1)**				
2. Does the organization develop a fair hearing and appeals process that has a mechanism to schedule a hearing of such requests? **A (EP 2)**				
3. Does the organization develop a fair hearing and appeals process that has identified the procedures for the hearings to follow? **A (EP 3)**				
4. Does the organization develop a fair hearing and appeals process that identifies or defines the composition of the hearing committee? **A (EP 4)**				
5. Does the organization develop a fair hearing and appeals process that provides for a mechanism to appeal an adverse decision through the governance function? **A (EP 5)**				

Key: 0 = Insufficient compliance; 1 = Partial compliance; 2 = Satisfactory compliance; NA = Not applicable; **A** indicates scoring category A; **C** indicates scoring category C; ▲2 indicates situational decision rules apply; △3 indicates direct impact requirements apply; Ⓜ indicates Measure of success is needed; ☆ indicates this standard also applies to organizations seeking Joint Commission's Medicare/Medicaid certification–based long term care accreditation

Standard HR.4.50 ★	Standard Score: ❑ Compliant ❑ Not Compliant			
Assessment Question	**Level of Compliance**	**Evidence of Compliance**	**Plan of Action/ Measure of Success (if needed)**	**Due Date**
1. Do policies and procedures or rules and regulations specify a period of no more than two years between appointments and reappointments and between granting, renewing, and revising clinical privileges? **A (EP 1)**				
2. Do credential files for licensed independent practitioners contain substantive information and indicate that clinical privileges are reviewed or revised at least every two years and are revised as needed; in addition, are appointments and reappointments made for a period of no more than two years? **C (EP 2) Ⓜ**				
3. Is a reappraisal conducted at the time of reappointment, renewal, or revision of clinical privileges? **A (EP 3)**				
4. Does the reappraisal address current competence and include the following: • Confirmation of adherence to organization policies and procedures, rules, or regulations • Relevant information from organization performance improvement activities when evaluating professional performance, judgment, and clinical or technical skills • Any results of review of the individual's clinical performance • Clinical performance in the organization that is outside acceptable standards? **A (EP 4)**				
5. Do the credentials files contain clear evidence that the full range of privileges has been included in the reappraisal? **A (EP 5)**				

Key: 0 = Insufficient compliance; 1 = Partial compliance; 2 = Satisfactory compliance; NA = Not applicable; **A** indicates scoring category A; **C** indicates scoring category C; ▲ indicates situational decision rules apply; △ indicates direct impact requirements apply; Ⓜ indicates Measure of success is needed; ☆ indicates this standard also applies to organizations seeking Joint Commission's Medicare/Medicaid certification–based long term care accreditation

Management of Information (IM)

Standard IM.1.10 ★	**Standard Score: ❑ Compliant ❑ Not Compliant**			
Assessment Question	**Level of Compliance**	**Evidence of Compliance**	**Plan of Action/ Measure of Success (if needed)**	**Due Date**
1. Does the organization base its information management processes on an assessment of internal and external information needs and does the assessment identify the following: • The flow of information throughout an organization, including information storage and feedback mechanisms • The data and information needed: within and among departments, services, or programs; within and among the staff, the administration, and the governance for supporting relationships with outside services and contractors; with licensing, accrediting, and regulatory bodies; with purchasers, payers, and employers; for supporting informational needs between the organization and the residents; and for participating in research and databases? **A (EP 1)**				
2. To guide development of processes for managing information used internally and externally, does the organization assess its information management needs based on the following: • Its mission • Its goals • Its services • Personnel • Resident safety considerations • Quality of care, treatment, and services • Mode(s) of service delivery • Resources • Access to affordable technology • Identification of barriers to effective communication among caregivers? **A (EP 2)**				
3. Does the organization base its management, staffing, and material resource allocations for information management on the scope and complexity of care, treatment, and services provided? **A (EP 3)**				
4. Do identified staff participate in assessment, selection, integration, and use of information management systems for clinical/service and organization information? **A (EP 4)**				

Key: 0 = Insufficient compliance; 1 = Partial compliance; 2 = Satisfactory compliance; NA = Not applicable; **A** indicates scoring category A; **C** indicates scoring category C; ▲ indicates situational decision rules apply; △ indicates direct impact requirements apply; Ⓜ indicates Measure of success is needed; ☆ indicates this standard also applies to organizations seeking Joint Commission's Medicare/Medicaid certification–based long term care accreditation

Standard IM.1.10 ★

Assessment Question	Level of Compliance	Evidence of Compliance	Plan of Action/ Measure of Success (if needed)	Due Date
5. Does the organization have an ongoing process to assess the needs of the organization, departments, and individuals for knowledge-based information? **A (EP 5)**				
6. Does the organization use the assessment for knowledge-based information as a basis for planning? **A (EP 6)**				

Standard IM.2.10 ★

Standard Score: ❑ Compliant ❑ Not Compliant

Assessment Question	Level of Compliance	Evidence of Compliance	Plan of Action/ Measure of Success (if needed)	Due Date
1. Does the organization have a written policy(ies) for addressing the privacy* and confidentiality† of information, that is based on and consistent with law or regulation? **A (EP 1)**				
2. Has the organization's policy, including significant changes to the policy, been effectively communicated to staff? **A (EP 2)**				
3. Does the organization implement the policy? **A (EP 3)**				
4. Does the organization monitor compliance with the policy? **A (EP 4)**				
5. Does the organization improve privacy and confidentiality of information by monitoring information and developments in technology? **A (EP 5)**				
6. Are individuals about whom identifiable health data and information are maintained or collected made aware of how the data will be used and whether it will be disclosed? **C (EP 6)** Ⓜ				

* **Privacy** An individual's right to limit the disclosure of personal information.

† **Confidentiality** The safekeeping of data/information so as to restrict access to individuals who have need, reason, and permission for such access.

Key: 0 = Insufficient compliance; 1 = Partial compliance; 2 = Satisfactory compliance; NA = Not applicable; **A** indicates scoring category A; **C** indicates scoring category C; ▲ indicates situational decision rules apply; △ indicates direct impact requirements apply; Ⓜ indicates Measure of success is needed; ☆ indicates this standard also applies to organizations seeking Joint Commission's Medicare/Medicaid certification–based long term care accreditation

Standard IM.2.10 ★				
Assessment Question	**Level of Compliance**	**Evidence of Compliance**	**Plan of Action/ Measure of Success (if needed)**	**Due Date**
7. Are personal identifiers removed to the extent possible for uses and disclosures of health information, consistent with maintaining the usefulness of the information? **A (EP 7)**				
8. Is protected health information* used for the purposes identified or as required by law or regulation and not further disclosed without resident authorization? **C (EP 8) Ⓜ**				
9. Does the organization preserve the privacy and confidentiality of data and information identified as sensitive? **A (EP 9)**				

Standard IM.2.20	Standard Score: ❑ Compliant ❑ Not Compliant			
Assessment Question	**Level of Compliance**	**Evidence of Compliance**	**Plan of Action/ Measure of Success (if needed)**	**Due Date**
1. Does the organization have a written policy(ies) for addressing information security, including data integrity† that is based on and consistent with law or regulation? **A (EP 1)**				
2. Has the organization's policy, including changes to the policy, been communicated to staff? **A (EP 2)**				
3. Does the organization implement the policy? **A (EP 3)**				
4. Does the organization monitor compliance with the policy? **A (EP 4)**				
5. Does the organization improve information security, including data integrity, by monitoring information and developments in technology? **A (EP 5)**				

* **Protected health information** Health information that contains information such that an individual person can be identified as the subject of that information.

† **Integrity** In the context of data security, data integrity means the protection of data from accidental or unauthorized intentional change.

Key: 0 = Insufficient compliance; 1 = Partial compliance; 2 = Satisfactory compliance; NA = Not applicable; **A** indicates scoring category A; **C** indicates scoring category C; ▲ indicates situational decision rules apply; △ indicates direct impact requirements apply; Ⓜ indicates Measure of success is needed; ☆ indicates this standard also applies to organizations seeking Joint Commission's Medicare/Medicaid certification–based long term care accreditation

Standard IM.2.20

Assessment Question	Level of Compliance	Evidence of Compliance	Plan of Action/ Measure of Success (if needed)	Due Date
6. Does the organization develop and implement controls to safeguard data and information, including the clinical record, against loss, destruction, and tampering? **A (EP 6)**				
7. Do controls to safeguard data and information include the following: • Policies indicating when the removal of records is permitted • Protection against unauthorized intrusion, corruption, or damage • Minimization of the risk of falsification of data and information • Guidelines for preventing the loss and destruction of records • Guidelines for destroying copies of records • Protection of records in a manner that minimizes the possibility of damage from fire and water? **A (EP 7)**				
8. Do policies and procedures, including plans for implementation, for electronic information systems address the following: data integrity, authentication,* nonrepudiation,† encryption‡ as warranted, and auditability,§ as appropriate to the system and types of information, for example, resident information and billing information? **A (EP 8)**				

* **Authentication** The validation of correctness for both the information itself and the person who is the author or user of information.

† **Nonrepudiation** The inability to dispute a document's content or authorship.

‡ **Encryption** The process of transforming plain text (readable) into cipher text that is unreadable without a special software key.

§ **Auditability** The ability to do a methodical examination and verification of all information activities such as entering and accessing.

Key: 0 = Insufficient compliance; 1 = Partial compliance; 2 = Satisfactory compliance; NA = Not applicable; **A** indicates scoring category A; **C** indicates scoring category C; ▲ indicates situational decision rules apply; △ indicates direct impact requirements apply; Ⓜ indicates Measure of success is needed; ☆ indicates this standard also applies to organizations seeking Joint Commission's Medicare/Medicaid certification–based long term care accreditation

Standard IM.2.30	Standard Score: ❑ Compliant ❑ Not Compliant			
Assessment Question	**Level of Compliance**	**Evidence of Compliance**	**Plan of Action/ Measure of Success (if needed)**	**Due Date**
1. Does the organization have a business continuity/disaster recovery plan for its information systems? **A (EP 1)**				
2. For electronic systems, does the business continuity/disaster recovery plan include the following: • Plans for scheduled and unscheduled interruptions, which includes end-user training with the downtime procedures • Contingency plans for operational interruptions (hardware, software, or other systems failure) • Plans for minimal interruptions as a result of scheduled downtime • An emergency service plan • A back-up system (electronic or manual) • Data retrieval, including retrieval from storage and information presently in the operating system, retrieval of data in the event of system interruption, and back up of data? **A (EP 2)**				
3. Is the plan tested periodically as defined by the organization (or in accordance with law or regulation) to ensure that the business interruption back-up techniques are effective? **A (EP 3)**				
4. Is the business continuity/disaster recovery plan implemented when information systems are interrupted? **A (EP 4)**				

Standard IM.3.10 ★	Standard Score: ❑ Compliant ❑ Not Compliant			
Assessment Question	**Level of Compliance**	**Evidence of Compliance**	**Plan of Action/ Measure of Success (if needed)**	**Due Date**
1. Are information technology industry standards or organization policies used and address the following: • Uniform data definitions • Data capture • Data display • Data transmission **A (EP 1)**				

Key: 0 = Insufficient compliance; 1 = Partial compliance; 2 = Satisfactory compliance; NA = Not applicable; **A** indicates scoring category A; **C** indicates scoring category C; ▲ indicates situational decision rules apply; △ indicates direct impact requirements apply; Ⓜ indicates Measure of success is needed; ☆ indicates this standard also applies to organizations seeking Joint Commission's Medicare/Medicaid certification–based long term care accreditation

Standard IM.3.10 ★

Assessment Question	Level of Compliance	Evidence of Compliance	Plan of Action/ Measure of Success (if needed)	Due Date
2. Is there a standardized list of abbreviations, acronyms, symbols, and dose designation that are not to be used throughout the organization? *(The preceding requirement is not scored here. It is scored at NPSG.02.02.01.)* **(EP 2)**				
3. Are minimum data sets, terminology, definitions, classifications, vocabulary, and nomenclature, including abbreviations, acronyms, symbols, and dose designations, standardized throughout the organization? **A (EP 3)**				
4. Are quality control systems used to monitor data content and collection activities? • Does the method used provide for timely and economical data collection with the degree of accuracy, completeness, and discrimination necessary for their intended use? • Does the method used minimize bias in the data and regularly assesses the data's reliability, validity, and accuracy? • Are those responsible for collecting and reviewing the data accountable for information accuracy and completeness? **A (EP 4)**				
5. Are storage and retrieval systems designed to support organization needs for clinical/service and organization-specific information? • Are storage and retrieval systems designed to balance the ability to retrieve data and information with the intended use for the data and information? • Are storage and retrieval systems designed to balance security and confidentiality issues with accessibility? • Are systems for paper and electronic records designed to reduce disruption or inaccessibility during such times as diminished staffing and scheduled and unscheduled downtimes of electronic information systems? **A (EP 5)**				
6. Are data and information retained for sufficient time to comply with law or regulation? **A (EP 6)**				

Key: 0 = Insufficient compliance; 1 = Partial compliance; 2 = Satisfactory compliance; NA = Not applicable; **A** indicates scoring category A; **C** indicates scoring category C; ▲ indicates situational decision rules apply; △ indicates direct impact requirements apply; Ⓜ indicates Measure of success is needed; ☆ indicates this standard also applies to organizations seeking Joint Commission's Medicare/Medicaid certification–based long term care accreditation

Standard IM.3.10 ★

Assessment Question	Level of Compliance	Evidence of Compliance	Plan of Action/ Measure of Success (if needed)	Due Date
7. Are knowledgable staff available for collecting, retrieving, and analyzing data and their transformation into information? **A (EP 7)**				
8. Are data organized and transformed into information in formats useful to decision makers? **A (EP 8)**				
9. Is dissemination of data and information timely* and accurate? **A (EP 9)**				
10. Are data and information disseminated in standard formats and methods to meet user needs and provide retrievability and interpretation? **A (EP 10)**				

Standard IM.4.10 ★

Standard Score: ❑ Compliant ❑ Not Compliant

Assessment Question	Level of Compliance	Evidence of Compliance	Plan of Action/ Measure of Success (if needed)	Due Date
1. Does the organization have the ability to collect and aggregate data and information to support care, treatment, and service delivery and operations, including the following: • Individual care, treatment, and services and care, treatment, and service delivery • Decision making • Management and operations • Analysis of trends • Performance comparisons over time throughout the organization and with other organizations • Performance improvement • Infection control • Resident safety? **A (EP 1)**				
2. To support clinical decision making, is information found in the resident record: • Readily accessible • Accurate • Complete • Organized for retrieval of data • Timely?* **A (EP 2)**				

* **Timely** Defined by organization policy and based on the intended use of the information.

Key: 0 = Insufficient compliance; 1 = Partial compliance; 2 = Satisfactory compliance; NA = Not applicable; **A** indicates scoring category A; **C** indicates scoring category C; ▲ indicates situational decision rules apply; △ indicates direct impact requirements apply; Ⓜ indicates Measure of success is needed; ☆ indicates this standard also applies to organizations seeking Joint Commission's Medicare/Medicaid certification–based long term care accreditation

Standard IM.4.10 ★

Assessment Question	Level of Compliance	Evidence of Compliance	Plan of Action/ Measure of Success (if needed)	Due Date
3. Are comparative performance data and information used for decision making, when available? **A (EP 3)**				

Standard IM.5.10 ★

Standard Score: ❑ Compliant ❑ Not Compliant

Assessment Question	Level of Compliance	Evidence of Compliance	Plan of Action/ Measure of Success (if needed)	Due Date
1. Does the organization provide access to knowledge-based information resources* needed by staff in any of the following forms: print, electronic, Internet, or audio? **A (EP 2)**				
2. Are knowledge-based resources available to clinical/service staff, through electronic means, after-hours access to an in-house collection, or other methods? **A (EP 3)**				
3. Does the organization have a process for providing access to knowledge-based information during times when electronic systems are unavailable? **A (EP 4)**				

Standard IM.6.10

Standard Score: ❑ Compliant ❑ Not Compliant

Assessment Question	Level of Compliance	Evidence of Compliance	Plan of Action/ Measure of Success (if needed)	Due Date
1. Do only authorized individuals make entries in the clinical record? **A (EP 1)**				
2. Does the organization define which entries made by nonindependent practitioners require countersigning consistent with law and regulation? **A (EP 2)**				
3. Are standardized formats used for documenting all care, treatment, and services provided to residents? **A (EP 3)**				

* Examples of knowledge-based information resources include current texts; periodicals; indexes; abstracts; reports; documents; databases; directories; discussion lists; successful practices; equipment and maintenance user manuals; standards; protocols; practice guidelines; clinical trials and other resources.

Key: 0 = Insufficient compliance; 1 = Partial compliance; 2 = Satisfactory compliance; NA = Not applicable; **A** indicates scoring category A; **C** indicates scoring category C; ▲ indicates situational decision rules apply; △ indicates direct impact requirements apply; Ⓜ indicates Measure of success is needed; ☆ indicates this standard also applies to organizations seeking Joint Commission's Medicare/Medicaid certification–based long term care accreditation

Standard IM.6.10

Assessment Question	Level of Compliance	Evidence of Compliance	Plan of Action/ Measure of Success (if needed)	Due Date
4. Are clinical record entries* dated, the author identified and, when necessary according to law or regulation or organization policy, authenticated either by written signature, electronic signature, or computer key or rubber stamp?† **C (EP 4)** Ⓜ				
5. Does the author authenticate either by written signature, electronic signature, or computer key or rubber stamp the following: • The history and physical examination • Medication orders • Practitioner orders • Discharge summary? **C (EP 5)** Ⓜ				
6. Does the clinical record contain sufficient information to identify the resident; support the diagnosis/condition; justify the care, treatment, and services; document the course and results of care, treatment, and services; and promote continuity of care among providers? **C (EP 6)** Ⓜ △3				
7. Does the organization have a policy on the timely entry of information into the resident's clinical record? **A (EP 8)**				
8. Does the organization define a complete record and the time frame within which the record must be completed after discharge, not to exceed 30 days after discharge? **A (EP 9)**				
9. Are clinical records reviewed on an ongoing basis at the point of care? **A (EP 12)**				

* For paper-based records, countersignatures entered for purposes of authentication after transcription or for verbal orders are dated when required by state or federal law and regulations and organization policy. For electronic records, electronic signatures will be date stamped.

† Authentication can be shown by written signatures or initials, rubber-stamp signatures, or computer key. Authorized users of signature stamps or computer keys sign a statement assuring that they alone will use the stamp or key.

Key: 0 = Insufficient compliance; 1 = Partial compliance; 2 = Satisfactory compliance; NA = Not applicable; **A** indicates scoring category A; **C** indicates scoring category C; ▲ indicates situational decision rules apply; △ indicates direct impact requirements apply; Ⓜ indicates Measure of success is needed; ☆ indicates this standard also applies to organizations seeking Joint Commission's Medicare/Medicaid certification–based long term care accreditation

Standard IM.6.10

Assessment Question	Level of Compliance	Evidence of Compliance	Plan of Action/ Measure of Success (if needed)	Due Date
10. Is the review of clinical records based on organization-defined indicators that address the presence, timeliness, readability (whether handwritten or printed), quality, consistency, clarity, accuracy, completeness, and authentication of data and information contained within the record? **A (EP 13)**				
11. Is the retention time of clinical record information determined by the organization based on law or regulation, and on its use for resident care, treatment, and services; legal, research, and operational purposes; and educational activities? **A (EP 14)**				
12. Are clinical records retained for five years from the resident's discharge date when there is no requirement in state law? **A (EP 15)**				
13. Are clinical records of minors retained for three years after the resident reaches legal age under the law? **A (EP 16)**				
14. Are original clinical records not released unless the organization is responding appropriately to laws or regulations, court orders, or subpoenas? **A (EP 17)**				
15. In the event of a change in the organization's own ership, do all residents' clinical records remain the organization's property and are transferred to the new owner unless otherwise indicated by law? **A (EP 19)**				

Key: 0 = Insufficient compliance; 1 = Partial compliance; 2 = Satisfactory compliance; NA = Not applicable; **A** indicates scoring category A; **C** indicates scoring category C; ▲ indicates situational decision rules apply; △ indicates direct impact requirements apply; Ⓜ indicates Measure of success is needed; ☆ indicates this standard also applies to organizations seeking Joint Commission's Medicare/Medicaid certification–based long term care accreditation

Standard IM.6.20	Standard Score: ❑ Compliant ❑ Not Compliant			
Assessment Question	**Level of Compliance**	**Evidence of Compliance**	**Plan of Action/ Measure of Success (if needed)**	**Due Date**
1. Does each clinical record contain, as applicable, the following clinical/case information: • Care, treatment, and services provided to the resident before his or her arrival, if any • Documentation and findings of assessments* • Initial medical assessment and conclusions or impressions drawn from medical history and physical examination • Diagnosis, diagnostic impression, or conditions • Reason(s) for admission or care, treatment, and services • Goals of the care and care plan • Orders for care, treatment, and service as required by law and regulation • Diagnostic and therapeutic orders • Diagnostic and therapeutic procedures, tests, and results • Progress notes made by authorized individuals • Reassessments and plan of care revisions • Relevant observations • Consultation reports • Allergies to foods and medicines • Medication ordered or prescribed • Dose of medications administered (including the strength, dose, or rate of administration) administration devices used, access site or route, known drug allergies, and adverse drug reaction • Medications dispensed or prescribed on discharge • Relevant diagnoses/conditions established during the course of care, treatment, and services? **C (EP 1)** Ⓜ				
2. Do clinical records contain, as applicable, the following demographic information: • Resident's name, address, date of birth, religion, marital status, social security number, gender, and the name of any legally authorized representative • The resident's legal status • The resident's langauge and communication needs? **C (EP 2)** Ⓜ				

* *See* the "Provision of Care, Treatment, and Services" (PC) chapter of the *CAMLTC*.

Key: 0 = Insufficient compliance; 1 = Partial compliance; 2 = Satisfactory compliance; NA = Not applicable; **A** indicates scoring category A; **C** indicates scoring category C; ▲ indicates situational decision rules apply; △ indicates direct impact requirements apply; Ⓜ indicates Measure of success is needed; ☆ indicates this standard also applies to organizations seeking Joint Commission's Medicare/Medicaid certification–based long term care accreditation

Standard IM.6.20

Assessment Question	Level of Compliance	Evidence of Compliance	Plan of Action/ Measure of Success (if needed)	Due Date
3. Do clinical records contain, as applicable, the following information: • Evidence of known advance directives • Evidence of informed consent when required by organization policy • Orders, renewal of orders, and documentation that resuscitative services are to be withheld or life-sustaining treatment withdrawn • Discharge plan, or the reason for lack of an ongoing plan when discharge potential does not exist • Referrals or communications made to external or internal care providers and community agencies • Physician's summary and the resident's final diagnosis when the resident is admitted from either a hospital or another health care organization? **C (EP 3) Ⓜ**				

Standard IM.6.50 ★

Standard Score: ❑ Compliant ❑ Not Compliant

Assessment Question	Level of Compliance	Evidence of Compliance	Plan of Action/ Measure of Success (if needed)	Due Date
1. Are qualified personnel identified, as defined by organization policy and in accordance with law or regulation, and authorized to receive and record verbal or telephone orders? **A (EP 1)**				
2. Are verbal orders dated and do they identify the names of the individuals who gave, received, and implemented the order? **C (EP 2) Ⓜ**				
3. When required by law or regulation, are verbal or telephone orders authenticated within the specified time frame? **A (EP 3)**				
4. For verbal or telephone orders or for telephonic reporting of critical test results, are the complete order or test results verified by having the person receiving the order or test result "read back" the complete order or test result? *(The preceding requirement is not scored here. It is scored at NPSG.02.01.01.)* **(EP 4)**				

Key: 0 = Insufficient compliance; 1 = Partial compliance; 2 = Satisfactory compliance; NA = Not applicable; **A** indicates scoring category A; **C** indicates scoring category C; ▲ indicates situational decision rules apply; △ indicates direct impact requirements apply; Ⓜ indicates Measure of success is needed; ☆ indicates this standard also applies to organizations seeking Joint Commission's Medicare/Medicaid certification–based long term care accreditation

Standard IM.6.60	Standard Score: ❑ Compliant ❑ Not Compliant			
Assessment Question	**Level of Compliance**	**Evidence of Compliance**	**Plan of Action/ Measure of Success (if needed)**	**Due Date**
1. Does the organization have a process to track the location of all components of the clinical record? **A (EP 1)**				
2. Does the organization use a system to assemble required information or make available a summary of information relative for resident care, treatment and services provided? **A (EP 2)**				

Standard IM.6.70	Standard Score: ❑ Compliant ❑ Not Compliant			
Assessment Question	**Level of Compliance**	**Evidence of Compliance**	**Plan of Action/ Measure of Success (if needed)**	**Due Date**
1. Are the provision of and response to the activities program based on the interdisciplinary care plan documented at least quarterly in the clinical record? **C (EP 1)** Ⓜ				
2. Do the activity providers document in the clinical record and report to the charge nurse any changes in the resident's response to the activity program? **C (EP 2)** Ⓜ				

Standard IM.6.80	Standard Score: ❑ Compliant ❑ Not Compliant			
Assessment Question	**Level of Compliance**	**Evidence of Compliance**	**Plan of Action/ Measure of Success (if needed)**	**Due Date**
1. Is the provision of and response to nutrition care services based on the interdisciplinary care plan documented at least quarterly in the clinical record? **C (EP 1)** Ⓜ				

Key: 0 = Insufficient compliance; 1 = Partial compliance; 2 = Satisfactory compliance; NA = Not applicable; **A** indicates scoring category A; **C** indicates scoring category C; ▲ indicates situational decision rules apply; △ indicates direct impact requirements apply; Ⓜ indicates Measure of success is needed; ☆ indicates this standard also applies to organizations seeking Joint Commission's Medicare/Medicaid certification–based long term care accreditation

Standard IM.6.80

Assessment Question	Level of Compliance	Evidence of Compliance	Plan of Action/ Measure of Success (if needed)	Due Date
2. Does documentation include the current status and changes in the resident's nutritional status, including the following information: • The resident's acceptance of prescribed diets • The resident's food and fluid consumption • Significant weight loss or gain, consistent with law or regulation • Hydration status • The resident's ability to eat independently • The resident's ability to use adaptive devices for eating • Current status and changes in the resident's physical or behavioral condition, including symptoms • Summary of the resident's condition, which includes the extent to which nutritional goals included in the interdisciplinary care plan are achieved? C (EP 2) Ⓜ				

Standard IM.6.90

Standard Score: ❑ Compliant ❑ Not Compliant

Assessment Question	Level of Compliance	Evidence of Compliance	Plan of Action/ Measure of Success (if needed)	Due Date
1. Is the provision of nursing care that is based on the interdisciplinary care plan and the resident's response to this care documented in the clinical record? C (EP 1) Ⓜ				
2. Does documentation include at least the following: • Medications and treatment given and untoward reactions • Nursing care provided • Current status and changes in the resident's physical or behavioral condition, including symptoms • Summary by licensed nursing staff of the resident's condition, which includes the extent to which nursing goals included in the interdisciplinary care plan are achieved, at least quarterly or more often if the resident's condition warrants? C (EP 2) Ⓜ				

Key: 0 = Insufficient compliance; 1 = Partial compliance; 2 = Satisfactory compliance; NA = Not applicable; **A** indicates scoring category A; **C** indicates scoring category C; ▲ indicates situational decision rules apply; △ indicates direct impact requirements apply; Ⓜ indicates Measure of success is needed; ☆ indicates this standard also applies to organizations seeking Joint Commission's Medicare/Medicaid certification–based long term care accreditation

Standard IM.6.100	**Standard Score:** ❑ Compliant ❑ Not Compliant			
Assessment Question	**Level of Compliance**	**Evidence of Compliance**	**Plan of Action/ Measure of Success (if needed)**	**Due Date**
1. Are the provision of medical treatment and care and the resident's response to medical treatment and care documented in the clinical record? **C (EP 1)** Ⓜ ⚠3				
2. Does documentation in the resident's clinical record include, before or on admission, the submission of the following: • Admitting diagnosis • Current medical findings • Diet prescribed • The resident's functional status? **C (EP 2)** Ⓜ				
3. Does documentation in the resident's clinical record include medical observations and recommendations made after the initial medical assessment, as well as progress notes that are reported at the time of observation and that describe significant changes in the resident's condition? **C (EP 3)** Ⓜ				
4. Does documentation in the resident's clinical record include progress notes recorded by the physician at each visit? **C (EP 4)** Ⓜ				
5. Upon the resident's discharge, does documentation in the resident's clinical record include the completion of the transfer form when appropriate, the discharge summary, and the resident's clinical record? **C (EP 5)** Ⓜ				

Key: 0 = Insufficient compliance; 1 = Partial compliance; 2 = Satisfactory compliance; NA = Not applicable; **A** indicates scoring category A; **C** indicates scoring category C; ▲2 indicates situational decision rules apply; ⚠3 indicates direct impact requirements apply; Ⓜ indicates Measure of success is needed; ☆ indicates this standard also applies to organizations seeking Joint Commission's Medicare/Medicaid certification–based long term care accreditation

Standard IM.6.100

Assessment Question	Level of Compliance	Evidence of Compliance	Plan of Action/ Measure of Success (if needed)	Due Date
6. If the resident expires in the organization, is the course of events leading up to the resident's death documented? C (EP 6) Ⓜ				
7. Does documentation in the resident's clinical record include evidence that the attending physician has reviewed the consulting physician's orders for consistency with the overall care plan? C (EP 7) Ⓜ				

Standard IM.6.110

Standard Score: ❑ Compliant ❑ Not Compliant

Assessment Question	Level of Compliance	Evidence of Compliance	Plan of Action/ Measure of Success (if needed)	Due Date
1. Are the provision of rehabilitation services provided based on the interdisciplinary care plan and are the resident's response to these services documented in the clinical record? C (EP 1) Ⓜ				
2. Does documentation describe the following: • The resident's and family's perception of and involvement in rehabilitation services • Reason for the referral to rehabilitation services or admission for comprehensive subacute services • Rehabilitation treatments, modalities, or procedures provided • The resident's response to treatment • The resident's involvement in rehabilitation services • The resident's progress toward treatment goals? C (EP 2) Ⓜ				
3. Are assessment of rehabilitation achievement and estimates of further rehabilitation potential entered at least weekly? C (EP 3) Ⓜ				

Key: 0 = Insufficient compliance; 1 = Partial compliance; 2 = Satisfactory compliance; NA = Not applicable; **A** indicates scoring category A; **C** indicates scoring category C; ▲2 indicates situational decision rules apply; △3 indicates direct impact requirements apply; Ⓜ indicates Measure of success is needed; ☆ indicates this standard also applies to organizations seeking Joint Commission's Medicare/Medicaid certification–based long term care accreditation

Standard IM.6.110				
Assessment Question	**Level of Compliance**	**Evidence of Compliance**	**Plan of Action/ Measure of Success (if needed)**	**Due Date**
4. Does documentation include a progress report and reassessment, including the following: • Summary of the resident's condition, which includes the extent to which rehabilitation goals included in the interdisciplinary care plan are achieved, every two weeks for the first quarter, every month for the second quarter, and quarterly thereafter or more frequently when the resident's condition changes • Estimates of the resident's further rehabilitation potential • Discharge plan? **C (EP 4) Ⓜ**				

Standard IM.6.120	Standard Score: ❑ Compliant ❑ Not Compliant			
Assessment Question	**Level of Compliance**	**Evidence of Compliance**	**Plan of Action/ Measure of Success (if needed)**	**Due Date**
1. Are the provision of and the resident's response to social service interventions documented in the clinical record? **C (EP 1) Ⓜ**				
2. Does documentation of social service interventions include at least the following: • Specified goals related to social services, including discharge planning, that are an integral part of the interdisciplinary care plan • Services provided and their outcomes • Summary of the resident's problems, services provided, goals, and condition, which includes the extent to which social services goals included in the interdisciplinary care plan are achieved, at least quarterly or more often if the resident's condition warrants • Referrals to outside agencies, resources, or individuals, as well as any follow-up actions or recommendations of outside agencies, resources, or individuals? **C (EP 2) Ⓜ**				

Key: 0 = Insufficient compliance; 1 = Partial compliance; 2 = Satisfactory compliance; NA = Not applicable; **A** indicates scoring category A; **C** indicates scoring category C; ▲ indicates situational decision rules apply; △ indicates direct impact requirements apply; Ⓜ indicates Measure of success is needed; ☆ indicates this standard also applies to organizations seeking Joint Commission's Medicare/Medicaid certification–based long term care accreditation

Standard IM.6.130 ★	**Standard Score:** ❑ Compliant ❑ Not Compliant			
Assessment Question	**Level of Compliance**	**Evidence of Compliance**	**Plan of Action/ Measure of Success (if needed)**	**Due Date**
1. Are the provision of and the resident's response to education documented in the clinical record? **C (EP 1) Ⓜ**				

Standard IM.6.140	**Standard Score:** ❑ Compliant ❑ Not Compliant			
Assessment Question	**Level of Compliance**	**Evidence of Compliance**	**Plan of Action/ Measure of Success (if needed)**	**Due Date**
1. Does clinical record documentation include significant changes in the resident's condition, care, and treatment? **C (EP 1) Ⓜ** △3				

Standard IM.6.150	**Standard Score:** ❑ Compliant ❑ Not Compliant			
Assessment Question	**Level of Compliance**	**Evidence of Compliance**	**Plan of Action/ Measure of Success (if needed)**	**Due Date**
1. Does clinical record documentation include treatment provided to the resident by off-site sources? **C (EP 1) Ⓜ**				

Standard IM.6.160	**Standard Score:** ❑ Compliant ❑ Not Compliant			
Assessment Question	**Level of Compliance**	**Evidence of Compliance**	**Plan of Action/ Measure of Success (if needed)**	**Due Date**
1. Does the clinical record include documentation of the following: • Resident's response to medications • Pharmacist's evaluation and consultation with the physician • The need for additional laboratory monitoring?* **C (EP 1) Ⓜ** △3				

* Documentation can be included in the resident's clinical record or in another location such as the pharmacist's report.

Key: 0 = Insufficient compliance; 1 = Partial compliance; 2 = Satisfactory compliance; NA = Not applicable; **A** indicates scoring category A; **C** indicates scoring category C; ▲2 indicates situational decision rules apply; △3 indicates direct impact requirements apply; Ⓜ indicates Measure of success is needed; ☆ indicates this standard also applies to organizations seeking Joint Commission's Medicare/Medicaid certification–based long term care accreditation

Standard IM.6.170	Standard Score: ❑ Compliant ❑ Not Compliant			
Assessment Question	**Level of Compliance**	**Evidence of Compliance**	**Plan of Action/ Measure of Success (if needed)**	**Due Date**
1. Does clinical record documentation include discharge information provided to the resident and/or to the receiving organization? **C (EP 1) Ⓜ**				
2. Does discharge information include the following: • Medical findings, diagnosis(es), and treatment orders • Summary of the care, treatment, and services provided and progress toward achieving goals • Diet orders and medication orders • Behavioral status, ambulation status, nutrition status, and rehabilitation potential • The resident's physical and psychosocial status • Nursing information useful in resident care • Advance directives • Referrals provided to the resident • The reason for transfer, discharge, or referral • The physician's orders for the resident's immediate care • Instructions given to the resident before discharge • The referring physician's name • The physician who has agreed to be responsible for the resident's medical care and treatment, if other than the referring physician? **C (EP 2) Ⓜ**				

Key: 0 = Insufficient compliance; 1 = Partial compliance; 2 = Satisfactory compliance; NA = Not applicable; **A** indicates scoring category A; **C** indicates scoring category C; ▲ indicates situational decision rules apply; △ indicates direct impact requirements apply; Ⓜ indicates Measure of success is needed; ☆ indicates this standard also applies to organizations seeking Joint Commission's Medicare/Medicaid certification–based long term care accreditation

Part 3
Knowing What to Expect at Survey

- ☑ Types of Surveys
- ☑ Presurvey Activities
- ☑ On-Site Survey Activities
- ☑ Postsurvey Activities
- ☑ Sample Survey Agendas

Types of Surveys

- ☑ **Traditional Long Term Care Accreditation Survey**
- ☑ **Medicare/Medicaid Certification–Based Long Term Care Accreditation Survey**
- ☑ **Initial Survey**
- ☑ **Early Survey Policy**
- ☑ **Unannounced Surveys**
- ☑ **Multiorganization Survey**
- ☑ **Complex Organization Survey**
- ☑ **Conditional Follow-Up Survey**
- ☑ **Extension Survey**
- ☑ **For-Cause Surveys**
- ☑ **Random Validation Survey of Evidence of Standards Compliance (ESC)**
- ☑ **On-Site Validation Survey Incorporated into the Clarification Process**

Your current accreditation decision determines the type and timing of your survey. Different survey types have specific application requirements, as explained in this section. For more detailed information on all types of surveys, refer to "The Accreditation Process" (ACC) chapter in the current edition of the Comprehensive Accreditation Manual for Long Term Care *(*CAMLTC*).*

☑ Traditional Long Term Care Accreditation Survey

The survey is based on the entire set of long term care accreditation standards in the *CAMLTC*. The survey can last for multiple days, depending on your average daily census. The multiple-day survey offers a comprehensive review of all long term care standards with focused education for improvement. Your Accreditation Survey Findings Report and certificate will reflect that your accreditation award is for long term care. For more information on traditional long term care accreditation, please see The Joint Commission's Web site at http://www.jointcommission.org.

☑ Medicare/Medicaid Certification–Based Long Term Care Accreditation Survey

If your organization is a Medicare/Medicaid–certified skilled nursing facility or nursing facility, you have the option of undergoing either a traditional long term care survey (as described above) or a survey for Medicare/Medicaid certification–based long term care accreditation. The latter is based on a subset of Joint Commission standards from the *CAMLTC* that go beyond the Conditions of Participation for Skilled Nursing Facilities/Nursing Facilities and address areas that usually are not evaluated during a state agency certification survey. *See* the *CAMLTC* for a list of these standards. The Joint Commission survey focuses on systems and processes that support organization safety, performance improvement, resident and family education, credentialing and privileging of licensed independent practitioners, pain management, and point-of-care testing.

If you elect this option, your on-site survey will be shorter than the length of the survey based on the traditional long term care accreditation survey, and the fee will be less than that for a traditional long term care accreditation survey. Your Accreditation Survey Findings Report and certificate will reflect that your accreditation award is substantially based on Medicare/Medicaid certification for long term care. For more information on the Medicare/Medicaid certification–based long term care accreditation option and standards, please *see* the "Medicare/Medicaid Certification–Based LTC Accreditation Standards" (MC) chapter in the *CAMLTC*.

☑ Initial Survey

The initial survey is an accreditation survey of a health care organization not previously accredited by The Joint Commission (or that has not been accredited/certified by The Joint Commission in at least four months), or an accreditation survey of an organization performed without reference to any prior survey findings. The length of the survey and the number and disciplines of the surveyors will vary based on the types and volume of services you provide.

The Joint Commission's policy for assessing and monitoring organizations new to the accreditation and certification process is as follows:

- If an organization new to the accreditation or certification process demonstrates compliance with Joint Commission standards, without consideration of track record requirements, the organization will receive Accreditation or Certification, respectively
- All organizations new to the accreditation or certification process that become accredited after their initial survey will be included in a 5% "pool" of organizations undergoing a Random Validation Survey of Evidence of Standards Compliance (ESC).
- The Joint Commission has reviewed requirements such as the minimum number of patients an organization must have in order to perform a credible survey. The outcome of this review has led to the approval of the following parameters:
    - The minimum number of patients/volume of services required for organizations seeking Joint Commission accreditation/certification for the first time
    - The high-risk/critical services in new organizations that will require a follow-up survey in one year following initial awarding of accreditation/certification
- The Random Validation Survey of ESC will provide a timely mechanism for monitoring continued standards compliance for organizations new to the accreditation or certification process, versus using the organization's prior track record to predict future performance.

An initial survey is conducted if your long term care organization fits one of the following profiles:

- Your organization is seeking Joint Commission accreditation for the first time
- Your organization has been unaccredited by The Joint Commission during the previous six months

The accreditation effective date for an organization that undergoes an initial survey is the date on which its ESC report was submitted, if the organization has a Requirement for Improvement (RFI). If there are no RFIs, the effective date is the date after the last day of the survey.

For organizations receiving a Conditional Accreditation decision after an initial survey, the effective date is the date of the Accreditation Committee meeting at which the decision was made, if the organization has submitted an acceptable ESC report. If the organization has yet to submit an acceptable ESC that resolves all RFIs at the time of the Accreditation Committee meeting, then the effective date for the accreditation decision is set retroactively as the date when the acceptable ESC is submitted. (*See* Table 1 on page 288 for more information on accreditation decisions.)

Note: *The information presented under "Presurvey Activities," "On-Site Survey Activities," and "Postsurvey Activities" applies primarily to full on-site surveys, rather than initial surveys.*

Table 1. Joint Commission Accreditation Decisions

The Joint Commission has six accreditation decision categories. Each decision and the conditions that lead to it are described here.

Accreditation Decision Category	Conditions That Lead to This Type of Decision
Accredited	The organization is in compliance with all applicable standards at the time of the on-site survey or has successfully addressed all RFIs in an ESC response.
Provisional Accreditation	The organization fails to successfully address all RFIs in an ESC report.
Conditional Accreditation	The organization was previously in Preliminary Denial of Accreditation due to an Immediate Threat to Health and Safety situation, or failure to resolve the requirements of a Provisional Accreditation, or is not in substantial compliance with the applicable standards, as usually evidenced by a single issue or multiple issues that pose a risk to patient care or safety that was present at the time of survey. The organization must remedy identified problem areas through preparation and submission of Evidence of Standards Compliance and subsequently undergo an on-site, follow-up survey. In addition, an organization may receive a Conditional Accreditation for failure to meet certain Joint Commission participation requirements, such as a Periodic Performance Review or timely submission of data.
Preliminary Denial of Accreditation	Justification to deny accreditation to the organization as evidenced by an Immediate Threat to Health and Safety situation, or failure to resolve the requirements of a Conditional Accreditation, or significant noncompliance with Joint Commission standards. The decision is subject to review and appeal prior to the determination to deny accreditation; the appeal process may also result in a decision other than Denial of Accreditation.
Denial of Accreditation	The organization has been denied accreditation. All review and appeal opportunities have been exhausted.
Preliminary Accreditation	The organization demonstrates compliance with selected standards in the surveys conducted under the Early Survey Policy.

☑ Early Survey Policy

Early Survey Policy Eligibility*

This policy is available to any long term care organization that is not currently accredited and has not been denied accreditation. If you want to be surveyed under this policy, you must indicate this on your application for accreditation.

Under the requirements for this policy, The Joint Commission will conduct two on-site surveys, both of which will be announced unless the organization is using accreditation to meet deemed status purposes.

The First Survey

The first survey may take place as early as two months before your organization begins operations, if the following conditions are met:

- Your organization is licensed or has a provisional license
- The building in which you will provide services is identified, constructed, and equipped to support such activities
- You have identified your CEO or administrator, director of clinical or medical services, and nurse executive, if applicable
- You have identified the date you will begin operations

Generally, the first survey uses a limited set of standards and assesses only your organization's physical facilities, policies and procedures, plans, and related structural considerations for care. For a long term care organization that is operating when the survey is conducted, the effective date for its Preliminary Accreditation decision is the day after the survey is conducted if the organization does not receive any RFIs. If the organization receives at least one RFI and therefore must submit an acceptable ESC report that resolves all RFIs, the effective date for Preliminary Accreditation is then set retroactively as the date of the acceptable ESC submission.

For an organization not in operation at the time of survey, the effective date for its Preliminary Accreditation decision is the day after it begins operating if it receives no RFIs. If the organization is not in operation at the time of survey, the organization must confirm in writing the date it begins operating.

A Preliminary Accreditation decision remains in effect until the organization completes a second, full survey or until The Joint Commission withdraws the Preliminary Accreditation.

Note: *You may want to contact your state authority that has jurisdiction regarding its recognition of Preliminary Accreditation for state licensure purposes.*

The Second Survey

The second survey is a full accreditation survey conducted approximately six months after your first survey and at least four months after your long term care organization has begun operations. Based on your survey results, your accreditation decision will be changed to Accredited, Provisional Accreditation, Conditional Accreditation, Preliminary Denial of Accreditation, or Denial of Accreditation.

The effective date of the accreditation decision is the day after the second survey if the organization does not receive any RFIs. If the organization receives at least one RFI and therefore must submit an ESC report to resolve all RFIs, the effective date of the preliminary accreditation decision is then set retroactively as the date the successful ESC report is submitted.

A Preliminary Accreditation decision remains in effect until the organization has completed a second, full survey or until The Joint Commission has withdrawn the Preliminary Accreditation. The Joint Commission may withdraw Preliminary Accreditation in the following situations:

- If an organization that was not providing services at the time of the first survey does not begin providing services when expected
- If an organization does not meet the survey eligibility criteria
- If an organization fails to accept the date of the second survey
- If an organization is found to be not in satisfactory compliance with the applicable standards and their EPs

* **Note:** *Early Survey Policy is not available to long term care organizations seeking accreditation under the Medicare/Medicaid certification–based accreditation option.*

☑ Unannounced Surveys

The Joint Commission's surveys have been unannounced since January 1, 2006, with a few exceptions.

The Joint Commission has implemented unannounced surveys for the following reasons:

- To enhance the credibility of the accreditation process by ensuring that surveyors observe organization performance under normal circumstances
- To reduce the unnecessary costs that health care organizations incur to prepare for survey
- To address public concerns that The Joint Commission receive an accurate reflection of the quality and safety of care
- To help health care organizations focus on providing safe, high-quality care at all times, and not just when preparing for survey
- To affirm the expectation of continuous standards compliance both by The Joint Commission of its accredited organizations and by these organizations of themselves

The Joint Commission exempted the following types of surveys from completely unannounced surveys:

- Initial surveys (that is, for long term care organizations that are undergoing their first Joint Commission surveys), including surveys conducted under the Early Survey Policy (unless requirements specify unannounced surveys)
- PPR Option 2 and Option 3 surveys (full length or limited)

The Joint Commission approved the exemption of the following types of *organizations* from completely unannounced surveys:

- Department of Defense facilities
- Bureau of Prisons facilities
- Foster care programs
- "Very small" organizations

An organization can have an unannounced survey between 18 and 39 months after its previous full unannounced survey. Pre-determined criteria based on Priority Focus Process (PFP) data across multiple quarters as well as trends in the performance of these data will determine the timing of an organization's full unannounced survey. For example, an organization that is due to have its next unannounced survey in January 2010 could have its survey as early as July 2008 or as late as April 1, 2010 (18 to 39 months). With an *unannounced survey,* an accredited long term care organization will receive *no notice* of its survey date prior to the start of the survey. In concert with the unannounced survey process, the following procedures will be implemented:

- Accredited organizations will be able to identify up to 10 days in their survey eligibility range (between 18 and 39 months after their last full unannounced survey) in which an unannounced survey should be avoided. These 10 days should not include federal holidays but may include regional events in which it may be difficult to conduct a survey. The Joint Commission will make every effort to accommodate the long term care organization regarding avoiding these 10 days. However, The Joint Commission reserves the right to conduct a survey during an "avoid period" if the reason(s) given to avoid a survey at that time is such that a survey can be reasonably accomplished.
- An annual subscription billing model will be implemented.
- Because an accredited organization cannot post its survey date, and, therefore, individuals cannot request a Public Information Interview (PII), an Accreditation Participation Requirement (APR) was established. This APR requires a long term care organization to demonstrate how it communicates to its public that if members of the public have any quality-of-care or safety concerns, they should notify The Joint Commission.
- On the day of the unannounced survey, by 7:30 A.M. in the organization's local time zone (for organizations within the United States and its territories), The Joint Commission will post on the organization's secure *The Joint Commission Connect*™ extranet site the letter of introduction, the survey agendas, and the biographies and pictures of the surveyors assigned to conduct the survey. For organizations outside of these locations, notifications will continue to be posted by 7:00 A.M. Eastern time. (*See* sample survey agendas on pages 352–354.)
- An organization will be invoiced approximately 7 to 10 days after its survey's completion to cover the direct costs of the survey (the indirect costs of the survey are covered in an organization's annual subscription payment).
- To avoid conflicts of interest, organizations are asked to identify on their electronic application (e-App) which surveyors work or worked at the long term care organization or a competing long term care organization or whether they have had personal experience with the surveyor that represents a potential conflict.

For more information on the new unannounced survey process, refer to "The Accreditation Process" (ACC) chapter of the *CAMLTC*.

Table 2. Exemptions to Unannounced Surveys

Program	Subject	Exception
ALL	Initial surveys	Announced (except deemed status surveys for Medicare certification)
	Early Survey Policy—1st and 2nd surveys	Announced
All programs	Department of Defense facilities	5 days within certain periods of time

☑ Multiorganization Survey

The Joint Commission offers multiorganization systems that own or lease at least two long term care facilities (or other health care organizations) the option of a modified survey process. This option has three components:

1. *A corporate orientation held at the beginning of the year*
2. *Survey of participating organizations with the same survey team leader*
3. *A corporate summation after the last organization in the system is surveyed*

Your system may choose to have a corporate orientation, a corporate summation, or both. The orientation session lets corporate staff orient the surveyor(s) to your system's structure and practices. The surveyor(s) also assesses centralized corporate services, documentation, and policies and procedures applicable to Joint Commission standards. The corporate summation gives you an overall analysis of your system's strengths and weaknesses. It also provides education related to accreditation survey findings across your system. The corporate orientation and corporate summation have separate fees.

Continuity in the composition of the survey team will be maintained by the survey team leader(s). The remaining members of the survey team rotate in and out of the system's unannounced schedule. The survey team leader compiles the information necessary to support the corporate summation.

With the multiorganization survey, The Joint Commission accredits individual health care organizations that are part of a larger system, not the system itself. Therefore, each organization within a system receives its own accreditation decision and report. The findings and decision for one organization within a system have no bearing on those of another organization within the same system.

☑ Complex Organization Survey

The Joint Commission defines a complex organization as one that requires the use of standards and their EPs from at least two accreditation manuals.

Those accreditation manual titles are as follows:

- *Comprehensive Accreditation Manual for Long Term Care*
- *Comprehensive Accreditation Manual for Critical Access Hospitals*
- *Comprehensive Accreditation Manual for Office-Based Surgery Practices*
- *Comprehensive Accreditation Manual for Ambulatory Care*
- *Comprehensive Accreditation Manual for Behavioral Health Care*
- *Comprehensive Accreditation Manual for Home Care*
- *Comprehensive Accreditation Manual for Hospitals: The Official Handbook*
- *Comprehensive Accreditation Manual for Laboratory and Point-of-Care Testing*

The complex organization survey is based on the services your organization provides as reported in your application for accreditation. The Joint Commission determines which manuals are relevant based on that application and provides your organization with a copy of all manuals to be used in the survey before it is conducted.

Note: *Any service or program that is a component of an accreditation-eligible organization may seek accreditation on its own if it can meet Joint Commission survey eligibility requirements. The results of such a separate accreditation survey will still apply to the overall organization's decision in accordance with applicable decision rules.*

If your complex organization acquires a new service component that needs to be surveyed using a new accreditation manual, that component should be surveyed within six months of its acquisition under an extension survey (*see* page 293). You will have 12 months from the time of acquisition before that service's performance is factored into your overall accreditation decision. (The extension survey takes place after six months, leaving an additional six months for the ESC report if necessary.)

Because of streamlining, the on-site evaluation process addresses the organization as an integrated whole rather than, as in the past, its individual components. To achieve this integration, the surveyor(s) needs to coordinate activities during the Preliminary Planning Session to accommodate the schedules of surveyors from different programs with different time commitments. This coordination includes the following:

- Selecting tracer residents who have been served across the settings covered by the different accreditation programs
- Identifying opportunities to integrate system tracers and other survey activities among accreditation programs, depending on the services provided, your organization's degree of centralization, and the distance between different locations
- Coordinating times for team meetings, special resolution sessions, and other mechanisms for sharing information with surveyors in different locations
- Identifying communication mechanisms, such as conference calls, for team members in different locations
- Arranging for at least one survey team member to attend the preliminary Exit Conference in the event that some members will be leaving early

Recommendations relative to specific services can come from any member of the survey team at any point in the survey. Even if a surveyor evaluating specific services (for example, home care) has completed his or her portion of the survey, the other staff is expected to continue to participate in any remaining survey activities led by the remaining surveyor(s). Such activities may include system tracers, the Leadership Session, or others. The remaining surveyor(s) includes all relevant staff members in discussions during these activities. In addition, the departing surveyor may ask his or her fellow surveyors to pursue certain issues during the remaining survey activities. Findings from any survey activities may identify continuity of care issues within your long term care organization. As a result, the remaining surveyors may include any not compliant standards on the Summary of Survey Findings report.

The on-site survey report has all programs' findings combined under each surveyor-cited priority focus area (PFA). (The highest number of not compliant standards across all programs determines how the PFAs are listed on the report.)

☑ Conditional Follow-Up Survey

If an organization receives Conditional Accreditation after a survey, the organization must submit an ESC to The Joint Commission and undergo an on-site, follow-up survey. An acceptable ESC is due within 45 or 60 calendar days (depending on whether the standard relates to a "Direct" or "Indirect" Impact Requirement) following the posting of your Accreditation Survey Findings Report to your secure extranet site.

The ESC report must include the action taken to correct deficiencies and the Measures of Success (MOS) you will use to evaluate your progress.

If your long term care organization has Conditional Accreditation after two failed ESCs, two failed MOS, or a failed ESC after a failed MOS, then a conditional follow-up survey is conducted. This survey determines whether your organization has taken sufficient action to upgrade your decision from Conditional Accreditation to Provisional Accreditation or Accredited.

☑ Extension Survey

An extension survey may be conducted at an accredited organization or a site that is owned and operated by an accredited organization.

This type of survey is performed if your organization's accreditation will not expire for at least nine months and at least one of the following conditions applies:

- You have begun offering a new service or program for which The Joint Commission has standards
- Your organization has changed ownership and significant changes in your management and clinical staff or operating policies and procedures have occurred
- You have begun offering at least 25% of your services in a new location or in a physical plant that has been significantly altered
- Your long term care organization's capacity to provide services has expanded by 25% or more (calculated by resident volume)
- You have begun providing a more intensive level of service or
- Your long term care organization has merged, consolidated with, or acquired an unaccredited site, service, or program for which The Joint Commission has standards and EPs

An extension survey may also be conducted if, due to unusual or compelling reasons, you have requested that your current accreditation be extended beyond the conclusion of your three-year cycle. The length of the survey is one to five days. The surveyor uses the same type of approach in an extension survey as a full survey.

Because of the varying circumstances for scheduling extension surveys, considerable variation may arise in the specific issues addressed by the surveyor(s).

☑ For-Cause Surveys

*The Joint Commission may perform a for-cause unannounced survey when it becomes aware of potentially serious standards compliance or resident care or safety issues, or when it has other valid reasons for surveying an accredited organization.**

Note: *For-cause unannounced surveys should not be confused with regular unannounced surveys.*

A for-cause unannounced survey can take place at any point in a long term care organization's accreditation cycle. No preliminary report is generated after a for-cause unannounced survey.

Note: *A long term care organization is charged for a for-cause unannounced survey, regardless of the outcome. An organization can determine the cost of such a survey by calling The Joint Commission's Pricing Unit at 630/792-5115.*

No advance notice is provided for a for-cause unannounced survey. Reasons for a for-cause unannounced survey include occurrence of any event or series of events in an accredited organization that creates either of the following significant situations:

- Concern that a continuing threat may exist to the safety or care of residents at risk
- Indication that the long term care organization is not or has not been in compliance with The Joint Commission's Information Accuracy and Truthfulness Policy

Such a survey can include all the organization's services or only those areas where a serious concern may exist.

The Joint Commission may deny accreditation if the organization does not allow The Joint Commission to conduct an unscheduled or unannounced survey.

☑ Random Validation Survey of Evidence of Standards Compliance (ESC)

To validate the statements made in ESC submissions, The Joint Commission will sample 5% of all organizations required to submit an ESC report, with or without MOS, for an unannounced, on-site validation survey. The surveyor conducting the validation survey will have access to the submitted ESC report and MOS. The surveyor will be surveying areas that were the subject of each RFI to determine whether the corrective actions were implemented as stated. The purpose of this survey is to maintain the credibility of the ESC process by validating statements made in the ESC submission.

Depending on whether an organization is required to submit an ESC only or an ESC and an MOS will determine whether the organization will be included in the "pool" for organizations to have a validation survey in short proximity to the ESC submission or following the MOS submission. If an organization is required to submit an ESC and an MOS, the organization will not be included in the "pool" until after the MOS is submitted.

* *See* the "Accreditation Participation Requirements" (APR) chapter of the *CAMLTC.*

☑ On-Site Validation Survey Incorporated into the Clarification Process

The Joint Commission has incorporated an on-site validation survey into the clarification process for those organizations that no longer meet a decision rule for either Preliminary Denial of Accreditation or Conditional Accreditation. The on-site validation survey will help maintain the integrity of the accreditation decision process and ensure that Joint Commission–accredited organizations are providing safe, high-quality care.

If an organization goes through survey and meets a decision rule for Preliminary Denial of Accreditation or Conditional Accreditation, it has 10 business days from the date that the survey findings are posted to the organization's secure extranet site to submit clarifying evidence to demonstrate that it was in compliance with one or more of the standards in question at the time of survey. (Organizations submit their clarifying evidence through an electronic form on the secure *The Joint Commission Connect* extranet site.)

After reviewing the organization's clarifying evidence and determining that the organization has no longer met the decision rule for Preliminary Denial of Accreditation or Conditional Accreditation, a Joint Commission surveyor will always follow up with an on-site validation survey to:

- Validate the clarifying evidence submitted and determine if such information or data was available to the previous on-site survey team
- Determine whether the organization does or does not meet a decision rule for Preliminary Denial of Accreditation or Conditional Accreditation

If the organization does not meet a rule for Preliminary Denial of Accreditation or Conditional Accreditation, it will be awarded accreditation (if it is compliant with all standards) or it will be required to submit an ESC report (if it still has RFIs). However, if the organization does meet a decision rule for Preliminary Denial of Accreditation or Conditional Accreditation, The Joint Commission staff will recommend to the Accreditation Committee that the organization remain in Preliminary Denial of Accreditation or Conditional Accreditation. If the results of the on-site validation survey suggest that the organization falsified its clarifying evidence, the staff member may recommend to the Accreditation Committee that the Information Accuracy and Truthfulness Policy should be invoked.

Currently the organization is not charged for having an on-site validation survey.

Presurvey Activities

- ☑ **Application for Accreditation**
- ☑ **Presurvey Information**
- ☑ **On-Site Survey Preparation**

Presurvey Activities

Application for Accreditation

If your organization has never been surveyed, you can contact The Joint Commission for an application for accreditation. You can obtain an application from The Joint Commission's Central Office at 630/792-5800 or by writing to the following address:

The Joint Commission
Customer Service
One Renaissance Boulevard
Oakbrook Terrace, IL 60181

You may also write to this address if you do not know your organization's password to your secure extranet site. Although you may request a paper copy of the application, which will arrive in approximately two weeks, the preferred method is to use the application for accreditation (e-App) available on *The Joint Commission Connect*™ extranet site. When you use the e-App, The Joint Commission provides your CEO with information about how to access and complete your application on the secure extranet site.

An organization needs to submit its e-App once, and it is required to provide updates within 30 days of a major change. You can complete the e-App via your organization's secure extranet site. After a long term care organization completes its application, it remains valid until the organization no longer wants to be Joint Commission accredited, as long as the organization completes and submits its updates to The Joint Commission. Initial applications are valid for six months.

Every year, The Joint Commission sends the organization the data, as previously reported in the e-App (and in annual updates, if there were any), in a pre-populated format, and asks the long term care organization to either update the information or confirm that no changes to the information are necessary.

Organizations that use the e-App type data directly into the application and submit the e-App to The Joint Commission electronically. In filling out the application, you need to provide a detailed description of your organization, including ownership, resident population(s), and types and volume of services provided. You should also specify at this time whether you wish to be surveyed under the Medicare/Medicaid certification–based long term care accreditation option. The application lists official records and reports of public or publicly recognized licensing (for example, a state license), examining, reviewing, or planning bodies that The Joint Commission may request. The application also authorizes The Joint Commission to obtain necessary records and reports not held by your organization and, on acceptance, establish the terms of the relationship between your organization and The Joint Commission.

An organization which chooses not to complete its application via its secure site on The Joint Commission extranet site may request a printed copy of the application by contacting its account representative. An organization can find out who its account representative is by calling 630/792-3007.

Accuracy of Information

The accuracy of the information you provide in your application is critical. This information helps determine the length of your survey, the standards according to which you will be surveyed, and the fee for survey. Please review all your information carefully, and contact your account representative at The Joint Commission with any questions you may have before submitting your application.

If at any time during the accreditation process your organization undergoes a change that modifies the information reported in your application, you must notify The Joint Commission in writing within 30 calendar days of the change. Information that must be reported includes the following:

- Change in ownership
- Change in location
- Significant increase or decrease in the volume of services
- Addition of a new type of health service or site of care
- Acquisition of a new component
- Removal of an existing health service or site of care
- Removal of an existing component

Business Associate Agreement

The Health Insurance Portability and Accountability Act of 1996 (HIPAA) established national standards for electronic health care transactions and addressed the security and privacy of health care data. The HIPAA regulations recognize that an accreditor's access to personally identified health information is both necessary and appropriate. Under the regulations, accreditors are considered business associates of health care organizations, and health care organizations are required to have agreements with their business associates to ensure that these associates appropriately safeguard health information that includes personal identifiers.

To comply with HIPAA's *Standards for Privacy of Individually Identified Health Information,* all health care organizations seeking or renewing accreditation must sign a business associate agreement with The Joint Commission. This agreement must be in place at the time your organization applies for accreditation.

A model business associate agreement to be used by all accredited health care organizations (*see* below) is available for review on The Joint Commission's Web site at http://www.jointcommission.org. (Click on "Accredited Organizations," then click on your accreditation program, then on "Accreditation Process," and finally on "Business Associate Agreement.") The actual agreement is integrated into your e-App.

Addendum to The Joint Commission Accreditation Contract

(Business Associate Agreement)

THIS ADDENDUM supplements and is made a part of **The Joint Commission** Accreditation Contract (hereinafter, the "Underlying Agreement") submitted to **The Joint Commission** by ("the Organization"). The Underlying Agreement, when accepted by **The Joint Commission**, establishes the terms of the relationship between **The Joint Commission** and the Organization.

Whereas, The Joint Commission and the Organization are parties to the Underlying Agreement pursuant to which **The Joint Commission** provides certain accreditation and related services to the Organization and, in connection with the provision of those services, the Organization discloses to **The Joint Commission** certain Protected Health Information ("PHI", as defined in 45 C.F.R. §164.501) that is subject to protection under the Health Insurance Portability and Accountability Act of 1996 ("HIPAA");

Whereas, the Organization is a "Covered Entity" as that term is defined in the HIPAA implementing regulations, 45 C.F.R. Part 160 and Part 164, Subparts A and E, the Standards for Privacy of Individually Identifiable Health Information ("Privacy Rule"); and 45 C.F.R. Part 164, Subpart C, the Security Standards for the Protection of Electronic Protected Health Information ("Security Rule");

Whereas, The Joint Commission, as a recipient of PHI from the Organization, is a "Business Associate" as that term is defined in the Privacy Rule;

Whereas, pursuant to the Privacy Rule and the Security Rule, all Business Associates of Covered Entities must agree in writing to certain mandatory provisions regarding the use and disclosure of PHI; and

Whereas, the purpose of this Addendum is to comply with the requirements of the Privacy Rule and the Security Rule, including, but not limited to, the Business Associate contract requirements at 45 C.F.R. §§164.314(a), 164.502(e), §164.504(e), and as may be amended.

NOW, THEREFORE in consideration of the mutual promises and covenants contained herein, the parties agree as follows:

1. **Definitions.** Unless otherwise provided in this Addendum, capitalized terms have the same meanings as set forth in the Privacy Rule or the Security Rule.
2. **Scope of Use and Disclosure by The Joint Commission of Protected Health Information**
   A. **The Joint Commission** shall be permitted to Use and Disclose PHI that is disclosed to it by the Organization as necessary to perform its obligations under the Underlying Agreement.

(continued)

B. Unless otherwise limited herein, in addition to any other Uses and/or Disclosures permitted or authorized by this Addendum or Required by law, **The Joint Commission** may:

i. Use the PHI in its possession for its proper management and administration and to fulfill any legal responsibilities of **The Joint Commission**;

ii. Disclose the PHI in its possession to a third party for the purpose of **The Joint Commission**'s proper management and administration or to fulfill any legal responsibilities of **The Joint Commission**; provided, however, that the Disclosures are Required by Law or **The Joint Commission** has received from the third party written assurances that (i) the information will be held confidentially and used or further disclosed only as Required by Law or for the purposes for which it was disclosed to the third party; and (ii) the third party will notify **The Joint Commission** of any instances of which it becomes aware in which the confidentiality of the information has been breached;

iii. Aggregate the PHI with that of other Organizations for the purpose of providing the Organization with data analyses relating to the Health Care Operations of the Organization. **The Joint Commission** may not Disclose the PHI of one Organization to another Organization without the written authorization of the Organizations involved; and

iv. De-identify any and all PHI created or received by **The Joint Commission** under this Addendum; provided, that the de-identification conforms to the requirements of the Privacy Rule.

3. **Obligations of THE JOINT COMMISSION.** In connection with its Use and Disclosure of PHI, **The Joint Commission** agrees that it will:

A. Use or further Disclose PHI only as permitted or required by this Addendum or as Required by Law.

B. Use reasonable and appropriate safeguards to prevent Use or Disclosure of PHI other than as provided for by this Addendum.

C. To the extent practicable, mitigate any harmful effect that is known to **The Joint Commission** of a Use or Disclosure of PHI by **The Joint Commission** in violation of this Addendum.

D. Report to the Organization any Use or Disclosure of PHI not provided for by this Addendum of which **The Joint Commission** becomes aware.

E. Require contractors or agents to whom **The Joint Commission** provides PHI to agree to the same restrictions and conditions that apply to **The Joint Commission** pursuant to this Addendum.

F. Make available to the Secretary of Health and Human Services **The Joint Commission's** internal practices, books and records relating to the Use and Disclosure of PHI for purposes of determining the Organization's compliance with the Privacy Rule, subject to any applicable legal privileges.

G. Within fifteen (15) days of receiving a request from the Organization, make available the information necessary for the Organization to make an accounting of Disclosures of PHI about an individual.

H. Within ten (10) days of receiving a written request from the Organization, make available PHI necessary for the Organization to respond to Individuals' requests for access to PHI about them in the event that the PHI in **The Joint Commission's** possession constitutes a Designated Record Set.

I. Within fifteen (15) days of receiving a written request from the Organization incorporate any amendments or corrections to the PHI in accordance with the Privacy Rule in the event that the PHI in **The Joint Commission's** possession constitutes a Designated Record Set.

J. Implement Administrative, Physical, and Technical Safeguards that reasonably and appropriately protect the confidentiality, integrity and availability of the Electronic PHI that it creates, receives, maintains or transmits on behalf of the Organization, and make its policies and procedures, and documentation required by the Security Rule relating to such safeguards, available to the Secretary of HHS for purposes of determining the Organization's compliance with the Security Rule;

K. Ensure that any agent, including a subcontractor, to whom it provides Electronic PHI agrees to implement reasonable and appropriate safeguards to protect that Electronic PHI; and

L. Promptly report to the Organization any security incident with respect to Electronic PHI of which it becomes aware.

4. **Obligations of the Organization.** The Organization agrees that it:

A. Has included, and will include, in the Organization's Notice of Privacy Practices required by the Privacy Rule that the Organization may disclose PHI for Health Care Operations purposes.

B. Has obtained, and will obtain, from Individuals consents, authorizations and other permissions necessary or required by laws applicable to the Organization for **The Joint Commission** and the Organization to fulfill their obligations under the Underlying Agreement and this Addendum.

C. Will promptly notify **The Joint Commission** in writing of any restrictions on the Use and Disclosure of PHI about Individuals that the Organization has agreed to that may affect **The Joint Commission's** ability to perform its obligations under the Underlying Agreement or this Addendum.

D. Will promptly notify **The Joint Commission** in writing of any changes in, or revocation of, permission by an Individual to Use or Disclose PHI, if such changes or revocation may affect **The Joint Commission's** ability to perform its obligations under the Underlying Agreement or this Addendum.

5. **Termination.**

A. Termination for Breach. The Organization may terminate this Addendum if the Surveyed Organization determines that **The Joint Commission** has breached a material term of this Addendum. Alternatively, the Organization may choose to provide **The Joint Commission** with notice of the existence of an alleged material breach and afford **The Joint Commission** an opportunity to cure the alleged material breach. In the event **The Joint Commission** fails to cure the breach to the satisfaction of the Organization, the Organization may immediately thereafter terminate this Addendum.

B. Automatic Termination. This Addendum will automatically terminate upon the termination of the Underlying Agreement.

C. Effect of Termination.

i. Termination of this Addendum will result in termination of the Underlying Agreement.

ii. Upon termination of this Addendum or the Underlying Agreement, **The Joint Commission** will return or destroy all PHI received from the Organization or created or received by **The Joint Commission** on behalf of the Organization that **The Joint Commission** still maintains and retain no copies of such PHI; provided that if such return or destruction is not feasible, **The Joint Commission** will extend the protections of this Addendum to the PHI and limit further Uses and Disclosures to those purposes that make the return or destruction of the information infeasible.

(continued)

6. **Amendment. The Joint Commission** and the Organization agree to take such action as is necessary to amend this Addendum from time to time as is necessary for the Organization to comply with the requirements of the Privacy Rule and the Security Rule.
7. **Survival.** The obligations of **The Joint Commission** under section 5.C (ii) of this Addendum shall survive any termination of this addendum.
8. **No Third Party Beneficiaries.** Nothing expressed or implied in this Addendum is intended to confer, nor shall anything herein confer, upon any person other than the parties and their respective successors or assigns, any rights, remedies, obligations or liabilities whatsoever.
9. **Effective Date.** This Addendum shall be effective on ______________.

Surveyed Organization	**THE JOINT COMMISSION**
Name: ______________________	Signature: ______________________
Title: ______________________	Print Name: ______________________
Date: ______________________	Title: ______________________
	Date: ______________________

Your Account Representative

On receiving your e-App, The Joint Commission assigns your organization an account representative, who serves as your primary contact at The Joint Commission. This person coordinates survey planning and handles your inquiries about policies, procedures, accreditation issues, or services, and inquiries throughout the accreditation cycle. If you have received your application, but have not been notified about your account representative, call 630/792-3007. You can also look at your organization information on the extranet site. The right-hand column lists your assigned account representative.

Survey Scheduling

If your organization is not yet accredited, The Joint Commission schedules your initial survey within six months of the time it receives your application. Please specify on your application in what month you would like your survey to be held. If your organization is accredited, it will have an unannounced survey (for more information about unannounced surveys, *see* page 290).

For initial surveys, requests to postpone an already scheduled survey are only considered in rare situations. An organization should direct a request for a postponement to its account representative. A request to postpone a survey may be granted if one or more of the following criteria are met:

- A natural disaster or other major unforeseen event has occurred that has totally or substantially disrupted operations
- The long term care organization is involved in a major strike, has ceased admitting residents, and is transferring residents to other facilities or organizations
- Residents and the long term care organization are being moved to a new building on the day or days of the survey

Note 1: *If a survey postponement is requested because of a natural disaster, strike, or movement to a new building, an on-site extension survey may be required if the organization is continuing to provide resident care services.*

Note 2: *If an organization is undergoing an unannounced survey and on the day of the survey the organization experiences one of these situations, the survey may be postponed.*

Sidebar 1. Priority Focus Areas

Priority focus areas (PFAs) are processes, systems, or structures in a health care organization that significantly affect the safety and quality of care provided. The list of PFAs was developed from information provided by The Joint Commission's Office of Quality Monitoring, expert literature, and expert opinions. Joint Commission categorized the different processes, systems, and structures leading to improved health care into 14 PFAs. The PFAs evolved from this process of identifying common patterns useful toward building positive health care outcomes and safe, quality health care.

The PFAs provide a consistent yet customized approach to providing an initial focus for the on-site survey process, and they may assist the health care organization at the time of its PPR.

The PFAs are the following:

- Assessment and Care/Services
- Communication
- Credentialed Practitioners
- Equipment Use
- Infection Control
- Information Management
- Medication Management
- Organizational Structure
- Orientation & Training
- Patient Safety
- Physical Environment
- Quality Improvement Expertise/Activities
- Rights & Ethics
- Staffing

PFAs guide the surveyor with assessing standards compliance in relation to the individual tracer activities. Outside formal conferences or interviews, much of the survey consists of reviewing issues in the form of tracer methodology. The tracer methodology incorporates the use of the PFP information, follows the care experience for individuals initially identified by CSGs, and allows the surveyor to identify performance issues that may be related to PFAs for your organization.

Presurvey Activities

Presurvey Information

Throughout the accreditation cycle, a long term care facility can access its PFP Summary on *The Joint Commission Connect* extranet site at the following times:

- 90 days before the annual Periodic Performance Review (PPR) is due
- The morning of an unannounced survey (during the preliminary planning meeting, long term care staff members will have time to check the extranet site for the PFP information)

Note: *Organizations that have an announced survey will be able to access the PFP Summary 14 days before an announced survey.*

The summary takes data from a variety of sources—including previous survey findings or recommendations, data from The Joint Commission's Office of Quality Monitoring, data from your e-App, ORYX® data (if applicable), and data from external sources. Examples of these sources

Sidebar 2. Clinical/Service Groups

Clinical/service groups (CSGs) categorize residents and services into distinct populations for which data can be collected. The Joint Commission created the list of CSGs based on data gathered from e-Apps from each accreditation program and on publicly available data from external sources. The list then underwent a thorough review to make sure that all categories were actually representative of populations served or services provided by the organizations surveyed by the individual accreditation programs. Joint Commission surveyors use a long term care organization's CSGs combined with other long term care-specific data to get a better understanding of the organization's systems and the residents it serves. Tracer residents are selected according to CSGs.

CSGs for Long Term Care:

- LTC-Hospital operated
- LTC-Freestanding
- Dementia care
- Geriatric psychiatric care
- Intermediate care
- Pediatric care
- Physical rehabilitation services
- Skilled nursing care/complex medical care
- Transitional care unit
- Traumatic brain injury services
- Ventilator services

Additional CSGs based on Centers for Medicare & Medicaid Services' Nursing Home Compare Data:

- Residents having delirium
- Residents having urinary tract infections
- Residents having loss of ability in activities of daily living
- Residents having mobility concerns
- Residents needing pain control
- Residents needing physical restraints
- Residents with declining physical activity
- Residents who lose too much weight
- Residents (short stay) with pressure sores
- Residents with high risk of pressure sores
- Residents with low risk of pressure sores
- Residents having depression
- Residents with low risk of bladder/bowel control problems
- Residents needing catheters
- Residents (short stay) given pneumonia vaccination
- Residents (short stay) given flu vaccination
- Residents given flu vaccination
- Residents given pneumonia vaccination

include Minimum Data Set (MDS) quality measures, and identifies the top four or five PFAs and clinical/service groups (CSGs) for your organization (*see* Sidebars 1 and 2 on page 303 and above). This is the same information that is available to the surveyors and on which they base the initial focus of survey activities.

How Is PFP Information Used in Survey Activities?

The surveyor(s) will review the PFP information on the surveyor extranet prior to the first day of survey and will use this information in the Preliminary Planning Session on the first day of survey as well as for other survey activities. The surveyor(s) will ask organization leaders for their perceptions of the organization's top system-level PFA and CSG priorities and will consider these areas in survey activities as well.

Information from prioritized PFAs and CSGs guide and focus other survey activities such as the following:

- Individual tracers
- Individual-based system tracers
- Review of the environment of care (EC)
- Credentialing

For example, if your PFP output lists your top four CSGs as dementia care, ventilator services, skilled nursing care, and rehabilitative services, the surveyor(s) tries to choose residents from these groups for inclusion in the initial individual tracers. As the survey progresses, the surveyor(s) may find other priority areas that need addressing and he or she may begin to focus less on the PFP suggested list and more on what he or she is finding.

ORYX Performance Measure Data

If an organization has chosen to participate in a listed performance measurement system and submit data to The Joint Commission, The Joint Commission posts an updated version of the organization's ORYX Performance Measure Report (*see* page 305) on the organization's secure extranet site after each submission of quarterly ORYX performance measurement data, approximately four weeks after each submission of measure data. (This does not apply if your organization will be undergoing an initial survey.) Cur-

Program	ORYX Policy
Long Term Care	LTC - 6 Measures - System

Summary of Active Measure Sets Based on 2007Q1 to 2007Q4						
Measure Set	Number of Active Measures	Standards Compliance Issues[1]	Undesirable Result[1]	Desirable Result[1]	Control Chart Not Stable[1]	Overall Set[2] (Ordered by priority)
Non-Core	6	0	2	1	6	

[1]The number of occurences for each measure set
[2]Overall set summary is based on detail measure performance as outlined in the ORYX Performance Measure Report Guide

Figure 1. *Measure set summary.*

rently, data are due to The Joint Commission on January 31, April 30, July 31, and October 31 of each year.

After organizations submit their ORYX performance measure data, reports will be posted to each organization's secure extranet site (click on "Reports" and select "ORYX Performance Measure Reports"). Organizations will receive an electronic message notifying them that their reports are available. Accredited organizations that have the option of meeting some or all of their ORYX performance measurement requirements without submitting data to The Joint Commission will continue to receive a report four times per year.

The ORYX Performance Measure Report does the following:

- Reminds organizations of their ORYX requirements for internally collecting and analyzing performance measure data for the appropriate required number of measures
- Better guides the survey process by informing surveyors to explore how the organization is using the information derived from internally collecting and analyzing its ORYX performance measure data in its ongoing performance improvement activities
- Lists the performance measures the organization has selected
- Summarizes the performance measure data the organization has submitted to meet Joint Commission ORYX performance measurement requirements
- Presents the data (for each selected measure) submitted by the organization's chosen performance measurement system to The Joint Commission in the form of comparison charts and control charts
- Identifies any months for which the organization had missing data and/or no cases to report (for each measure selected), performance outliers, and unusual data patterns

The Summary of Measures page in the Performance Measure Report (Figure 1, above) lists the performance measures an organization has selected to meet the ORYX requirements. The measures are identified by the following:

- An accreditation program code (for example, LTC= long term care)

Key	Definition
	Statistically Significant Performance Issue(s) Identified -- Detailed Internal Measure Review Recommended
	Warning: Undesirable Issue(s) Identified -- Internal Measure Review Recommended
Blank	No Issue Identified. Review any unstable Control Charts
	Desirable Performance. Review any unstable Control Charts

Key	Definition
	Control Chart not stable. Interpret Comparison Analysis with caution
NC	Health Care Organization had **no cases** for all measures within the measure set
ND	Unable to perform comparison and control chart analysis using current Joint Commission methodologies.

Figure 2. *Measure set legend.*

Summary of Active Measures Based on 2007Q1 to 2007Q4						
Non-Core	Measure Collection Begin Date	Standards Compliance Issues	Control Chart	Comparison Chart	Missing Data	Data Quality Issues
Falls with injury. (3448)	1/1/2003					
Rate of documented falls. (3457)	1/1/2000					
Rate of lower respiratory infections treated. (3465)	7/1/1998					
Rate of LTC patients/residents with indwelling catheters with symptomatic UTI. (9650)	1/1/1999					
Rate of LTC residents with symptomatic UTIs. (9637)	1/1/1999					
Unplanned weight loss in LTC residents/patients (9399)	1/1/2000					

Figure 3. *Measure level summary.*

- A measure identification number
- An abbreviated measure name
- The month/year the organization began collecting data for each measure
- The last month/year the organization submitted data for each measure it no longer uses
- The number of months each measure has been used

The summary also indicates whether there were any data points that were statistically out of control, outlier data points, missing data points, and/or potential data quality concerns (aberrant data) for each of the performance measures.

The control and comparison charts in the report are created using the data your organization submits to your performance measurement system, which in turn transmits aggre-

HCO	
Measure Set	Non-Core
Measure	Rate of documented falls. (3457)
Direction of Improvement	Decrease in rate/value
Type of Measure	Proportion

Measure Issue Summary				
Standards Compliance Issues	Control Chart	Comparison Chart	Missing Data	Data Quality Issues

Numerator Total number of documented falls (for the reporting period).

Denominator Total number of resident/patient days for the reporting period.

Control chart (P-chart)

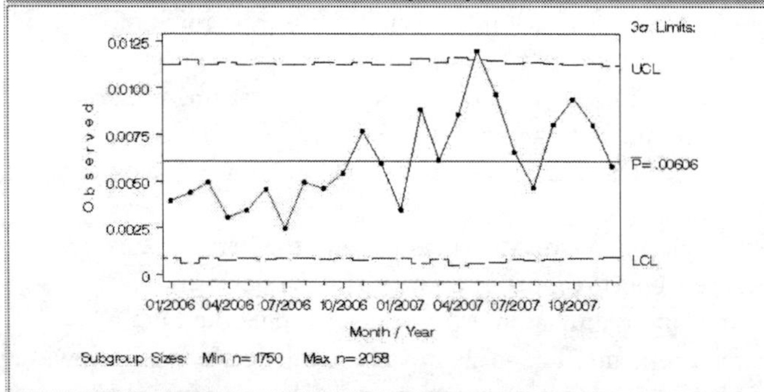

Comparison chart

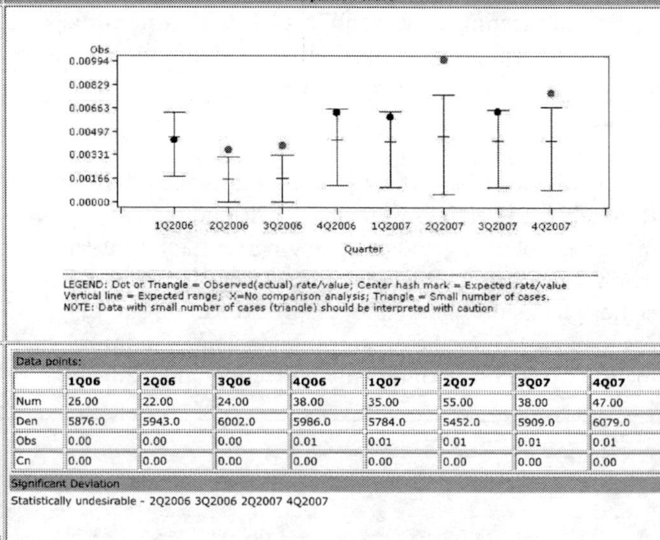

LEGEND: Dot or Triangle = Observed(actual) rate/value; Center hash mark = Expected rate/value
Vertical line = Expected range; X=No comparison analysis; Triangle = Small number of cases.
NOTE: Data with small number of cases (triangle) should be interpreted with caution

Data points:

	1/06	2/06	3/06	4/06	5/06	6/06	7/06	8/06	9/06	10/06	11/06	12/06
Num	8.00	8.00	10.00	6.00	7.00	9.00	5.00	10.00	9.00	11.00	15.00	12.00
Den	2027.0	1823.0	2026.0	1946.0	2031.0	1966.0	2021.0	2027.0	1954.0	2025.0	1951.0	2010.0
Obs	0.00	0.00	0.00	0.00	0.00	0.00	0.00	0.00	0.00	0.01	0.01	0.01
	1/07	2/07	3/07	4/07	5/07	6/07	7/07	8/07	9/07	10/07	11/07	12/07
Num	7.00	16.00	12.00	15.00	22.00	18.00	13.00	9.00	16.00	19.00	16.00	12.00
Den	2024.0	1806.0	1954.0	1750.0	1836.0	1866.0	1979.0	1941.0	1989.0	2022.0	1999.0	2058.0
Obs	0.00	0.01	0.01	0.01	0.01	0.01	0.01	0.00	0.01	0.01	0.01	0.01

Out of Statistical Control Tests (e.g., Special Cause Variation)

One data point above +3 sigma or below -3 sigma - 5/2007
Eight consecutive data points on the same side of the mean - 8/2006 9/2006 10/2006

Data points:

	1Q06	2Q06	3Q06	4Q06	1Q07	2Q07	3Q07	4Q07
Num	26.00	22.00	24.00	38.00	35.00	55.00	38.00	47.00
Den	5876.0	5943.0	6002.0	5986.0	5784.0	5452.0	5909.0	6079.0
Obs	0.00	0.00	0.00	0.01	0.01	0.01	0.01	0.01
Cn	0.00	0.00	0.00	0.00	0.00	0.00	0.00	0.00

Significant Deviation

Statistically undesirable - 2Q2006 3Q2006 2Q2007 4Q2007

Missing Data Issues

There are no missing data issues

Data Quality Issues

There are no data quality issues

Figure 4. *Measure level detail.*

gate monthly data to The Joint Commission. The Joint Commission analyzes each of your selected performance measures (displayed in the control chart) in monthly increments. Control charts are provided for each measure after it has been used for at least 12 months; comparison charts are provided regardless of how long the measure has been used. Both control and comparison charts note the name of the measure, provide a brief description of its focus, and show the "direction" in which data for the measure would demonstrate improvement.

Redesigned Performance Measure Reports

The reports have been redesigned to better support and help guide accredited organizations in their performance assessment and improvement activities. In addition, the reports will help surveyors assess the organization's use of performance measure data in performance improvement activities. (*See* page 305 for an example of the redesigned ORYX Performance Measure Report.)

The redesigned ORYX Performance Measure Report provides a user-friendly format with summary "dashboards," comprehensive measure details, automated links to specific sections, and selective printing capabilities.

The newly redesigned ORYX Performance Measure Report highlights desirable and undesirable data trends. Key enhanced features include the following:

- A dashboard of color-coded symbols at both the measure set and individual measure level provide a quick and easy graphical summary of an organization's performance on its measures. Each measure set and individual measure on the dashboard provides a hyperlink that the user can click to access more detailed information.
- An easy-to-use legend that defines each of the color-coded symbols
- At the measure set level the dashboard displays the total number of measures within the set used by the organization and highlights the set(s) for which standards compliance issues may arise (for example, compliance issues with Standard PI.2.20, EP 13), desirable or undesirable data trends, and/or statistical process control issues.
- At the individual measure level, the dashboard identifies measures for which standards compliance issues may arise, desirable or undesirable data trends, and/or statistical process control issues.
- Control and comparison charts for each measure along with the actual data values behind the graphical chart displays
- Individual measures that require an organization's attention are highlighted when potential standards compliance issues and/or undesirable trends are identified.

Future enhancements include a user's guide that will address frequently asked questions.

If you have any questions about your ORYX report, call the ORYX Information Line at 630/792-5085 or send an e-mail to oryx@jointcommission.org.

Presurvey Activities

On-Site Survey Preparation

Notifying the Public about a Joint Commission Survey

Because of the unannounced survey process, an organization cannot post its survey date and therefore individuals cannot request a Public Information Interview (PII). To address this situation, an APR relating to continuous public involvement was established (*see* the "Accreditation Participation Requirements" [APR] chapter of the *CAMLTC*). APR.09.01.01 requires an organization to demonstrate how it communicates to its public that if members of the public have any quality-of-care or safety concerns, they should notify The Joint Commission. The organization may notify the public by posting an accreditation certificate, posting information on its Web site and in resident admission brochures, or using any other effective means of its choice.

The public includes, but is not limited to, the following:

- Residents and their families
- Resident advocates and advocacy groups
- Members of the community for whom services are provided
- Staff members

Conducting a Public Information Interview

Because all surveys are now unannounced, PIIs are conducted only if someone contacts the surveyor(s) during an on-site survey to request a PII and the survey process can accommodate the PII. Should this occur, the surveyor(s) identifies an appropriate time during the survey to schedule this session.

Survey Logistics

Organizations should have an unannounced survey logistics plan in place for all staff members to follow. Be sure to address the following items in your plan:

- Prepare an instruction sheet for staff at the information desk, reception area, or security desk for staff to follow when surveyors arrive. Include
  - An internal calling tree, with backups identified in the event staff members are unavailable
  - A location to which staff may direct the surveyor(s) to wait
  - Procedures for issuing temporary passes or IDs to the surveyor(s), if applicable
  - Procedures for surveyor visitor book sign-in, if applicable
- Plan for a workspace that the surveyor(s) will need designated as his or her "headquarters" for the survey. A desk or table, telephone, and access to an electrical outlet will be needed, if possible.
- Identify who will be the surveyors' contact person during the survey, including backups in case that person is not available when the surveyors arrive.

To help create your survey logistics plan, please see *the "Joint Commission Survey Planning Master List" worksheet on pages 362–363 in Appendix 2.*

Verification of Surveyor Identification

Organizations will need to access their Joint Commission extranet site upon arrival of the surveyor(s) for an unannounced survey. This is accomplished by accessing the Internet and The Joint Commission's Web site (http://www.jointcommission.org) and clicking on "Joint Commission Connect." You will need to enter your login ID and password to enter the organization's secured Joint Commission Web site. Access the "Notification of Scheduled Events" link on your extranet site.

IMPORTANT: *Your unannounced survey procedures should include the login ID and password to access the organization's* The Joint Commission Connect™ *extranet site.*

By 7:30 A.M. in the organization's local time zone on the first day of the unannounced survey, the organization's extranet site will contain:

- An introductory letter signed by the executive vice president of Accreditation and Certification Operations authorizing the surveyors' presence for the unannounced survey
- Surveyor names and biographies
- Survey dates
- PFP output

Agenda Planning

The organization's agenda for survey will be present on its extranet site in advance of the unannounced arrival. Use the agenda and this activity guide as a planning tool for the unannounced survey by:

- Identifying key participants and their backups for various sessions
- Including phone numbers for these key individuals so they can be contacted quickly by the survey coordinator or other staff
- If applicable, including representative and backup representative names and phone numbers from all components of the organization (that is, long term care, behavioral health care, home care, ambulatory care)
- Identifying surveyor working space, group meeting locations, and alternatives in the event original space is occupied

Information Needed for the Surveyor(s)

The first hour of the survey is designated for a Preliminary Planning Session. This time allows the organization and the surveyor(s) to get organized for the survey. Organizations should direct the surveyor(s) to an appropriate working space and should also have a method prepared for notifying all departments and units that the surveyor(s) has arrived for an unannounced survey.

In addition, the organization will need to put staff members in charge of gathering the following information so that it is available for the surveyor(s) as soon as possible after arrival:

- Performance improvement data from the past 12 months
- Infection control surveillance data from the past 12 months
- EC data including the electronic Statement of Conditions™ (e-SOC) and Plans for Improvement, if applicable; management plans and annual evaluations; and EC multidisciplinary team meeting minutes for the 12 months prior to survey
- An organization chart
- A map of the organization, if available
- List of departments/units/areas/programs within the organization, if applicable
- Staffing effectiveness data
- Any reports or lists of residents (for example, MDS resident roster) that will help identify individuals to trace

- Name of key contact person who can assist surveyors in planning tracer selection
- MOS identified in the Plan of Action from the PPR
- ORYX Performance Measurement data/MDS Quality Indicator Reports/MDS Quality Measure Reports
- Most recent state agency survey reports including Centers for Medicare & Medicaid Services certification reports, licensure reports, and complaint investigation reports

Note: *If this information is not immediately available, the surveyor(s) will begin with an individual tracer.*

Advance planning to generate data reports on demand or to locate the latest internal reports for surveyor review is recommended. Use the list as a tool and indicate next to each item the data source, the frequency of updates, and the person responsible for the information and his or her backup with phone numbers, and the format for the information (computer or print out). This will facilitate the gathering process for your staff.

To help compile the necessary documents and assign staff members in charge of collecting those documents, consult the "Documents for Preliminary Planning Session" worksheet on pages 364–365 in Appendix 2.

The Document Review Session is no longer a scheduled part of the on-site survey process. However, some activities will require certain types of records to be available. As you review the descriptions of activities that follow, you may find it helpful to keep a list of any information, records or files (in addition to the items listed above) that the surveyor(s) may request so you can have them on hand.

On-Site Survey Activities

- ☑ Surveyor Arrival and Preliminary Planning Session
- ☑ Opening Conference
- ☑ Orientation to the Organization
- ☑ Special Issue Resolution
- ☑ Daily Briefing
- ☑ Surveyor Team Meeting/Planning Session
- ☑ Credentialing
- ☑ Competence Assessment: Credentialing of Licensed Independent Practitioners
- ☑ Individual Tracer Activities
- ☑ Program-Specific Tracer Activities: Resident-Centered Care
- ☑ Program-Specific Tracer Activities: Staffing
- ☑ Example Questions for Long Term Care Tracers
- ☑ Narrative Example: Individual Tracer of a Long Term Care Resident
- ☑ Individual-Based System Tracer: Medication Management*
- ☑ Individual-Based System Tracer: Infection Control*
- ☑ Individual-Based System Tracer: Data Use*
- ☑ Physical Environment
- ☑ Leadership Session
- ☑ Criticality and the Accreditation Decision Process
- ☑ Surveyor Report Preparation
- ☑ CEO Exit Briefing and Organization Exit Conference

* For surveys longer than two days.

On-Site Survey Activities

Surveyor Arrival and Preliminary Planning Session

This one-hour survey activity takes place immediately after the surveyor(s) arrives. At this time, you should provide the surveyor(s) with the data listed in the previous section titled "Information Needed for the Surveyor(s)" on pages 308–309.

Purpose

This session is for the surveyor(s) to plan individual tracer activity, review materials, and discuss the focus among other survey team members, when applicable.

Where Will the Activity Take Place?

This session will take place in the location you have chosen for surveyor use during the survey. The surveyor(s) will need workspace designated as his or her "headquarters" for the duration of the survey. A desk or table, telephone, and access to an electrical outlet are desirable.

Who Will Participate From Your Organization?

- Organization staff members who need to prepare all data listed in the section titled "Information Needed for the Surveyor(s)" on page 308.
- Otherwise, staff members will be contacted when needed, but no one directly participates in the planning session.
- Please provide the name and phone number of a key contact person who can assist the surveyor(s) in planning tracer selection.

What Will Occur?

- The surveyor(s) must begin survey activity while the organization is communicating the surveyor's arrival and gathering for the Opening Conference. (This is a one-hour time frame.) If immediately made available, the surveyor(s) will begin with a review of information, outlined in the section titled "Information Needed for the Surveyor(s)" on pages 308–309. The surveyor(s) will begin an individual tracer if the information is not immediately made available.
- Discuss any changes that need to be made to the survey agenda with the surveyor(s) during this session. Changes made to the agenda should be limited and are at the discretion of the surveyor.
- A surveyor will sign off on your electronic Statement of Conditions™ (e-SOC) and Plans for Improvement (PFIs). If your organization has not developed a PFI, the surveyor will sign a blank PFI form, drawing a line through it to indicate that he or she is signing a blank form, and leave this with your survey coordinator to keep for future surveys. Surveyors send a copy of all signed PFIs to The Joint Commission Central Office.*
- Based on your PFP information, the surveyor(s) will identify representative CSGs and some general information about your active residents. If the resident list you have provided includes diagnoses/conditions, the surveyor(s) will select residents from the list for tracers. If the list does not include diagnoses/conditions, either the surveyor(s) will describe the type of resident he or she wishes to trace and ask your survey coordinator for help in choosing individuals, or he or she will visit a unit or department to select individuals and request help from the staff there.
- If any requests for Public Information Interviews (PII) should occur, the surveyor(s) will schedule time for them in your survey agenda.

Information for Complex Organizations

The on-site evaluation addresses the organization as an integrated whole as opposed to the fragmented focus on individual components in the current process. Organizations being surveyed under multiple accreditation programs should have information from all programs available at the Preliminary Planning Session. If your organization is part of a complex organization survey, the surveyor(s) will coordinate activities during the planning session to accommodate the schedules of surveyors from different programs with different time commitments. This includes the following:

- Selecting tracer residents who have been served across the settings covered by the different accreditation programs
- Identifying opportunities to integrate individual-based system tracers and other survey activities among accreditation programs, depending on the services provided, your organization's degree of centralization, and the distance between different locations
- Coordinating times for team meetings, special resolution sessions, and other mechanisms for sharing information with surveyors in different locations
- Identifying communication mechanisms, such as conference calls, for team members in different locations

* The discussion of the Statement of Conditions PFI does not apply to organizations seeking the Medicare/Medicaid certification–based long term care accreditation option.

- Arranging for at least one survey team member to attend the Exit Conference in the event that some members will leave early

On-Site Survey Activities

Opening Conference

This conference, which is held on the first day of the survey, is a meeting among the organization leaders, key staff, and the surveyor(s). The meeting lasts 15 minutes.

Purpose

- Introduction of the surveyor(s)
- Introduction of organization leaders and key staff
- Description of the survey

Where Will the Activity Take Place?

The conference may take place in the location of your choice.

What Will Occur?

The surveyor(s) facilitates this session by first introducing The Joint Commission participants, then the organization is asked to make its introductions. The surveyor(s) then briefly describes the structure of the survey and may need clarification about the material submitted or the organization's services. As a result of the resident-centered approach to the survey process, surveyor(s) need to interview residents privately for some tracers. Surveyor(s) will explain this to your organization. This private interview is intended to put residents at ease. Surveyor(s) will debrief with the staff members. A list of required data and information appears in the previous section titled "Information Needed for the Surveyor(s)" on pages 308–309. The organization may ask questions about the survey, the agenda, or other related topics at this time.

On-Site Survey Activities

Orientation to the Organization

The Orientation to the Organization activity directly follows the Opening Conference. This 45-minute session is an interactive discussion facilitated by the surveyor(s). Prepared presentations by the organization are not necessary.

Purpose

To give you the opportunity to describe your organization's basic structure; mission; vision; scope of care, treatment, and services; resident population(s); and strategic planning approach to the surveyor(s). For complex organizations, this will include all programs and services.

Where Will the Activity Take Place?

The meeting usually takes place in the same room where the Opening Conference was held.

Who Will Participate From Your Organization?

If possible, senior leaders representing all programs/settings in a complex organization (such as home care, long term care) should attend. Individuals should be able to address leaders' responsibilities for planning, resource allocation, management, oversight, performance improvement, and support in carrying out the organization's mission and strategic objectives.

Senior leaders typically include but are not limited to representatives from the following areas (not all organizations will have representatives from each area, depending on organization structure, care, and services provided):

- At least one member of the governing body or organization trustee (in single-owner organizations, this individual may also be the CEO)
- Senior organization leaders (for example, CEO, medical director, COO, CFO, CIO, vice-president for clinical services, nurse executive, director of resident services, chief administrator/director of each program) from all programs (for example, hospital, long term care)
  Note: *Participation of department directors is not required; however, senior leaders of all other programs in a complex organization that independently would be eligible for an accreditation survey should participate.*

What Will Occur?

During the orientation, the surveyor(s) or the survey team leader will ask staff members to talk about your organization, focusing on management and important processes and functions. Discussion topics may include the following:

Leaders' Role in Governance and Operations

- Mission, vision, goals, and strategic directions
- Organization structure
- Operational management
- Contract management
- Health care errors reduction and/or resident safety including use of root cause analysis
- National Patient Safety Goals
- Community involvement
- Leaders' roles in emergency management planning
- Initiatives for resident-centered care, if any

Leaders' Role in Priority Focus Areas

This is a facilitated discussion between organization members and Joint Commission surveyor(s) (a formal presentation is not necessary because it would not support discussion). Leaders may be asked to identify the organization's PFAs, as well as the clinical care and services groups with the highest volumes. The top PFAs may be discussed with the organization based on its PFP output including:

- Information about the organization's strengths and weaknesses at the PFA level
- Information gathering and baseline assessment of organization systems/processes from a leadership, management oversight perspective and other leader responsibilities
- Leaders' approach to the PPR and methods used to address areas needing improvement (discussed within a performance improvement context)
- Ongoing initiatives to improve delivery of health care as well as prioritize future projects
- Leaders' idea of variations in what your organization considers your top PFAs and CSGs

Leaders' Role in Improving Performance

- How leaders set expectations, plan, assess, and measure initiatives to improve the quality of services
- Organization approach to safety, including selection of proactive risk assessment, resulting improvements, and Board involvement in safety issues
- Provision of personnel and resources including time, information systems, data management, and staff training

Note: *The surveyor(s) may request examples of performance improvement initiatives including evidence that performance was achieved and sustained.*

Long Term Care Medicare/Medicaid Certification Option Discussion Topics

- Organization's Minimum Data Set (MDS) Quality Measure Reports, Facility MDS Quality Indicator Profile, or Quality Measure Reports
- Most recent state agency survey reports including Centers for Medicare & Medicaid Services (CMS) certificate reports (that is, CMS form 2567), licensure reports, and complaint investigation reports
- Follow-up activities relevant to these reports

For assistance in preparing for this conference, please consult the "Opening Conference and Orientation to the Organization" worksheet on pages 366–367 in Appendix 2.

On-Site Survey Activities

Special Issue Resolution

This activity is performed when the surveyor(s) needs to resolve issues that have been identified during other survey activities or when more time is needed to address a specific topic. For surveys lasting more than one day, this session is about 30 minutes at the end of the day.

Purpose

To allow the surveyor(s) to pursue issues that have arisen during the course of the survey that could not be resolved.

Where Will the Activity Take Place?

The location will depend on the issue(s) to be addressed.

Who Will Participate From Your Organization?

This also depends on the issues(s) to be addressed. The surveyor will let you know.

What Will Occur?

Depending on the circumstances, this might involve:

- Review of policies and procedures
- Review of additional resident records to confirm a tracer finding
- Discussions with selected staff, if necessary
- Review of data, such as performance improvement results
- Review of clinical record delinquency data
- Other issues requiring more discussion

What Documents Will You Need?

The surveyor conducting the activity will provide direction to the organization about the documents he or she will need.

On-Site Survey Activities

Daily Briefing

The Daily Briefing occurs every morning of a multiday survey, with the exception of the first day. The session is approximately 15 to 30 minutes. When multiple surveyors are on site, the briefing is conducted jointly with a predetermined session facilitator.

Purpose

- To offer a concise summary of survey process activities completed from the previous day's activities
- To highlight positive findings
- To identify patterns or trends of significant concern that could lead to a determination of noncompliance
- To help leaders understand the survey process and the issues that may contribute to your organization's accreditation decision
- To give your staff an opportunity to provide information that may have been missed during the previous survey day
- To review the survey agenda for the present day, including determining where individual tracers will take place and making any necessary adjustments based on organization requests for education or consultation or the need for more intensive assessment of a specific issue
- To schedule time for more extensive discussion or review additional evidence of compliance for issues that arise

Where Will the Activity Take Place?

The briefing will take place in the location of your choice.

Who Will Participate From Your Organization?

- CEO/administrator
- Other senior leaders identified by the CEO/administrator, including physician leaders
- Other staff at the discretion of the organization
- Members of the governing body, if available
- Individual who is coordinating for The Joint Commission survey

What Will Occur?

During the Daily Briefing, the surveyor(s) will:

- Facilitate leaders' understanding of the survey process and the findings that contribute to the accreditation decision
- Offer a concise summary of the survey process activities completed on the previous day
- Make general comments regarding significant issues resulting from the previous day's activities
- Note any positive findings
- Emphasize patterns or trends of significant concern that could lead to noncompliance
- Inform the organization that final findings for any given standard will be possible only when all activities are complete and results are aggregated
- Allow the organization to provide information that may have been missed during the previous survey day
- Address organization requests for consultation on findings and indicate when such consultation can take place
- Schedule time for more extensive discussion or review of additional evidence of compliance on issues that arise
- Review the agenda for the survey day ahead (including identifying individual tracers) and make any necessary adjustments based on organization needs or the need for more intensive assessment of an issue

Special Situations

Times may arise when a surveyor is scheduled for an activity that does not take place at the same location where a Daily Briefing would normally occur. Situations may also arise in which a surveyor is brought in for a day or two and departs earlier than the rest of the team. If one or more surveyors cannot physically be present for the daily briefing, a surveyor may ask the organization for assistance with arrangements to join all surveyors via conference call.

On-Site Survey Activities

Surveyor Team Meeting/ Planning Session

If your survey is conducted by more than one surveyor, this meeting is held daily for all surveyors who are on site to allow them to share information and observations and plan for upcoming survey activities. If your survey is conducted by one surveyor, this time is used for planning. The meeting is scheduled for 30 minutes at the end of each survey day except the last. If your survey lasts longer than two days, an additional 30-minute session is scheduled before or after lunch on each survey day.

Purpose

- To identify areas that have been visited during tracer activities
- To coordinate locations, services, and so on that will be visited during subsequent tracer activities
- To share observations on organization performance
- To identify key findings
- To coordinate follow-up on potential issues
- To identify issues or areas that all surveyors should be looking at during individual and individual-based system tracers

Where Will the Activity Take Place?

This session takes place in the location you have chosen for surveyor use during the survey.

Who Will Participate From Your Organization?

No one from your organization is present at this meeting.

What Will Occur?

The surveyor(s) discusses survey observations and plans for subsequent activities with each other. The surveyor(s) also identifies issues that require further exploration in subsequent individual and systems tracers. Surveyors will review some of the documents identified on pages 308–309 to help plan survey activities and target residents for tracers.

If surveyors are at different sites or locations when team meetings are to be held, they may ask for assistance in setting up communication among all members of the team (for example, the availability of a speakerphone for a conference call). If only one surveyor conducts your survey, he or she uses this time to plan upcoming activities, including the selection of additional individual tracers.

On-Site Survey Activities

Credentialing

The surveyor facilitates a discussion of your organization's credentialing and privileging process for the medical director and licensed independent practitioners. He or she also reviews credentials files to assess compliance with the standards.

Purpose

The organization and surveyor discuss organization-specific issues relative to:

- The process the organization uses to collect relevant data to make decisions for appointment
- Consistent implementation of the credentialing and privileging process for licensed independent practitioners and other professionals
- Processes for granting, and appropriate delineation of, privileges
- Whether practitioners practice within the limited scope of delineated privileges
- Linkage of results of peer review and focused monitoring to the credentialing and privileging process
- Identification of potential concerns in the credentialing, privileging, and appointment process

The surveyor may request peer review and focused monitoring records for the session.

Where Will the Activity Take Place?

The discussion may take place in the location of your choice.

Who Will Participate From Your Organization?

Individuals from the organization selected for participation should be able to address issues related to the credentialing and privileging process. These individuals may include the following:

- Medical director, if applicable
- Person responsible for maintenance of credentials records
- CEO or administrator
- Director of Nursing
- Individuals responsible for human resources processes
- Other individuals with the authority to access information contained in personal and credential files

What Will Occur?

The surveyor will engage the group in a discussion about the role of the medical director and governing body in the credentialing/privileging function and then review credentials files for selected licensed independent practitioners and members of the medical staff. Topics for discussion and for verification through the file review include the following:

- The design of the credentialing/privileging process to determine if the specific steps required by the standards are in place
- The scope of the process to determine if all licensed independent practitioners and other practitioners are reviewed by the credentialing and privileging process
- Consistent implementation of the process among all practitioners
- Whether privileges are appropriate to the qualifications and competencies
- Whether a mechanism is available to communicate practitioner privileges, and whether practitioners practice within the defined privileges

What Documents Will You Need?

During this activity the surveyor will engage in a discussion of the effectiveness of the credentialing/privileging function. The organization will bring credentials files identified by the surveyor to this session for review based on the practitioners identified from the tracers and other sources. The surveyor will identify the specific credential files he or she would like to review, which may include some or all of the following files:

- Nonphysician licensed independent practitioners
- Unusual procedures
- Practice outside usual scope of specialty
- Medical director

The surveyor and the organization will summarize identified weaknesses or concerns in the medical staff credentialing and privileging function. Information from this session will be shared with other survey team members (if applicable) so that any issues identified can be incorporated into subsequent tracers for verification.

On-Site Survey Activities

Competence Assessment: Credentialing of Licensed Independent Practitioners

During this session, surveyor(s) will use data gathered during individual tracer activity to learn about your organization's competence assessment process for staff, licensed independent practitioners, and other credentialed practitioners. As the surveyor conducts the survey, he or she identifies the credential files he or she will review. The types of credential files are nonphysician licensed independent practitioners, staff members participating in unusual procedures, individuals possibly practicing outside the scope of their licenses, and the medical director. The duration of this session is about an hour.

Purpose

- To learn about your organization's competence assessment process for staff, licensed independent practitioners, and other credentialed practitioners
- To learn about your organization's orientation, education, and training processes
- To discuss competence assessment process–related strengths and potential risk points
- To learn about the clinical staff credentialing and privileging process

Where Will This Activity Take Place?

These discussions may take place in the area of your choice.

Who May Participate from Your Organization?

- Individuals responsible for human resources processes
- Individuals responsible for the orientation and education of staff
- Individuals responsible for assessing staff competency
- Individuals responsible for assessing licensed independent practitioners and other credentialed practitioner competency
- Other individuals who have authority to access information contained in personnel and credential files

What Will Occur?

Surveyor(s) will use data gathered during the individual tracer activity and will engage participants in the following topics:

- Internal processes for determining compliance with the organization's policies and procedures, applicable law and regulation, and Joint Commission standards
- Methods used to determine staffing adequacy (staffing effectiveness), frequency of measurement, what is done with the results
- Performance improvement initiatives related to competency assessment for staff, licensed independent practitioners, and other credentialed practitioners
- Orientation of staff, licensed independent practitioners, and other credentialed practitioners to your organization, job responsibilities, and/or clinical responsibilities
- Experience, education, and abilities assessments
- Ongoing education and training
- Competency assessment, maintenance, and improvement
- Competency assessment process for contracted staff, as applicable
- Process for granting of privileges to licensed independent practitioners

On-Site Survey Activities

Individual Tracer Activities

A tracer is used to evaluate your organization's performance against standards as viewed and experienced by the resident and as provided and coordinated by your organization.

Purpose

- To follow the course of care, treatment, and services provided to the resident within the organization using current records whenever possible
- To assess the interrelationships between disciplines, departments, programs, services, or units (where applicable), and the important functions in the care and services provided
- To evaluate the performance of processes, with particular focus on the integration and coordination of distinct but related processes
- To identify potential concerns in the relevant processes

Who Will Participate from Your Organization?

Staff members and management who have been involved in the resident's care, treatment, and services.

Where Will the Activity Take Place?

The surveyor(s) may visit all areas of your organization that affect the delivery of care, treatment, and services.

What Will Occur?

Selecting the Tracer

Selecting tracers begins on the first day of survey during the Surveyor Arrival and Preliminary Planning Session. The surveyor(s) selects tracers based on top CSGs identified in the PFP. The surveyor(s) also uses the criteria to select tracer individuals who cover all populations, settings, and services.

As the survey progresses, the surveyor(s) may also use survey findings to assist in tracer selection. The surveyor(s) may consider selecting individuals with more complex situations and more contact with various parts of the organization. This will provide the opportunity to assess continuity-of-care issues.

Using Individual Tracers for Continuous Evaluation

Many organizations find tracer activity helpful in the continuous evaluation of their services. If you choose to conduct mock tracers, in addition to CSGs, consider the following criteria in selecting the resident.

Selection Criteria

- Residents related to system tracers such as infection control and medication management
- Residents recently admitted
- Residents due for discharge or recently discharged
- Residents that cross programs, such as home care to nursing home or nursing home to a hospital
- Residents due for discharge that day or the next day
- Residents who cover multiple additional criteria listed below:
  - Resident receiving health services coordination (that is, medication management, skin integrity, complex medical services)
  - Resident not receiving health services coordination
  - Resident with limited mobility
  - Resident who smokes
  - Resident from a special population (dementia, pediatrics, neurological ITBI, MR/DD)
  - Resident receiving supervised assistance with one or more ADLs

Medical/Dental Services

- Maternal/child care
- Pediatric or less than 18-year-old care
- Geriatric care
- Equipment maintenance

Other Services

- Pain management (uncontrolled pain)
- High-risk areas
- Equipment maintenance
- Organization's quality indicators from MDS, if available

Criteria for Medicare/Medicaid Certification–based accreditation option

- Pain management
- Home goals
- End-of-life care
- Point-of-care testing/CLIA Waived Testing
- Rehabilitation therapy

Conducting the Individual Tracer

The tracer methodology is an evaluation method in which the surveyor(s) selects a resident and uses that individual's record as a roadmap to move through an organization to assess and evaluate the organization's compliance with selected standards and the organization's systems of providing care and services. Tracers will often be conducted in the following manner:

- The surveyor(s) has approximately two hours to conduct a tracer. It may be shorter or longer depending on the complexity of the resident's needs and other circumstances.
- The tracer begins in the setting/unit in which the clinical record is located. The surveyor(s) begins the tracer by reviewing the cause of care in the clinical record and traces the entire care or service from preadmission through postdischarge (as applicable). No mandated order is in effect for visits to care areas or departments. One approach to conducting a tracer is to sequentially follow the course of care received by the resident.
- Multiple resident records may be reviewed during a tracer activity. The purpose of using a record is not to audit its contents, but to use it as a tool in following care, treatment, and services.
- A surveyor may arrive in a setting/unit and need to wait for staff members to become available. In these cases, the surveyor will use this time productively (for example, to tour the unit, program, or service and to address EC issues, or observe care, treatment, and service processes).
- Issues identified from the tracer activities may lead to further exploration in the systems tracers or other survey activities such as the Environment of Care (EC) and Leadership Sessions
- Findings from tracer visits provide focus for other tracers and may influence the selection of other tracers. They may also identify issues related to coordinating and communicating information relevant to the safety and quality of care services.

Performing the Individual Tracer

- Evaluating the top four to five PFAs for the organization throughout the initial tracer activities
- Reviewing the resident's record with the staff person responsible for the individual's care, treatment, or service provided to the resident. If the responsible staff person is not available, the surveyor may speak with other staff members. Staff participation in this part of the tracer should be limited. Other staff involved in the individual's care will meet with the surveyor as the tracer proceeds. For example, the surveyor will speak to a dietician if the individual being traced has nutritional issues.
- Observing direct resident care
- Observing clinicians, including physicians providing direct resident care
- Observing the medication management process (for example, preparing and administering medications, storing and controlling medications)
- Observing infection control issues (for example, techniques for hand hygiene, sterilization of equipment, disinfection, food sanitation, housekeeping)
- Observing the care planning process (for example, timing of assessments)
- Discussing data use in individual units—performance improvement measures used, what has been learned, improvements made using data, data dissemination
- Observing the impact of the environment on individual safety and staff roles in minimizing environmental risk
- Interviewing the individual and/or family (if it is appropriate and the resident and/or family grants permission). The discussion should focus on the course of care, the plan for discharge, and, as appropriate, attempt to verify issues identified during the tracer.
- Following any interview with the individual and/or family, discussing additional issues that have arisen in the tracer, with other staff if necessary. The surveyor may pull and review two to three additional records to verify issues that may have been identified. The surveyor may ask staff members in the unit, program, or service to assist with reviewing the additional records. The following criteria are used to guide the selection of additional records:
  - Similar or same diagnosis or tests
  - Individual close to discharge
  - Same diagnosis but different physician/practitioner
  - Same test but different location
  - Same age or sex
  - Length of stay
- Discussing ORYX/Quality Measurement—staff level interaction, when applicable
- Interviewing staff
- Reviewing minutes and procedures as needed

At the conclusion of the tracer, the surveyor communicates to the program/unit manager(s) and care providers any specific observations made and explains that overall evaluation of standards will reflect the results from all tracers and assessment activities.

On-Site Survey Activities

Program-Specific Tracer Activities: Resident-Centered Care

The focus of this tracer is primarily on resident rights. The surveyor will shadow a resident through his or her normal daily activities. The duration of this session is about an hour and a half. The surveyor may return to this resident for activities scheduled in subsequent days of the survey.

Purpose

- To learn how your organization supports the long term care resident's quality of life through direct and indirect observation and interviews
- To evaluate the implementation of resident rights by tracing and experiencing what the resident experiences
- To identify long term care processes and system issues contributing to a lack of resident-centered care

Where Will This Activity Take Place?

The surveyor will need access to anywhere the resident travels in the course of a normal day.

Who May Participate from Your Organization?

The resident, family, resident council, and staff and leaders involved in the resident's care, treatment, or services

What Will Occur?

The focus of this tracer is primarily on resident rights. The surveyor shadows a resident through his or her normal daily activities (includes bathing, treatments, rehab, beautician/barber, lunch, and so forth). While shadowing a resident, the surveyor will need some private time with the resident to discuss:

- His or her cultural background
- Beliefs about health and health care
- Spiritual preferences
- Self-rating of his or her level of independence in the facility
- Expectations for health care
- Interests and hobbies
- Need for companionship from another human being
- Choices relative to care and treatment decisions, types of food, eating time preferences
- The atmosphere of your organization

Note: *When observing personal care activities (such as bathing), the surveyor is sensitive to the resident's right to privacy.*

On-Site Survey Activities

Program-Specific Tracer Activities: Staffing

The focus of this tracer is to identify breaches in continuity of care and explore operational processes in the presence of staff or administrative turnover. The duration of this session is about an hour.

Purpose

- To evaluate actions taken by your organization during staff turnover to ensure positive outcomes to resident care
- To identify processes and possibly system issues contributing to negative resident outcomes in light of staff or administrative turnover

Where Will This Activity Take Place?

These discussions may take place in the area of your choice. Documents that are requested include staffing plans, staff variance reports, and meeting minutes.

Who May Participate from Your Organization?

- Certified nursing assistants, as applicable
- Agency staff
- Non-nursing ancillary staff
- Administrator
- Family council members, if available
- Other leaders or participants at the direction of the surveyor

What Will Occur?

The surveyor will conduct individual interviews with staff members that include the following discussions:

- Processes pertaining to the care of residents to prevent negative outcomes
- Barriers to those processes
- Staff's knowledge of the residents for which it is assigned
- Perception of issues leading to turnover
- Staff communication
- Recruitment and hiring practices
- Orientation and training
- Changes in policy, procedure, vision, expectations

The surveyor will conduct interviews with residents and/or their family members (family interviews can be conducted by telephone) to ask questions about:

- The care received and the perceived barriers to that care
- Communication regarding administrative and staff turnover
- Changes in the provision of care when there is administrative or staff turnover

The surveyor will also conduct individual interviews with leaders (for example, governing body member, administrator, director of nursing, etc.) to discuss their knowledge regarding the following:

- MDS outcomes
- Association of negative outcomes with staff issues (staffing effectiveness)
- Follow-up actions taken
- Communication of changes in mission, vision, process, and so forth
- Methods used to stabilize or prevent turnover

On-Site Survey Activities

Example Questions for Long Term Care Tracers

The following are examples of questions that *could* be asked during a tracer in the long term care setting. A health care organization can consider using these questions or variations of these questions in conducting its own tracers in preparation for an on-site survey and as an improvement tool. Keep in mind that while not all of the following questions will apply in all types of long term care settings, they do represent a number of situations and issues that can typically arise in long term care settings and can provide a starting point into systems and processes that may be traced during an on-site survey.

In addition, please note that tracers are unique to each organization and are chosen based on the organization's PFAs, CSGs, and so forth. Therefore, these example questions are not guaranteed to be asked during a survey. These questions are only a small representation of the numerous possible questions a surveyor may ask while conducting a tracer.

- Can you tell me about the admission assessment process for (resident's name)? How often does your organization require reassessments? When will you reassess this resident?
- How did you assess for the risk of pressure ulcers for (resident's name)? What process do you follow for residents admitted with pressure ulcers? How do you prevent them from becoming worse?
- How did you orient and educate (resident's name) and her family members to your organization? What resident safety issues did you cover? Were any education materials provided?
- What information did your staff members receive when (resident's name) arrived at your organization from the hospital? How did your organization obtain the information on this resident?
- How did social services share information about advance directives with (resident's name) and her family? How did social services follow up after the initial conversation?

- When (resident's name) had an advance directive, how was the care staff informed? How did staff members communicate with each other about this advance directive?
- How did you involve (resident's name) in the planning and/or delivery of his care?
- What initial education and ongoing competency assessment do you as a nurse receive?
- (Questions a surveyor may ask after he or she receives permission to speak with a resident and explains why he or she is there.) Did anyone talk with you about your rights and responsibilities as a resident? How are you involved in decisions regarding your care? Are you receiving the assistance you need with hygiene and self-care needs?
- How did you involve (resident's name) in the medication reconciliation process? What steps did you take to update that list? How often does that occur?
- What process did you use to identify (resident's name) when administering medications and treatments or drawing blood? What did you use as the two resident identifiers?
- How did you prepare and dispense medication for (resident's name)?
- How did you monitor the effects of medications on (resident's name)? How did you inform (resident's name) about the potential side effects?
- Show me how (resident's name) was assessed for pain. How often were pain reassessments made?
- What education and training have you received in the past year on resident safety? Can you give me some examples of this?
- What process did you follow to handle verbal orders? What was your communication process?
- Tell me about your last emergency drill. When did it take place and what happened? Have you had any training since the last drill? If so, when was that?
- Do you collect data for any quality improvement projects? If so, tell me about your project and how you are using the data.
- May I see your blood glucose instrument maintenance log to assure it is tested and working properly each day it is used for (resident's name)? What is your policy on maintenance?
- Tell me about the end-of-life care plan for (resident's name). How was this resident involved in this planning? How were staff members informed about the care plan?

On-Site Survey Activities

Narrative Example: Individual Tracer of a Long Term Care Resident

Surveyors conduct tracers during an on-site accreditation survey to assess how well a long term care organization's systems and processes function to deliver safe, high-quality care, treatment, and services. By following a patient's experience or a system's function through a health care organization, surveyors are provided with an in-depth look at day-to-day operations and can ask staff relevant questions about how they deliver care. While the surveyor is making the necessary links between actual care delivery and Joint Commission standards during tracer activity, staff members only need to understand and communicate clearly about their own work and how they carry it out.

In the following tracer narrative, a surveyor follows a resident at a long term care facility. The narrative includes some example questions (placed in pull-out boxes) that could be asked at specific points during the tracer. Please keep in mind that while the following narrative does represent a tracer that could take place in one type of a long term care setting, tracers are unique. No two are the same. The following tracer is provided as an example only and may not represent all the tracers that may occur during your on-site survey. **Note:** *The following tracer example is written from the perspective of a surveyor and, as such, is provided in the first-person narrative.*

I conducted a tracer in a 76-bed nursing home that had 26 short-term rehabilitation residents and 50 long term care residents. The PFAs were Communication, Patient Safety, and Physical Environment. The priority CSG was skilled nursing/complex medical care.

On the first day I selected a short-term rehabilitation resident to follow for an individual tracer. The resident selected was a 70-year-old woman admitted six weeks earlier with a primary diagnosis of bilateral fractures of her upper arms. Her secondary diagnoses were adult-onset diabetes, hypertension, and high cholesterol. I began the tracer on the unit by reviewing the resident's medical record with the nurse assigned to care for her. We reviewed her initial assessments including the medical history and physical. I asked the nurse how information is transferred from the hospital to the nursing home and how medications are reconciled.

> Tell me about your assessment process and this particular resident's assessments. What time frame does each department have to complete its assessment? Show me how this resident was assessed for pain. How often do you require reassessments?

> Let's look at the resident's diagnoses and orders. How did you receive information when this resident came into your organization from the hospital? How were her medications reconciled across the continuum?

The resident's chart included an order for physical therapy five times a week for increased range of motion of both upper extremities and for strengthening of her lower extremities. Occupational therapy also was ordered five times a week to improve her level of function of activities of daily living. Prior to her accident the resident lived alone and was able to care for herself. She did not have any immediate family. Her main support system was two friends who visited her several times a week. The friends were elderly and, although very supportive, they would not be able to help her when she returned home.

Her record showed she was prescribed several medications, including a pain reliever. I noticed that the medication orders were telephone orders. I asked the nurse to explain the process for taking telephone orders. Her response was to write the order and then read it back to the practitioner, which is consistent with the National Patient Safety Goal. The physician cosigned the order the next day. I asked the nurse about the organization's list of unapproved abbreviations. They were readily available.

> Tell me about your process for receiving telephone orders.

> Do you have a list of unapproved abbreviations? If so, may I see a copy? What process do you follow if an order contains an incorrect abbreviation?

I then asked the nurse to ask the resident if I might interview her. The resident agreed and I talked with her in her room. She was alert, oriented, and appeared younger than her stated age. She told me she was making progress in therapy, but she was discouraged because she still was unable to lift her arms high enough to comb her hair or to brush her teeth. I asked her if she feels any pain and how that is addressed when it occurs. She said that she had occasional pain that was addressed with a mild pain reliever. She said she always requested the pain reliever prior to going to physical therapy because it made her comfortable during her session. I inquired about her other medications and asked her what she was taught about them. She stated that she knew what some were for as she had been taking them prior to her accident, but there were some she was not familiar with. She volunteered that if she was not well enough to go home soon she wanted to transfer to a facility closer to her home and friends.

> Are you satisfied with your care? What kind of progress are you making in therapy? What are your limitations? What kind of education are you receiving throughout your therapy?

> Do you experience any pain during or after your therapy? How do you inform the staff about this? What is done to relieve your pain?

> Do you know why you are taking these medications? What were your instructions about these medications? What do you know about any potential medication side effects?

After interviewing the resident, I proceeded to the therapy room to meet with the physical therapist. The physical therapist stated that her progress was good but slower than anticipated. The therapist spoke with her orthopedic doctor who informed her that her injuries to her upper arms and shoulders were extensive and that he doubted that she would ever have full range of motion, but thought she could regain additional range of motion with continued therapy. The therapist told me that the resident was soon going to receive instruction on how to do some independent exercises in the evening and on the weekends. She shared with me the printed exercises that the resident was to be instructed on. Once the resident was able to do a return demonstration she would be given the go-ahead to do the exercises independently. I asked the therapist how she communicates with nursing about the resident's progress and what she is allowed to do outside the therapy room. The therapist showed me the communication sheet they used. In addition, nursing, a social worker, and the therapist meet weekly to discuss this and other residents. When necessary, a demonstration is given to staff members.

> How was this resident's care or treatment plan determined? Which staff members were involved? How was this resident involved? What kind of progress is this resident making in physical therapy? What kind of education did she receive? Tell me how you communicate her progress and abilities to her direct caregivers.

> How do you evaluate a resident's progress and determine readiness for the independent exercises? How do you prepare the resident for this additional responsibility? How do you follow up with the resident about the independent exercises?

> How do direct caregivers know what the resident is able to do and what her limitations are?

I then met with the occupational therapist. She stated that the resident is still not able to raise her arms high enough to groom her hair and complete dressing herself. The resident was motivated and worked hard to reach her goal of independence. In addition to kitchen skills, the therapist has worked with the resident in her room to supervise her daily bathing, grooming, dressing, and undressing. They have modified her wardrobe to accommodate her limited upper extremity range of motion. Both therapists thought the resident might eventually be able to go home safely but they did not see that happening in the next 60 days.

> What kind of progress is this resident making in occupational therapy? What are her limitations? What follow up is being done with this resident to address her needs?

I returned to the nursing home to interview the certified nursing assistant caring for the resident to determine her understanding of the resident's limitations and needs. The certified nursing assistant told me what she did for the resident and what she encouraged the resident to do for herself. She said both nursing and the therapist gave her direction on caring for the resident. She had a good understanding of the resident's strengths and limitations. She stated that if the resident expresses any pain or develops pressure areas she reports her findings to the nurse in charge. The certified nursing assistant indicated she has been employed by the facility for six months. I asked her about her orientation. I also asked her what she was taught about hand washing. Her answer was appropriate and in keeping with The Joint Commission's National Patient Safety Goal on hand washing. I selected this employee as one of the human resource file records to look at during the Competency session.

> As the direct caregiver, how do you know what the resident is able to do and what her limitations are? How are you informed of the resident's progress regarding therapy?

> How do you assess pain in a resident? How do you assess pressure areas? What type of training have you received regarding these topics?

> As a new employee, tell me about your orientation. What education did you receive about hand washing?

Next on the list was the social worker. I had some concerns about this resident's finances and what progress was being made to transfer her to another nursing home closer to her home and friends. The social worker told me that the resident was a very active woman right up until the time she had her accident. She was able to resurface a driveway and do other heavy chores. She wanted to move because the other nursing home is closer to her friends. The resident and her friends are part of the Mennonite community.

What kind of social services support have you provided this resident? How have you helped her with financial concerns? What is the plan for transferring this resident to another nursing home closer to her home and friends?

On-Site Survey Activities

Individual-Based System Tracer: Medication Management

This survey activity begins during one of the individual tracers when the surveyor identifies a resident who is receiving a high-risk medication. The surveyor may complete a data collection tool and may request assistance from the organization in completing the form. Medication processes that are evaluated include selection and procurement, storage, ordering and transcribing, administration, and monitoring. If you are surveyed under the Medicare/Medicaid certification–based long term care accreditation option, this activity will not take place except as applicable in evaluating compliance with the pertinent National Patient Safety Goals.

Purpose

- To explore your organization's medication process
- To evaluate the continuity of medication management from procurement of medications through the monitoring of their effects on residents
- To review the National Patient Safety Goals related to medication management
- To establish a baseline assessment of your organization's compliance with relevant standards
- To identify potential medication management system concerns and issues requiring further exploration during subsequent individual tracers and other survey activities
- To provide education (if time permits)
- To discuss relevant standards-based issues related to USP–NF 797*

Where Will the Activity Take Place?

The group discussion may take place in the location of your choice. The surveyor may also visit any area of your facility related to medication management.

Who Will Participate From Your Organization?

- Tracer participants: tracer-visited unit and department staff responsible for medication management processes
- Summation participants: discuss with the surveyor but generally the survey coordinator, pharmacist if applicable, others who were interviewed or responsible for areas surveyed

What Will Occur?

The surveyor moves through the organization, much the same as during an individual tracer. The focus of this tracer is on medication management with the objectives of each visit or interview being to:

- Learn about the organization's medication management processes
- Evaluate the continuity of medication management from procurement of medications through monitoring
- Evaluate the medication reconciliation process during "handoffs" from one level of care to another

The surveyor traces the medication through the system, while exploring critical subprocesses. This may include a visit to the following places or check of services:

- The unit
- The pharmacy (if applicable)
  - Explore this medication's procurement, storage and dispensing while investigating important issues, such as drug security, look-alike/sound-alike issues, collaboration with other disciplines/departments
  - Ascertain the process for pharmacy review of this specific medication

* USP–NF 797 refers to the 2004 United States Pharmacopeia–National Formulary chapter titled "USP Tests and Assays Chapter 797, Pharmaceutical Compounding, Sterile Preparations." The Joint Commission began surveying compliance with these requirements in 2004. *See* October 2004 or April 2006 issues of *The Joint Commission Perspectives*® for more information.

  - Evaluate the oversight of this drug—formulary and pharmacy and therapeutics committee reviews
  - Review the pharmacy after-hours processes including observation of a night cabinet, if applicable
- The lab, if applicable
  - Explore the role of the laboratory in evaluating the medication
  - Identify the use of evaluative tools, such as an antibiogram or resident laboratory testing
  - Ascertain interdepartmental communication processes
- Dietary service
  - Explore the role of the dietary service in evaluating the medication
  - Identify the use of evaluative tools, such as an antibiogram or resident laboratory testing
  - Ascertain interdepartmental communication processes
- Warehouse/Materials Management for review of equipment or devices, if applicable to the medication being traced

Interviews with:

- The consultant pharmacist
- The medical director
- Director of nursing
- Nursing staff
- Various staff to explore communication exchange during handoffs from one shift to the next
- Explore the critical steps in medication management: selection and procurement, storage, ordering and transcribing, preparing and dispensing, administering and monitoring

Conference room discussion (10 minutes)

- Summarize identified strengths and risk points or vulnerabilities
- Clarify any information for the surveyor or organization
- Share with other team members (as applicable) issues that need to be further explored in subsequent individual tracers

Other issues that may be addressed during this or other tracer time include:

- Implementing USP–NF 797 requirements related to standard requirements
- Process for reporting errors/system breakdowns/near misses/overrides
- Data collection, analysis, systems evaluation, and performance improvement initiatives
- Medications brought into the organization by the resident
- Education of staff and resident
- Information management systems related to medication management
- Resident involvement in safe medication management

For assistance in preparing for this activity, please consult the "Individual-Based System Tracer: Medication Management" worksheet on page 373 in Appendix 2.

On-Site Survey Activities

Individual-Based System Tracer: Infection Control

This session begins during one of the individual tracers when the surveyor identifies a resident with an infectious disease. The surveyor moves through the organization, much the same as an individual tracer. If you are surveyed under the Medicare/Medicaid certification–based long term care accreditation option, this activity will not take place except as applicable to evaluating compliance with the pertinent National Patient Safety Goals.

Note: *When a separate Infection Control (IC) system tracer is not on the agenda (for example, on shorter surveys), the surveyor will address IC throughout individual tracers and during the Individual-Based System Tracer: Data Use (*see *page 329).*

Purpose

- To identify strengths and potential concerns in your IC program
- To determine actions that may be necessary to address any identified risks
- To assess your organization's degree of compliance with relevant standards
- To identify IC issues that require further exploration during subsequent individual tracers and other survey activities

Where Will the Activity Take Place?

The surveyor may visit any area of your facility where IC activities occur during the tracer component. The group discussion may take place in the location of your choice.

Who Will Participate From Your Organization?

- Part One: IC program coordinator and a physician, if applicable
- Part Two: Tracer-visited unit and staff responsible for IC practices

What Will Occur?

Part One

The session begins with a meeting that includes introductions and an overview of the following goals for the IC system tracer:

- Evaluate the planning, implementation, and evaluation of the organization's IC program
- Learn about the process used throughout the organization to reduce infection using a resident selected during the individual tracer
- Discuss the process for plan development, outcome of the annual evaluation process and oversight of opportunities for improvement

Part Two

This session occurs throughout the organization. The activity begins in a resident care, treatment, and service area (for example, the resident's room or rehabilitation area) identified by the surveyor during the individual tracer. In complex organizations, each surveyor conducts an individual tracer for a resident with an infection. The surveyor may move to other areas as appropriate and applicable to trace IC processes across the organization. The surveyor observes staff members and engages with them in discussion focused on IC practices in any area that is visited. Organizations may use IC data during this part of the activity if they are relevant to the discussion.

Topics of Discussion

The surveyor will draw from tracer activity experience, organization IC surveillance data, other IC–related data, and PFP information, when available, to create scenarios to discuss with the organization. Participants will be asked to discuss the following aspects of the organization's IC program as it relates to the scenarios:

- How the organization identifies individuals with infections
- What process exists for laboratory confirmation (for example, physician's request for testing, physician order, communication to the lab, collection of specimen, transportation to the lab, turn-around time of results, communication of results from lab to physician)
- How individuals with infections are considered within the context of the IC program
- Current and past surveillance activity (taking place in the last 24 months for unannounced surveys only)
- Type of analysis conducted on IC data, including comparisons
- Reporting IC data (frequency and audience)
- Prevention and control activities (for example, staff training, housekeeping procedures, organizationwide hand hygiene, food sanitation, and the appropriate storage, cleaning, disinfection, sterilization, other disposal of supplies and equipment)
- Interventions for licensed independent practitioners, staff, students/trainees, and volunteers that include screening for exposure and/or immunity to infectious diseases they come in contact with, the referral for assessment, potential testing, immunization and/or prophylactic treatment and counseling of those who have potentially been identified with an infectious disease
- Physical facility changes, either completed or in progress, that have an impact on IC
- Actions taken as a result of surveillance and the outcomes of those actions

Discussion can revolve around individuals already included in IC surveillance and reporting activities, or those not yet confirmed as meeting a definition or criteria for entry into and monitoring through the IC surveillance system. In addition to surveyor-identified scenarios, the organization is encouraged to present examples of cases that will highlight various aspects of the IC program. Some of the scenarios the surveyor(s) will want to discuss, as applicable to the organization, include the following:

- Individuals seen with fever of unknown origin
- Individuals with a postoperative infection (if appropriate)
- Individuals admitted to the organization postoperatively (if appropriate)
- Individuals placed on an antibiotic new to the list of available medications (preferably one with corresponding C&Ss, blood levels, and/or other labs used for dosing)
- Individuals placed on some form of isolation or precaution because of diagnosis of infectious disease. If not easily identifiable, consider individuals with any of the following diagnoses (this is not an exhaustive list): varicella, pulmonary tuberculosis, invasive *Hemophilus influenzae,* meningococcal disease, drug-resistant pneumococcal disease, pertussis, mycoplasma, mumps, rubella, MRSA, VRE, *Clostridium difficile,* RSV, enteroviruses, skin infections (impetigo, lice, scabies)
- IC practices related to emergency management
- Individuals placed on some form of isolation or precaution because of being immunocompromised

- Recent changes in a physical facility that has an impact on IC
- Individual with known case of active tuberculosis

The surveyor and organization will conclude by summarizing identified strengths and potential areas of concern in the IC program.

For assistance in preparing for this activity, please consult the "Individual-Based System Tracer: Infection Control" worksheet on pages 374–375 in Appendix 2.

On-Site Survey Activities

Individual-Based System Tracer: Data Use

This interactive discussion and evaluation focuses on how your organization uses data to improve resident safety and care. This session lasts approximately one hour.

Purpose

To discuss the following topics:

- How your organization analyzes, interprets, and uses data—in particular, how your leaders use data to prioritize decisions about improving resident care and safety
- Strengths and concerns in the processes you use to meet your internal and external information needs
- The techniques you use to protect the confidentiality and security of all types of data
- Your organization's data gathering and preparation processes, including measure selection, data collection and analysis, dissemination and use of information, and monitoring performance improvement (PI)
- Your organization's approach to assessing staffing effectiveness, how you use the data/information obtained from these assessments, and PI data
- Performance issues related to the ORYX performance core measurement requirements

Where Will the Activity Take Place?

This session may take place in the location of your choice.

Who Will Participate From Your Organization?

The surveyor will inform the organization after the initial planning meeting which staff members should attend as active participants. Whenever possible and based on the focus, physician involvement is desired.

Note: *Position names and responsibilities vary from organization to organization. Individuals responsible for planning will be asked to attend if the focus is on planning; individuals responsible for data collection will be asked to attend if the focus is on data collection, and so forth.*

What Will Occur?

The review of the organization's data prior to this session provides focus for the surveyor on one of the following subprocesses:

- **Planning and Selecting Measures:** Understanding your organization's planning process for data use including how your organization identifies and prioritizes measures
- **Data Collection:** Understanding your organization's methodology for ensuring that all data are collected as planned
- **Data Aggregation and Analysis:** Understanding your organization's processes for turning data into useful information
- **Data Use:** Understanding how your organization uses the information obtained from data analysis

This surveyor may also discuss the following:

- ORYX data or MOS Quality Indicator measures data
- Medication management
- Infection control
- Staffing effectiveness
- Proactive risk assessment
- National Patient Safety Goals (including monitoring of Centers for Disease Control and Prevention and World Health Organization hand hygiene compliance)
- Other data collection, as applicable to the individual organization or program

For assistance in preparing for this activity, please consult the "Individual-Based System Tracer: Data Use" worksheet on pages 376–378 in Appendix 2.

On-Site Survey Activities

Physical Environment

The three important components of the physical environment are:
- Environment of Care (EC)
- Life Safety (LS)
- Emergency Management (EM)

Purpose

EC

The purpose of this session is to provide guidance for evaluating the organization's system and performance for managing risk in the environment of care. This includes identifying areas of concern and strengths in the organization's processes, identifying or determining the action(s) necessary to address any identified areas of concern, or assessing or determining the organization's actual degree of compliance with relevant standards.

LS

The purpose of this session is to provide guidance for conducting a tour of your organization's buildings that are required to be designed and maintained according to Life Safety requirements. **Note:** *This session is devoted entirely to evaluation of the "Life Safety" (LS) chapter requirements and not other issues.*

EM

The purpose of this session is to provide guidance on your organization's emergency management processes and its performance in addressing the emergency management requirements of standards. This includes its role in relation to the community's, county's, or region's emergency management program.

Where Will the Activity Take Place?

The group discussion may take place in the location of your choice. However, the discussion should take place in your Incident Command Center to facilitate the Emergency Management discussion. The surveyor may visit any area of your organization during the observation component, depending on what potential risks are identified in the preceding discussion.

Environment of Care Session

Who Will Participate in the EC Session From Your Organization?

Individuals from your organization selected for participation should be able to address issues related to the management of the EC in all major departments or areas within your organization. This group should include representatives from the following services (in some organizations, individuals may be responsible for multiple roles):
- Person(s) designated by leaders to coordinate safety management activities
- Person(s) designated by leaders to coordinate security management activities
- Person who manages the organization's facility(ies)
- Person who manages the organization's building utility systems
- Person responsible for maintaining the organization's medical/laboratory equipment
- Leader of the EC team or safety committee
- Organizational leaders

Note: *To facilitate a beneficial exchange between the surveyor and your organization, your organization should identify a relatively small group of active participants for discussions and interviews. Other staff may attend as observers.*

What Will Occur?

Group Discussion Guidelines

This activity represents approximately **30% of the session** and occurs after the surveyor has had the opportunity to review for orientation purposes the following documents:
- The annual evaluations of the EC management plans
- EC multidisciplinary team meeting minutes and activities (previous 12 months)

It is also important that observations related to the EC made by other members of the survey team (if there is a team) and any EC–related issues identified in PFP information be discussed during this session.

The surveyor reviews the objectives of the EC session with your organization's participants. During this time the surveyor should draw discussion from your organization that will give insight into the following steps of your EC risk management cycle. (*See* Figure 5 on page 331.)

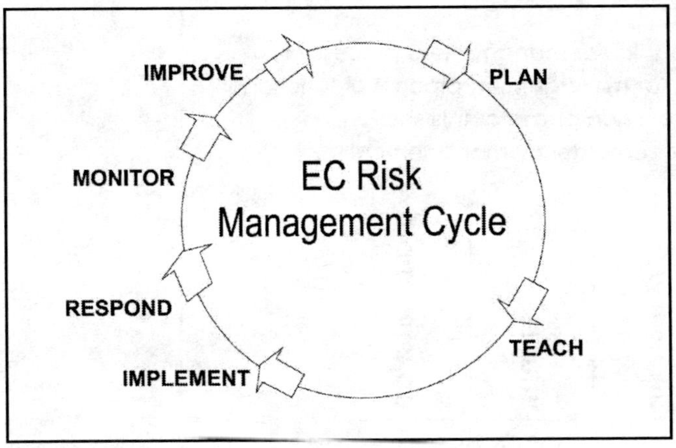

Figure 5. *Environment of care risk management cycle.*

Step 1. Plan: What specific risks related to its environment of care has the organization identified?
Step 2. Teach: How has the organization communicated roles/responsibilities for staff/volunteers? (The human resources department may be involved in this step.)
Step 3. Implement: What procedures and controls (both human and physical components) does the organization implement to minimize the impact of risk to patients, visitors, and staff?
Step 4. Respond: What procedures does the organization implement to respond to an EC incident/failure? How, when, and to whom are EC problems, incidents, and/or failures reported within the organization? Are contingency plans current and accurate?
Step 5. Monitor: How does the organization monitor EC performance (both human activities and physical components)? What monitoring activities have taken place within the last 12 months?
Step 6. Improve: What EC issues are currently being analyzed? What actions have been taken as a result of EC monitoring activities?

Your organization should discuss how the six EC functional areas have been addressed in each of the management processes listed above. The categories include:

- General safety and security
- Hazardous materials and waste
- Fire safety
- Medical/laboratory equipment
- Utilities
- Other environmental considerations

Observation Guidelines

The surveyor observes and evaluates your organization's performance in managing EC risk. This activity represents approximately **70% of the session** and occurs after the group discussion portion of the session.

The particular management process or risk selected for observation and further evaluation is based on the following:

- EC documents previously reviewed
- Observations by other survey team members
- Knowledge gained during the group discussion portion of this session

The surveyors will observe the implementation of those particular management processes determined to be potentially vulnerable, or will trace a particular risk(s) in one or more of the EC risk categories your organization manages by:

- Beginning where the risk is encountered or first occurs (that is, a starting point might be where a particular safety or security incident occurs, a particular piece of medical equipment is used, or a particular hazardous material enters the organization)
- Having staff members describe or demonstrate their roles and responsibilities for minimizing the risk, what they are to do if a problem or incident occurs, and how to report the problem or incident
- Assessing any physical controls for minimizing the risk (that is, equipment, alarms, contingency plans)
- If equipment, alarms, or building features are present for controlling the particular risk, reviewing implementation of relevant inspection, testing, or maintenance procedures
- If others in the organization have a role in responding to the particular problem or incident, having them describe or demonstrate that role, and reviewing the condition of any equipment they use in responding

If the risk moves around in your organization's facility (that is, a hazardous material or waste), the surveyor will follow the risk from "cradle to grave."

What Documents Will You Need?

The annual evaluations of your EC management plans and the meeting minutes from your EC multidisciplinary team meetings for the past 12 months should still be available from the Preliminary Planning Session.

Information for Complex Organizations

In complex organizations that have decentralized EC management activities at remote sites, those persons responsible for managing the activities listed above at those sites should be available (that is, in person or by conference call).

For assistance in preparing for this activity, please consult the "Environment of Care" worksheet on pages 368–372 of Appendix 2.

The following matrix is a screening tool for use in selecting a particular management process or functional area to explore in this session. Selection of a particular management process or functional area should be based on information gathered during the discussion phase of this session, EC-related information in PFP, and any unusual EC, Life Safety, or emergency management observations made during survey prior to this session.

	SAFETY & SECURITY*	HAZMAT	EMERGENCY MANAGEMENT	FIRE *	Medical/ Laboratory/ Equipment.	UTILITIES	CONSTRUCTION
PLAN							
TEACH							
IMPLEMENT							
RESPOND							
MONITOR							
IMPROVE							

Figure 6. *Matrix for functional areas.*

Life Safety Session

Who Will Participate in the LS Session From Your Organization?

- The person who manages the organization's facility(ies)
- Other staff at the discretion of the organization

What Needs to be Provided?

- Blueprints of the building that show features of life safety (for example, fire and smoke barriers)
- Ladder
- Flashlight
- Keys or tools necessary to gain access to spaces above the ceilings

What Will Occur?

This activity occurs after the e-SOC PFI has been reviewed and accepted (during the Preliminary Planning Session). The surveyor asks you for a ladder and flashlight, as well as any necessary keys or tools, to gain access to spaces above ceilings in each location he or she visits during the tour. At the conclusion of this session, the surveyor and the organization will be able to do the following:

- Identify areas of concern in the organization's processes for designing buildings to "Life Safety" (LS) chapter requirements in the *CAMLTC*
- Identify areas of concern in the organization's processes for maintaining buildings to "Life Safety" (LS) chapter requirements in the *CAMLTC*
- Identify areas of concern in the organization's processes for identifying and resolving "Life Safety" (LS) chapter problems
- Determine the organization's degree of compliance with relevant "Life Safety" (LS) chapter requirements
- Determine the action necessary to address any identified "Life Safety" (LS) chapter problems

To effectively evaluate compliance with the "Life Safety" (LS) chapter, the surveyor will assess the following:

- Hazardous areas, such as soiled linen rooms, trash collection rooms, and oxygen storage rooms
- Any required fire separations
- Any required smoke separations (at least two)
- At least two exits per building and verify that they are continuous from the highest level they serve to the outside of the building
- The main fire alarm panel to verify that it is functional and protected
- The automatic fire pump (if any) to verify that it is functional

At each location, the surveyor will conduct an "above the ceiling" survey by observing the space above the ceiling to identify any of the following:

- Penetrations of smoke, fire, or corridor walls
- Smoke or fire walls that are not continuous from slab to slab and outside wall to outside wall

- Penetrations or discontinuities of rated enclosures including hazardous areas, stairwells, chutes, shafts, and floor or roof slabs
- Corridor walls that are not slab-to-slab or do not terminate at a monolithic ceiling (if the building is fully sprinklered and the ceiling is smoke tight, the walls may terminate at the ceiling line)
- The presence or absence of required smoke detectors or fire dampers
- The presence or absence of required fire proofing on structural members such as columns, beams, and trusses

Facility Orientation

1. Review the organization's electronic Statement of Conditions (e-SOC) and any PFIs accepted by the survey team.
2. Meet with the appropriate organizational staff to become oriented to the following:
   - Layout of the building (including arrangement of compartments, location of any suites, age of building additions, areas without automatic sprinklers, areas under construction, and any equivalencies granted by The Joint Commission)
   - Organization processes for Interim Life Safety Measures (ILSMs)

Issues observed by the Life Safety specialist related to EC standards will be communicated to other members of the survey team for further review during the survey.

How will the Surveyor's Findings Be Documented?

If a deficiency in the "Life Safety" (LS) chapter requirements is not noted as a previously approved PFI, it will be recorded as a finding in the accreditation report. A "below-the-ceiling" Life Safety deficiency identified by other survey team members that are not noted as a PFI are documented as a finding in the summary report.

Emergency Management Session

Who Will Participate from Your Organization?

- Person(s) responsible for the organization's emergency management activities
- Person(s) designated by leaders to coordinate security management activities
- Organizational leaders

What Will Occur?

During this session, your organization's performance in addressing the emergency management requirements of standards will be reviewed, including its performance in the following:

- The organization's ability to create an emergency operations plan, monitor six critical functions during an emergency, and evaluate the planning process and the plan itself
- Conducting the required Hazard Vulnerability Analysis (HVA)
- Identifying its role in relation to the community's, county's, or region's emergency management program
- Identifying an "all hazards" command structure that links with the community's command structure
- Making any necessary improvements to its emergency management based on critiques of emergency management drills
- Reviewing at least one exercise per year to evaluate how effectively the organization performs when it cannot be supported by the community

Because many emergencies have similarities in terms of their effects on the organization (for example, loss of power may result from a lightning strike, an ice storm, or a brownout), focusing on performance in six critical functions can help an organization more adequately prepare for emergencies and take an all-hazards approach. These six critical areas are the following:

- Communication
- Resources and assets
- Safety and security
- Staff responsibilities
- Utilities management
- Resident clinical and support activities

Discussion should focus around the management processes. Surveyors should *not* be the primary speakers during this time, but rather listeners to the discussion. This is intended to be a discussion.

Observation Guidelines

The surveyor observes and evaluates your organization's performance in emergency management. The particular management processes selected for observation and further evaluation include the following:

- Assessing the emergency management plan for mitigation, preparedness, response, and recovery strategies, actions, and responsibilities for each priority emergency
- Assessing the emergency plan for responding to utility system disruptions or failures (for example, alternative source of utilities, notifying staff, how and when to perform emergency clinical interventions when utility systems fail, and obtaining repair services)
- Evaluating the emergency operations plan through exercises

What Documents Will You Need?

The annual evaluations of your emergency management plans and the meeting minutes from your multidisciplinary team meetings for the past 12 months should still be available from the Preliminary Planning Session.

On-Site Survey Activities

Leadership Session

The surveyor(s) meets with organization leaders near the end of the survey after most of the Individual and Individual-based System Tracer activities are completed.

Purpose

- To provide leaders of the organization and the surveyor an opportunity to meet, explore, assess, and discuss the leaders' role in relationship to the organization's performance in PFAs and organizationwide functions observed during survey
- To provide an opportunity to discuss linkages between observations, standards-based issues, and leaders' responsibility for improvement in the organization (that is, making connections between survey observations and leaders' responsibility for the organization's performance)

Where Will the Activity Take Place?

This discussion may take place in the location of your choice.

Who Will Participate From Your Organization?

Leaders with responsibility and accountability for design, planning, and implementing organization processes. These leaders typically include but are not limited to representatives from the following (not all organizations will have representatives from each area, depending on organization structure and care and services provided):

- At least one member of the governing body/trustee (in single-owner organizations, this individual may also be the CEO)
- Senior organization leaders (for example, the CEO, COO, CFO, CIO, vice president for clinical services, administrator, nurse executive, or director of resident services)
- Elected and appointed leaders of the medical staff (if applicable)

To facilitate a beneficial exchange between the surveyor and the organization, the organization should identify a relatively small group of active participants for discussions and interviews. Other staff may attend as observers.

What Will Occur?

The surveyor(s) will facilitate a discussion with organization leaders and explore their roles related to the performance of organizationwide processes and functions. Discussion will be guided by observations made throughout the survey within the context of PFAs and organizationwide processes and functions. For example, survey findings might suggest opportunities for improvement in key areas, such as planning, data use, performance improvement, communication, or staff competence/effectiveness.

Although survey findings can provide context for the discussion, surveyors and leaders will explore key characteristics of the PFA or function. Leaders should provide the surveyor with their views and perspectives about an area or topic being discussed. Discussion topics might include the following:

- The planning process used
- How data are used after they are collected
- The approach used to change processes and workflow
- How information about newly implemented processes is communicated throughout the organization
- How leaders envision the performance of the PFA or function under discussion
- Leaders' support and direction, including planning and resource allocation
- The degree to which the implementation is comprehensive and organizationwide
- The relationship of the PFA or function to resident safety and quality
- How the effectiveness of the performance of the PFA or function is evaluated

Information for Complex Organizations

On integrated or complex surveys, a single Leadership Session will include discussion of all programs and services accredited at the time of this survey. All surveyors on site at the time of this session may participate. The organization should have leader representation from all programs undergoing survey.

The surveyor(s), with the assistance of the organization, will review and summarize the subjects discussed and potential opportunities for improvement that may have surfaced. The surveyor(s) will also review any topics that may be further explored in subsequent system or resident tracers.

For assistance in preparing for this session, please consult the "Leadership" worksheet on page 379 in Appendix 2.

On-Site Survey Activities

Criticality and the Accreditation Decision Process

Beginning in 2009, the new accreditation decision process will focus on critical standards and EPs. Accreditation decisions will consider the criticality of findings and the number of Requirements for Improvement that the organization receives. The more critical the standard, the more there is a potential risk to patient care or safety and the more immediate the issue of noncompliance needs to be resolved.

Criticality is defined as the immediacy of risk to patient safety or quality of care as a result of noncompliance with a Joint Commission requirement. The levels of criticality fall into the following four categories:

1. Immediate Threat to Health and Safety
2. Situational Decision Rules
3. Direct Impact Requirements
4. Indirect Impact Requirements

The immediacy of risk to the patient and to the organization's accreditation status increases as one moves from noncompliance with standards which have an "indirect" impact on patient care (the base or "blunt end" of the pyramid in Figure 7 on page 336) to Immediate Threat to Health and Safety (the top or "sharp end" of the pyramid). The time frame within which organizations are expected to demonstrate resolution of instances of noncompliance increases as one moves from the "sharp end" to the "blunt end" of the pyramid. The four levels of risk are defined as follows:

1. Immediate Threat to Health and Safety

The top (sharp end) of the pyramid represents the most immediate risk. While not linked to any specific standards or EPs, Immediate Threat to Health and Safety situations are identified on site and have or may potentially have serious adverse effects on patient health and safety. Upon resolution of an Immediate Threat to Health and Safety situation, the organization's accreditation status will change from Preliminary Denial of Accreditation to Conditional Accreditation and remain as such until a Conditional Accreditation follow-up survey is conducted to assess the organization's sustained implementation of appropriate corrective actions.

Examples of Immediate Threat to Health and Safety findings are as follows:

- Inoperable fire alarm
- Adult-strength medications on pediatric crash cart
- Lack of master alarms for medical gas systems
- Patients with known antibodies receiving transfusions without the units being typed for the corresponding antigens

2. Situational Decision Rules

This criticality level is the second level of the pyramid. These situations involve a recommendation for Preliminary Denial of Accreditation or Conditional Accreditation based on such issues as loss of facility licensure, provision of care by unlicensed individuals who require such a license, and failure to implement corrective action in response to identified *Life Safety Code* deficiencies. In follow-up to these situations, organizations must demonstrate resolution of the situation through the ESC process. An on-site survey is conducted to validate implementation of corrective action.

Examples of Situational Decision Rule findings are as follows:

- Evidence of an unlicensed facility
- Unlicensed individual who requires a license
- Failure to implement corrective action in response to identified *Life Safety Code* deficiencies

In the revised 2009 comprehensive accreditation manuals, EPs are "tagged" with a ▲ indicating Situational Decision Rules apply to the requirement.

3. Direct Impact Requirements

This criticality is the third level of the pyramid. A "Direct Impact" Requirement (standard, EP, National Patient Safety Goal, or APR) is a requirement that has a "direct impact" if noncompliance is likely to create an immediate risk to patient safety or quality of care. *The immediate risk usually results because there are no or few processes—or no or few protective defenses—intervening between the noncompliance and the impact on the safety or quality of a patient's care.*

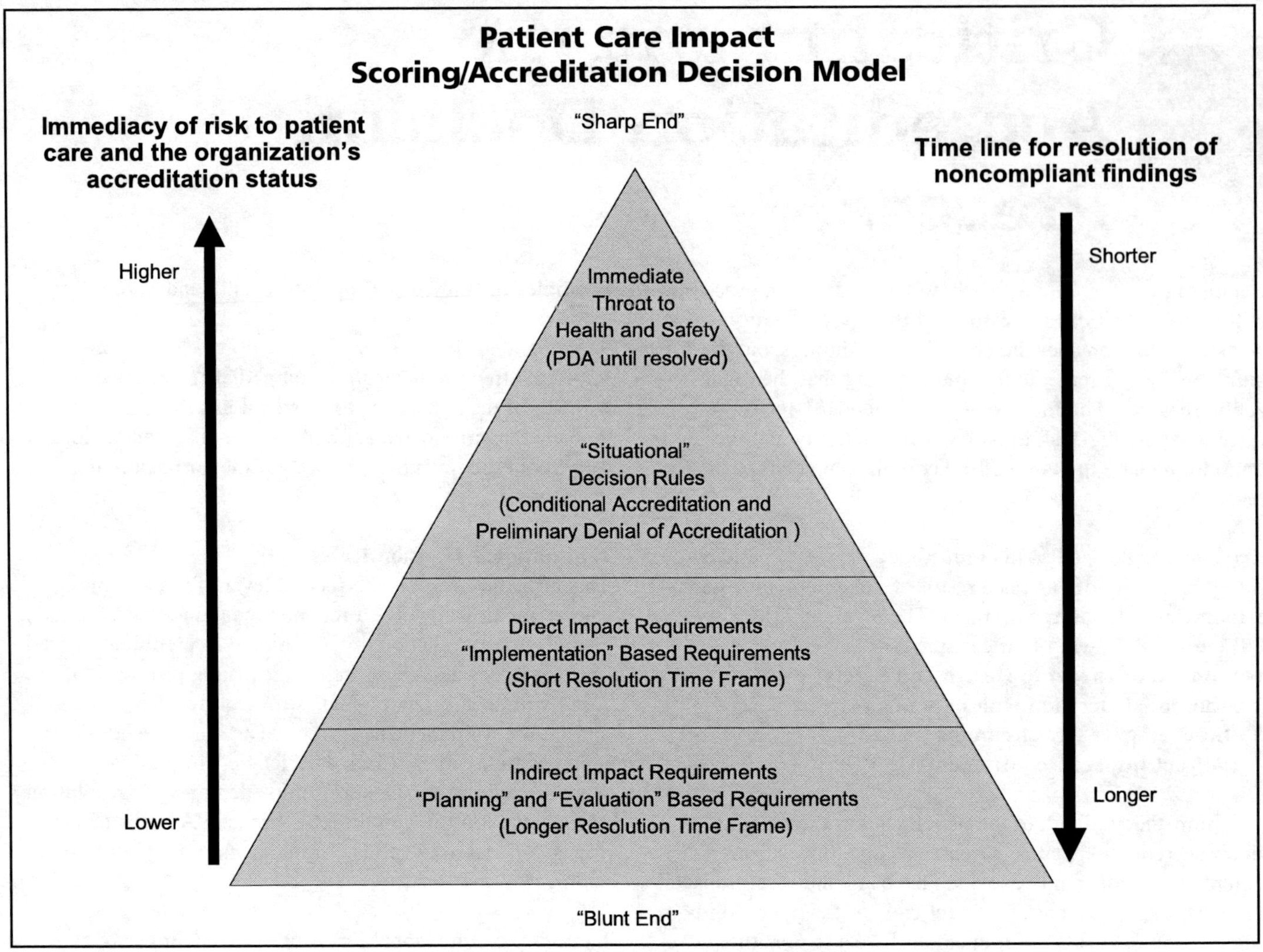

Figure 7. *Patient Care Impact Scoring/Accreditation Decision Model*

Evaluation of compliance with these requirements will be prioritized in the survey process. All instances of identified partial compliance or insufficient compliance with EPs which are associated with the Direct Impact Requirements need to be resolved through the ESC process **within 45 days.** The organization's accreditation decision would be held in abeyance pending demonstration of ESC within the established time frame. Failure to resolve the instances of partial compliance or insufficient compliance with the associated EPs will lead to progressively more adverse accreditation decisions (Provisional Accreditation, Conditional Accreditation, and Preliminary Denial of Accreditation).

Examples of Direct Impact findings are as follows:

- Sedation—Standard PC.13.20, EP 2: *The resident is reevaluated immediately before moderate or deep sedation and before anesthesia induction.*
- Pain—Standard PC.8.10, EP 7: *When pain is identified, the resident is treated by the long term care organization or referred to treatment*
- Emergency Medications—Standard MM.2.30, EP 3: *Emergency medications are available in unit-dose, and ready-to-administer forms whenever possible.*
- Other general areas include time-out, site marking, and look-alike/sound-alike drugs.

In the revised 2009 comprehensive accreditation manuals, EPs are "tagged" with a ⚠(3) indicating that Direct Impact Requirements apply to the requirement.

4. Indirect Impact Requirements

This level of criticality is at the bottom (blunt end) of the pyramid. These requirements pose less immediate risk to patient care and safety than "Direct Impact" Requirements, but noncompliance increases risk to patient safety and quality of care over time. This risk may ultimately even exceed in scope or severity a "direct impact."

All instances of identified partial compliance and insufficient compliance with EPs under these requirements must be resolved through the ESC process **within 60 days.** As above, the organization's accreditation decision will be held in abeyance pending demonstration of ESC within the established time frames. As with the Direct Impact Requirements, failure to resolve instances of partial compliance or insufficient compliance will lead to progressively more adverse accreditation decisions.

Examples of Indirect Impact findings are as follows:

- Rewritten Leadership Standard LD.01.01.01: *The organization has a leadership structure.*
- Human Resources—Standard HR.2.10, EP 2: *The organization orients staff and licensed independent practitioners to the identified key elements prior to the provision of care, treatment, and services.*
- Infection Control—Standard IC.1.10, EP 2: *Individuals and/or positions with the authority to take steps to prevent or control the acquisition and transmission of infectious agents are identified.*

All partially compliant and insufficiently compliant EPs must be addressed via the ESC submission process. There will no longer be supplemental findings. The time line for completing the ESC submission will depend on the "criticality" of findings and immediacy of risk. EPs that are identified as having a direct impact on patient care as a result of partial or insufficient compliance will require the submission of an ESC within 45 days. EPs that are identified as having an indirect impact will require an ESC within 60 days. In addition, if the number of noncompliant standards at the time of survey exceeds a predetermined threshold, a follow-up on-site survey will be required to validate implementation of the ESC.

On-Site Survey Activities

Surveyor Report Preparation

The surveyor or survey team uses this time to compile, analyze, and organize the data collected throughout the survey into a report that reflects your organization's compliance with the standards. This activity may last between 90 minutes and 2 hours.

Purpose

- To integrate survey findings in preparation for the CEO Exit Briefing and Organization Exit Conference
- To prepare your Summary of Survey Findings Report

Where Will the Activity Take Place?

This session is held in the location you have chosen for surveyor use during the survey. The surveyor(s) needs a room that includes a conference table, power outlets, and telephone.

Who Will Participate From Your Organization?

No one from your organization is present at this meeting, although the surveyor(s) may ask your survey coordinator or other staff members for additional information during the session to confirm or disprove a finding.

What Will Occur?

The surveyor(s) reviews findings from all the activities conducted during your survey to determine standards compliance. The surveyor(s) uses a laptop computer to prepare the Summary of Survey Findings report and plan for the CEO Exit Briefing and Organization Exit Conference.

When determining compliance, the surveyor(s) begins with the EPs for each standard. EPs are the specific performance expectations and structures or processes that must be in place for an organization to provide safe, high-quality care. EPs are evaluated on a three-point scale:

0	=	Insufficient compliance
1	=	Partial compliance
2	=	Satisfactory compliance
NA	=	Not applicable

Two components are scored for all EPs: compliance with the actual requirement and your track record of compliance. (**Note:** *The track record is not applicable when assessing compliance in the PPR.*) Track records represent the amount of time your organization has been in compliance with an EP, a standard, or some other requirement, and they vary depending on whether you are being surveyed for the first time or are undergoing a resurvey.

Score	Re-Survey
2	12 months or more
1	6 to 11 months
0	Fewer than 6 months

For National Patient Safety Goals, you need to have complied with the goal and its EPs since its effective date to receive a score of 2. If you have not been compliant for the full time the goal and its EPs have been in effect, you receive a score of 0.

There are also two EP scoring criteria categories (A and C), which influence the way an EP is scored in relation to the two scoring components. A brief description of these categories and the rules for scoring each of them is presented in Table 3 beginning below.

After all EPs for a standard are scored, the standard itself can be judged compliant or not compliant. A standard is not compliant if any of its EPs are scored 0 or 1. For more information about scoring guidelines, *see* the "How to Use This Manual" chapter in the *CAMLTC*.

Table 3. Scoring Criteria Categories for Elements of Performance

Category A

- These EPs relate to structural requirements, such as policies or plans, which either exist or do not exist, and are scored either 0 or 2.
- They also may address an issue that may be fully compliant even though it focuses on performance or outcome, such as the National Patient Safety Goals.
- These EPs may also be related to a Medicare Condition of Participation that must always be fully compliant.

Category C

C EPs are scored 0, 1, or 2 based on the number of times your organization does not meet the EP. These EPs are frequency based and require totaling the number of occurrences (that is, results of performance or nonperformance) related to a particular EP. Each situation discovered by a surveyor(s) is counted as a separate occurrence.

Note: *Multiple events of the same type related to a single resident and single practitioner or staff member are counted as one occurrence only.*

Use the following rules to determine your EP score:

- Your EP score is 2 if there are one or no occurrences of noncompliance with the EP.
- Your EP score is 1 if there are two occurrences of noncompliance with the EP.
- Your EP score is 0 if there are three or more occurrences of noncompliance with the EP.

If an EP in the C category has multiple requirements designated by bullets, the following scoring guidelines apply:

- If there are fewer than two findings in all bullets, the EP is scored 2.
- If there are three or more findings in all bullets, the EP is scored 0.
- In all other combinations of findings, the EP is scored 1.

When there are fewer than three possible findings for a Category C EP, the entire population is used as the sample for scoring purposes. In these cases, two findings (as opposed to three) would result in insufficient compliance and one finding would result in partial compliance. The surveyor(s) needs to document that a small sample exists.

Track Record Achievements for Organizations Undergoing Re-Survey

In addition to meeting the requirement(s) in each EP, regardless of category, your organization must also meet the following track record achievements:

Score	**Re-Survey**
2	12 months or more
1	6 to 11 months
0	Fewer than 6 months

Sample Sizes

If during an on-site survey your organization has been found to be not compliant or partially compliant with one or more EPs, you must demonstrate ESC for each standard that is not compliant. The ESC report must address compliance at the EP level. When an EP within a noncompliant standard requires an MOS, your organization must demonstrate whether each MOS identified in the ESC was met.

Note: *Not every EP requires an MOS. EPs that do require an MOS are clearly marked in each standards chapter.*

When demonstrating achievement with an MOS during the ESC process, your organization is required to use the following sample sizes, which were established because of their statistical significance, their relative simplicity in application, and their sensitivity to an organization's population size:

- For a population size of fewer than 30 cases, sample 100% of available cases.
- For a population size of 30 to 100 cases,* sample 30 cases.
- For a population size of 101 to 500 cases, sample 50 cases.
- For a population size greater than 500 cases, sample 70 cases.

Note: *Organizations are encouraged, but not required, to follow this sample size when demonstrating achievement with an MOS for an EP.*

(continued)

* "Case" refers to a single instance in which a situation related to a survey finding occurs. For example, if a survey finding was related to pain assessment, then a "case" would be any resident record. If a survey finding was related to pain management, a "case" would be any resident record for residents receiving pain management.

When conducting a PPR (optional use) or demonstrating an ESC (mandatory use), use the following percentages to determine your EP score: 90% through 100% of your sample size is in compliance = score 2; 80% through 89% of your sample size is in compliance = score 1; less than 80% of your sample size is in compliance = score 0.

In addition, the following information should guide your organization's selection of samples:

- The appropriate sample size should be determined by the specific population(s) related to the survey findings.
- The sampling approach should involve either systematic random sampling (for example, your organization selects every second or third case for review) or simple random sampling (for example, your organization uses a series of random numbers generated by a computer to identify the cases to be reviewed).
- If your organization chooses not to use these sample sizes while conducting PPR Options 1 or 2, you should make sure that your sample size is sufficiently large enough to ensure statistical significance.
- When submitting a clarifying ESC report, if your organization selects records as part of its sample, the records should be from a period of no more than three months before the last date of the survey.
- Assessment of MOS compliance is conducted for a four-month period following the date of ESC approval. Your organization should select records as a part of your sample following the date of ESC approval and use the required sample sizes. MOS percentage compliance rates are derived from the average of all four months.

CEO Exit Briefing and Organization Exit Conference

CEO Exit Briefing

On the last day of your survey, just before the Organization Exit Conference, the surveyor may meet with your CEO to apprise him or her of the survey results. This meeting will last 10 to 15 minutes.

Purpose

- To review the standards and EPs not fully in compliance and survey team observations with your CEO
- To present the Summary of Survey Findings Report to your CEO and discuss any concerns he or she may have with the findings
- To determine whether the Summary of Survey Findings Report will be distributed at the Organization Exit Conference

Where Will the Activity Take Place?

The briefing may take place in the location of your choice.

Who Will Participate From Your Organization?

Your CEO or administrator, if applicable

What Will Occur?

The surveyor(s) meets with your CEO to provide him or her with a copy of the Summary of Survey Findings Report. Your CEO decides whether the report will be shared verbally or in writing with staff members attending the Organization Exit Conference. If the report is distributed, your CEO arranges for its reproduction and distribution. (A very short time is available before the Organization Exit Conference to complete this task.)

Organization Exit Conference

The surveyors proceed to meet with your organization's leaders and other staff members to present the survey findings and address questions and comments from the staff. This meeting should last no longer than 30 minutes.

Purpose

- To report the summary of survey findings to your senior leaders
- To allow your staff a final opportunity to question the survey findings or present additional evidence of compliance while the surveyors are on site
- To review any follow-up actions that will be required

Where Will the Activity Take Place?

The conference may take place in the location of your choice.

Who Will Participate From Your Organization?

- Your CEO or administrator (or designee)
- Senior leaders from your organization
- Other organization staff members designated by your CEO

What Will Occur?

All surveyors who are on site at the time will attend this conference. They will use the Summary of Survey Findings Report as the basis for conducting this activity. The report is organized by the order of chapters in the accreditation manual.

The surveyor(s) will recap all standards and EPs that require you to submit an ESC report and, in some cases, an MOS to The Joint Commission.

If you have presented additional information to the surveyors during this conference, they may need to revise the Summary of Survey Findings Report and print an updated copy for your CEO.

The Joint Commission Central Office accepts no additional documentation except your ESC submission, so be sure to bring up any concerns you have about survey findings during this conference.

Information for Complex Organizations

If you are undergoing a complex organization survey, some surveyors may not be present for the entire duration of the survey. If a surveyor is departing early, he or she holds an interim exit conference to tell the staff about his or her findings. These findings are preliminary and may be affected by results from subsequent survey activities; the program's survey still continues even though the assigned surveyor has left early. Another surveyor from the team also attends this meeting so he or she can address the departing surveyor's findings and any questions your staff poses when your final exit conference takes place.

Postsurvey Activities

- ☑ Summary of Survey Findings Report
- ☑ Submitting Clarifications
- ☑ Evidence of Standards Compliance
- ☑ Quality Report

Postsurvey Activities

Summary of Survey Findings Report

Following evaluation of an organization's performance of functions and processes, the surveyor or survey team reviews the results of integrated individual findings. Then, with the use of laptop-based decision support software, the surveyor or survey team meets with the organization's CEO prior to the closing conference and provides him or her with a copy of the Summary of Survey Findings Report. The surveyor or survey team uses this report contents in making his or her closing conference presentations.

The Summary of Survey Findings Report is sorted by manual chapters and includes standards, EPs, and other requirements found to be less than fully compliant at the time of survey as well as survey team observations. However, the report left on site **does not** include the potential accreditation decision.

Shortly after the survey, the organization's official report is posted on the organization's secure *The Joint Commission Connect* extranet site and includes RFIs as appropriate.

If an organization does not receive any RFIs, the organization's accreditation decision is rendered at the same time that the organization's official report is posted, and it is effective the day after the completion of the survey.

Postsurvey Activities

Submitting Clarifications

In accordance with a continuous accreditation process, organizations (1) conduct PPRs, (2) adjust policies, procedures, and practices to be in line with the APRs, standards, EPs, and National Patient Safety Goals (as necessary), (3) collect data on core measures, and so on. But what happens after the survey? What should organizations do if they receive an RFI but believe they were compliant at the time of survey? What should they expect if they meet a decision rule for Conditional Accreditation or Preliminary Denial of Accreditation? This article provides the answers to those questions and explains the postsurvey process.

Next Steps Following a Survey

Accreditation Decision: Accredited

If an organization has RFIs but does not meet a decision rule for Conditional Accreditation or Preliminary Denial of Accreditation, it has 45 days to submit a corrective ESC for Direct Impact Requirements and 60 days to submit ESC for Indirect Impact Requirements. For organizations that can demonstrate ESC at the time of survey, an optional clarification may be submitted within 10 days of posting the accreditation decision on the organization's secure extranet. (*See* Sidebar 3, on page 345, for an explanation of the difference between corrective and clarifying ESCs.)

Accreditation Decision: Conditional Accreditation or Preliminary Denial of Accreditation

If an organization has RFIs and meets the decision rule for Conditional Accreditation or Preliminary Denial of Accreditation, then Joint Commission staff will review the findings from the survey to determine whether the RFIs were valid. The Joint Commission will post its accreditation decision on the organization's secure extranet site within 30 days of the last day of survey.

If the accreditation decision is Conditional Accreditation or Preliminary Denial of Accreditation, the organization

Sidebar 3. The Difference Between Providing Clarifications and Corrective Evidence of Standards Compliance

A Clarification

- Presurvey, factual evidence that clearly demonstrates that the organization was compliant at the time of survey
- ESC clarification is due within 10 business days if the organization met a decision rule for Conditional Accreditation or Preliminary Denial of Accreditation
- Clarification does *not* describe something that was corrected since the survey
- **Examples:** A description of the policy or procedure that was present prior to the survey, a description of how the process was designed well and implemented consistently, or an audit of records that proves the organization was more than 90% compliant at the time of survey

Corrective Evidence of Standards Compliance

- Postsurvey changes made (completed) to become compliant with standards found not compliant during survey
- Corrective Evidence of Standards Compliance (ESC) due within 45 and/or 60 days if the organization did *not* meet a decision rule for Preliminary Denial of Accreditation
- Corrective ESCs should be
  - Precise (focus on the failed element)
  - Concise
  - Affirmative in evidence
  - A story told in past tense to describe what has been done (not what will be done)
- When submitting corrective ESCs, organizations should include the following:
  - **Who:** The title of the person who approved the action, policy, or procedure and the title of the person who was trained
  - **What:** A description of the action taken and how the element of performance was addressed
  - **When:** The date each action, policy, procedure, and/or training was completed
  - **How:** A description of how employees were taught the changes
  - **Measure of Success,** if required

has 10 business days to submit a clarification through its secure extranet site. (The Joint Commission will call the organization before posting the report to the extranet site.) The organization's account representative will go over the 10-day clarification instructions with the organization to help it through the clarification process.

After an organization submits a clarification, The Joint Commission staff will review the evidence and recommend one of the following outcomes:

- If the organization's clarification is judged to have no residual areas of standards noncompliance, the organization may then experience an on-site validation survey. If the on-site validation survey validates the clarification submitted and determines that the information or data was available to the previous on-site survey team, the organization will be awarded Accreditation.
- The organization's clarification is judged to have fewer areas of standards noncompliance and it no longer meets a decision rule for Preliminary Denial of Accreditation or Conditional Accreditation (which is confirmed with an on-site validation survey), but still has RFIs that will necessitate an appropriate ESC submission. (The ESC report would be due 45 days from when the revised accreditation decision is posted on the extranet site, after the 10-day clarification window.) A surveyor will follow up with an on-site validation survey.
- The organization's clarification continues to be not compliant with the standards and it will be recommended to the Accreditation Committee that the organization remains in Conditional Accreditation. The organization must submit corrective ESCs for the remaining RFIs within 45 days from when the revised accreditation decision is posted on the organization's extranet site (after the 10-day clarification window) *and* undergo an on-site survey.
- The organization's clarification continues to be not compliant with the standards and it will be recom-

mended to the Accreditation Committee that the organization remains in Preliminary Denial of Accreditation. This decision is often subject to review and appeal prior to the determination of a final Denial of Accreditation.

See Figure 8, page 347, for a visual explanation of an organization's potential next steps after a survey.

Clarifying Different Categories of Elements of Performance

When an organization submits evidence, it will vary based on the category of EP that was found to be not compliant at the time of survey. The information following provides some guidance for submitting clarifying evidence for EPs in different categories, but an organization should also follow the guidance given in the 10-day clarification instructions, which are provided by its account representative.

Category A Elements of Performance

Category A EPs relate to the presence or absence of the requirement(s) and are scored either yes (2) or no (0).

If an organization believes it was compliant at the time of survey with a Category A EP that was scored not compliant, it should submit the following information in a 10-day clarification to The Joint Commission:

- **What:** A description of the policy or procedure that was present prior to survey or how the policy or procedure was implemented consistently throughout the organization
- **Who:** The title of the person who approved the policy or procedure
- **When:** The date of approval of the policy or procedure and the effective date
- **How:** The description of how the information was disseminated to staff members
- **Why:** An explanation as to why the surveyor(s) did not have access to the information or why it was not provided to the surveyor(s) at the time of survey.

Category C Elements of Performance

Category C EPs are scored 0, 1, or 2 based on the number of times the organization did not meet the EP. These EPs are frequency based and require totaling the number of occurrences (that is, results of performance or nonperformance) related to the particular EP. Each situation discovered by a surveyor(s) will be counted as a separate occurrence. (However, multiple events of the same type related to a single resident and single practitioner or staff member are counted as one occurrence only.)

If an organization believes it was compliant at the time of survey with a Category C EP that was scored not compliant, it should conduct an audit and submit its findings to The Joint Commission as a 10-day clarification. Organizations should adhere to the following guidelines for auditing:

- The audit should use records from no more than 30 days prior to survey.
- The sampling of the audit should be random (systematic random sampling involves selecting every second or third case for review; simple random sampling involves a series of random numbers generated by a computer to identify cases for review).
- The specific population directly related to the surveyor's findings should determine the sample size (*see* the box below for sampling criteria for auditing Category C EPs).

Sampling Criteria for Auditing Category C Elements of Performance

Population Size	Sample Size
Fewer than (<) 30 cases	100% of cases
30 to 100 cases	30 cases
101 to 500 cases	50 cases
Greater than (>) 500 cases	70 cases

After conducting an audit, if an organization finds that it was 90% to 100% compliant at the time of survey, it would submit that information as a clarification to The Joint Commission. (If the organization finds that it was 80% to 89% compliant, it is partially compliant with the requirement; if the organization is compliant 79% or less, it is insufficiently compliant with the requirement.) The percentage of compliance is determined by the ratio of the number of times the requirement was found to be compliant to the total number of times this requirement occurred.

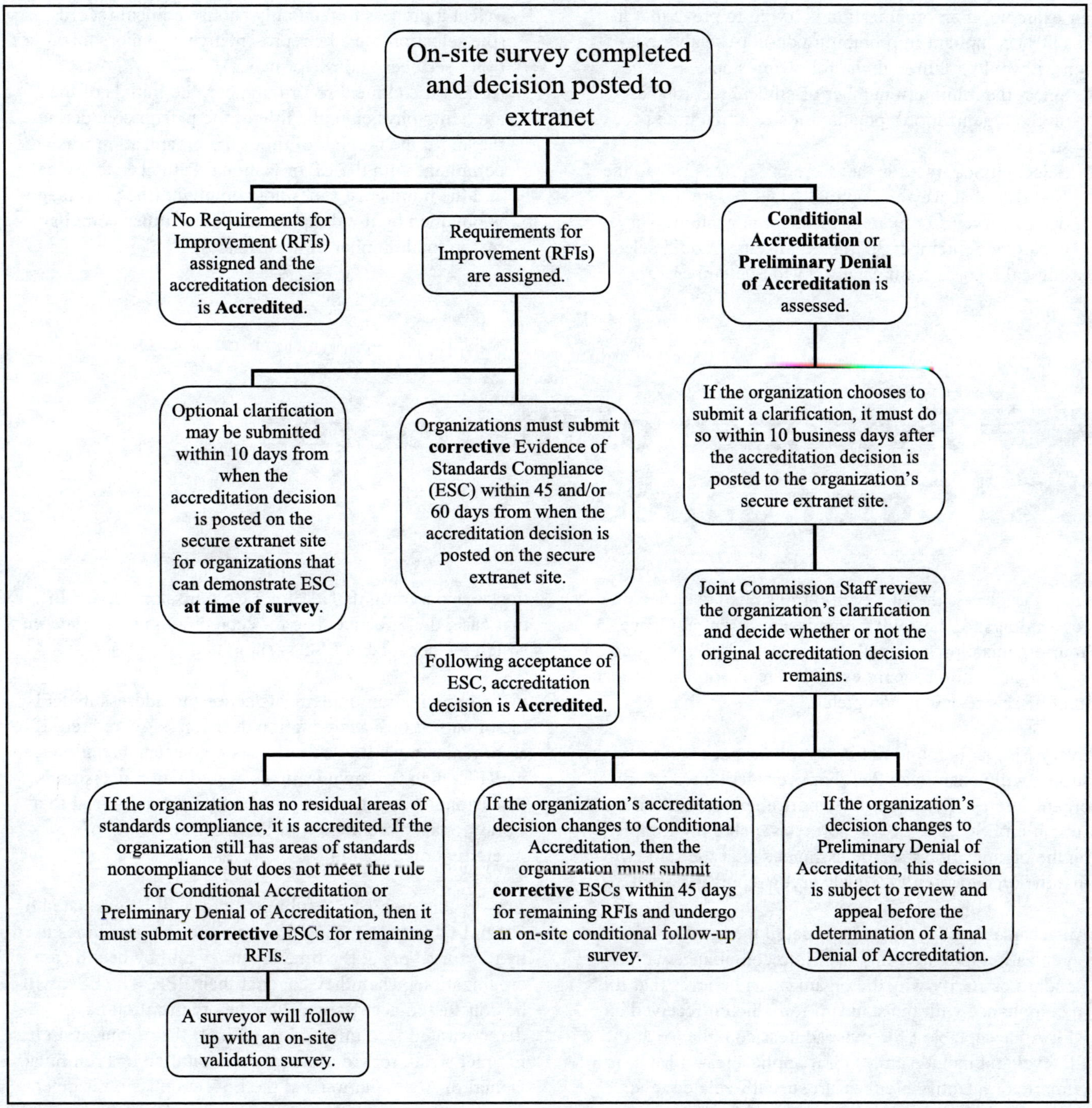

Figure 8. *Potential next steps after survey.*

For example, if an organization is trying to prove that it was 90% compliant in prohibiting do-not-use abbreviations, it would go through the following steps:

- Select the minimum number of clinical records based on the organization's population size at the time of survey.
- Select clinical records that were in service prior to the first day of survey and up to 30 days before the first day of survey (for example, if an organization's survey began on September 30, the organization could select clinical records from August 31 to September 29).
- Select a process to randomly choose clinical records (the selection must be representative of the organization's services and performance).
- Collect the clinical record number, the initials of the attending physician, the title of the person conducting the audit, the number of times the organization was compliant with the EP or National Patient Safety Goal and the number of times not compliant (the percentage is obtained by dividing the number of times compliant by the total number of occurrences).

Postsurvey Activities

Evidence of Standards Compliance

After the survey, the surveyor(s) transmits his or her survey findings to The Joint Commission's Central Office. Your organization's official survey report will be posted on your organization's secure extranet site as soon as the Central Office's review is completed.

Every EP that is found not in compliance at the time of the survey will generate an RFI. For every RFI cited in an organization's official survey report, the organization must submit an ESC. The ESC report is available for completion on the organization's secure extranet site at the same time that the organization's official survey report is posted.

An acceptable ESC report must detail the action(s) that the organization took to bring itself into compliance with a standard or clarify why the organization believes that it is in compliance with the standard for which it received an RFI. An acceptable ESC must address compliance at the EP level and include an MOS, if applicable. An MOS is a numeric or quantifiable measure, usually related to an audit, which determines whether an action is effective and sustained.

An acceptable ESC report is due within 45 days if the EP relates to a Direct Impact Requirement and 60 calendar days if the EP relates to an Indirect Impact Requirement following the posting of the official survey report. The required time frame will be specified in your report. Following a successful submission of the ESC report, the organization receives an accreditation decision. However, the organization's accreditation decision is retroactive to the day after the last day of the survey, unless the organization is undergoing its first Joint Commission survey. In that case, the effective date for accreditation is the date on which the acceptable ESC is submitted.

If the organization implements actions to address its RFIs, the organization's accreditation decision is Accredited. If an organization's ESC report does not acceptably address its RFIs, then the organization's accreditation decision is Provisional Accreditation, which can eventually lead to a Conditional Accreditation or Preliminary Denial of Accreditation decision.

The organization's ESC submission(s) will be evaluated by Central Office staff using the same scoring guidelines used by the surveyors at the time of survey and by health care organizations when they conduct their PPR. The ESC will be considered acceptable when the organization has demonstrated resolution of all RFIs. If the organization has not met a rule for Conditional Accreditation or Preliminary Denial of Accreditation and the ESC submission is determined to be acceptable, its decision will be Accredited, and it will be required to submit the data for applicable MOS, if required, for each EP four months later.

If the organization has not met a rule for Conditional Accreditation or Preliminary Denial of Accreditation and it is determined that an organization's ESC submission is unacceptable, its accreditation decision will be Provisional Accreditation, and it will be required to submit an acceptable ESC within 30 days. If the second ESC is determined to be acceptable, the organization's accreditation decision will remain Provisional Accreditation until it has submitted acceptable results of the corresponding MOS four months later. If the second ESC is determined to be unacceptable, a recommendation for Conditional Accreditation will be presented to the Accreditation Committee.

Central Office staff will evaluate the MOS results, when required. If it is determined that the MOS results are acceptable, no further action will be required of the organization. If the organization had a Provisional Accreditation decision, its accreditation decision will be changed to Accredited. If it is determined that an organization's MOS submission is unacceptable and its accreditation decision is not currently Provisional Accreditation, its accreditation decision will be changed to Provisional Accreditation; the organization will be required to submit a second set of MOS results in another four months. If an organization whose accreditation decision is Provisional Accreditation because of an unacceptable first ESC submission submits an unacceptable first MOS submission, a recommendation for Conditional Accreditation will be presented to the Accreditation Committee.

If the organization's first ESC submission is determined to be acceptable and the second MOS submission is determined to be acceptable, its accreditation decision will be changed to Accredited, and no further action will be required of the organization. If the second MOS submission is determined to be unacceptable, a recommendation for Conditional Accreditation will be presented to the Accreditation Committee.

The organization's ESC submission and sustained implementation of it, including the MOS, are subject to review in random unannounced surveys.

A final decision letter will be posted to the organization's secure, password-protected area of *The Joint Commission Connect* extranet Web site when its ESC has been reviewed and an accreditation decision has been rendered. A Quality Report will then be posted on Quality Check® on The Joint Commission's Web site.

Postsurvey Activities

Quality Report

Your Quality Report provides information about your performance on standards related to the safety and quality of care you provide. It gives accreditation information from your organization as well as comparative information gathered from organizations surveyed nationwide. The Joint Commission provides Quality Reports to your organization and to the public.

The Quality Report contains the following elements:

- The date of the most recent survey
- An organization's current accreditation decision
- A summary of quality distinctions, or "merit badges," that have been awarded to your organization, such as the following:
  - Ernest A. Codman Award, which recognizes achievement by health care organizations and individuals in the use of process and outcomes measures to improve organization performance
  - The John M. Eisenberg Patient Safety Award, which recognizes major achievement by individuals and health care organizations in improving resident safety
  - Malcolm Baldrige National Quality Award, which recognizes quality and business achievements in all types of U.S. organizations
  - Cheers Award, which recognizes individuals, organizations, regulatory agencies, professional organizations, researchers, pharmaceutical, and other health care–related businesses for setting standards of excellence in preventing medication errors
  - American Health Care Association (AHCA) Quality Award—This award recognizes AHCA member organizations that demonstrate their commitment to continuous quality improvement. Adapted for long term care organizations, organizational members of the AHCA apply for this award. This award is modeled after the Malcolm Baldrige National Quality Award.

  - Nursing Homes/Long Term Care Management OPTIMA Award—The OPTIMA award recognizes innovative and outcome-oriented team work that improves the care and quality of life of the residents in long term care facilities.
- A comparison of your organization's performance to that of other Joint Commission–accredited organizations related to quality indicators, such as National Patient Safety Goals, National Quality Improvement Goals, and the resident care experience
- A list of your organization's services and programs
- A description of accreditation and its importance, including background information on The Joint Commission, a description of the accreditation process, and care delivery issues addressed in the accreditation process

When you receive your Quality Report, you also receive a user's guide that explains accreditation and the various elements of the report, provides a glossary of the terms used, and describes the methodology that was used to determine the organization comparisons shown.

Quality Reports are available for organizations on Quality Check®. A complete directory of all Joint Commission–accredited organizations is available through Quality Check on The Joint Commission's Web site (http://www.qualitycheck.org). For reports prior to 1996, call The Joint Commission's Customer Service Department at 630/792-5800. Also call Customer Service with any queries regarding the availability of Quality Reports for organizations and lists of all available reports.

Guidelines for using your Quality Report in marketing and communication activities are provided in "The Joint Commission Quality Report" (QR) chapter of the *CAMLTC*.

Response to a Quality Report

The Joint Commission gives you an opportunity to respond to the information shown in your Quality Report by submitting a commentary of up to two pages. (This commentary is completely optional.) If you choose to submit a commentary, you may do so by completing an online form that is posted to your extranet site. The commentary cannot be longer than two pages and may not mention a surveyor(s) by name or use defamatory or libelous language. Only one commentary per organization is permitted, regardless of the number of services that were evaluated in the survey.

After your organization submits the form, The Joint Commission staff will review the commentary for appropriateness and then accept the document for posting with your organization's Quality Report on Quality Check®. If your commentary does not meet the required guidelines, The Joint Commission notifies you and allows you to submit a revised copy.

Sample Survey Agendas

- ☑ **Two-Day Long Term Care Survey Conducted by One Surveyor**
- ☑ **One-Day Medicare/ Medicaid Certification–Based Long Term Care Survey Conducted by One Surveyor**

The following sample agendas represent the possible scheduling of activities during the two most common types of long term care surveys: a two-day survey by one surveyor for Long Term Care and a one-day survey by one surveyor for Medicare/Medicaid Certification–Based Long Term Care. They are provided here to give you an idea of how the on-site survey is conducted relative to time distribution across departments and care areas. However, your organization-specific survey agenda will be based on the size of your organization; the resident population you serve; and the scope of care, treatment, and services you offer. Your agenda may have slight differences from this "template" agenda, even if the number of days and surveyors match those identified for your survey.

Sample Agenda: Two-Day Long Term Care Survey Conducted by One Surveyor

Information Needed for the Preliminary Planning Session and Survey Planning Meeting

- Performance Improvement data from the past 12 months
- Facility Quality Indicator Profile
- Infection Control surveillance data from the past 12 months
- Environment of Care data as follows:
  - Statement of Conditions (SOC) and Plans for Improvement, if applicable
  - Management plans and annual evaluations, if applicable
  - Environment of Care multidisciplinary team meeting minutes for the 12 months prior to survey, if applicable
- Organization chart
- Map of the organization, if available
- List of departments/units/areas/programs/services within the organization, if applicable
- Any reports or lists of residents (e.g., Resident Level Quality Indicator Summary or resident census) that will help in identifying individuals to trace
- Name of key contact person who can assist surveyors in planning tracer selection

DAY 1

Time	Surveyor
8:00–8:30 A.M.	Surveyor Arrival and Preliminary Planning Session
8:30–9:00 A.M.	
9:00–9:30 A.M.	Opening Conference and Orientation to Organization
9:30–10:00 A.M.	Continued Surveyor Planning Session
10:00–10:30 A.M.	*Life Safety Code*® Building Assessment
10:30–11:00 A.M.	
11:00–11:30 A.M.	Individual Tracer Activity
11:30–12:00 P.M.	
12:00–12:30 P.M.	
12:30–1:00 P.M.	Surveyor Lunch
1:00–1:30 P.M.	Individual Tracer Activity
1:30–2:00 P.M.	
2:00–2:30 P.M.	
2:30–3:00 P.M.	Individual Based System Tracer – Data Use
3:00–3:30 P.M.	
3:30–4:00 P.M.	Special Issue Resolution
4:00–4:30 P.M.	Surveyor Team Meeting / Planning Meeting

DAY 2	
Time	**Surveyor**
8:00–8:30 A.M.	Leadership Session
8:30–9:00 A.M.	
9:00–9:30 A.M.	Individual Tracer Activity
9:30–10:00 A.M.	
10:00–10:30 A.M.	
10:30–11:00 A.M.	
11:00–11:30 A.M.	
11:30–12:00 P.M.	Environment of Care Session
12:00–12:30 P.M.	
12:30–1:00 P.M.	Surveyor Lunch
1:00–1:30 P.M.	Competence Assessment Process
1:30–2:00 P.M.	Credentialing
2:00–2:30 P.M.	Surveyor Report Preparation
2:30–3:00 P.M.	
3:00–3:30 P.M.	
3:30–4:00 P.M.	CEO Exit Briefing and Organization Exit Conference
4:00–4:30 P.M.	

Sample Agenda: One-Day Medicare/Medicaid Certification–Based Long Term Care Survey Conducted by One Surveyor

Information Needed for the Preliminary Planning Session and Surveyor Planning Meeting

- Organization chart
- Name and phone number of contact person who will assist the surveyors during survey
- Map of your organization, if available
- List of all sites eligible for survey
- List of services provided at each site
- Performance Improvement data
- MDS report, if you are Medicare certified
- Infection-related data
- Environment of Care data
- Environment of Care meeting minutes
- Resident roster
- Measure of Success (MOS) data identified in the Plan of Action from your Periodic Performance Review

Time	Surveyor
8:00–8:30 A.M.	Surveyor Arrival and Preliminary Planning Session
8:30–9:00 A.M.	
9:00–9:30 A.M.	Opening Conference and Orientation to Organization
9:30–10:00 A.M.	
10:00–10:30 A.M.	Continued Surveyor Planning Session
10:30–11:00 A.M.	Individual Tracer Activity
11:00–11:30 A.M.	
11:30–11:45 P.M.	
11:45--12:00 P.M.	Environment of Care Session
12:00–12:30 P.M.	
12:30–1:00 P.M.	Surveyor Lunch
1:00–1:30 P.M.	Individual Based System Tracer—Data Use
1:30–1:45 P.M.	
1:45–2:00 P.M.	Competence Assessment Process/Credentialing
2:00–2:30 P.M.	
2:30–3:00 P.M.	Surveyor Report Preparation
3:00–3:30 P.M.	
3:30–4:00 P.M.	
4:00–4:30 P.M.	CEO Exit Briefing and Organization Exit Conference

Appendix 1
Elements of Performance That Are Attached to Measures of Success

In an effort to help health care organizations organize their resources when conducting the Periodic Performance Review (PPR), this appendix lists all the elements of performance that require submission of a Measure of Success when found not compliant.

	National Patient Safety Goals (NPSG)
NPSG.01.01.01	EP 1–EP 4, EP 6
NPSG.01.02.01	EP 2
NPSG.02.01.01	EP 1–EP 3
NPSG.02.02.01	EP 3
NPSG.02.05.01	EP 1–EP 3, EP 5
NPSG.03.05.01	EP 3, EP 5, EP 8
NPSG.07.01.01	EP 1
NPSG.07.02.01	EP 1
NPSG.07.04.01	EP 5–EP 7
NPSG.08.01.01	EP 1–EP 4
NPSG.08.02.01	EP 1–EP 2
NPSG.08.03.01	EP 1
NPSG.08.04.01	EP 1–EP 6
NPSG.09.02.01	EP 2, EP 4–EP 5
NPSG.10.01.01	EP 2
NPSG.10.02.01	EP 2
NPSG.10.03.01	EP 2
NPSG.13.01.01	EP 1–EP 2, EP 4
	Ethics, Rights, and Responsibilities (RI)
RI.2.10	EP 2–EP 4
RI.2.20	EP 3–EP 6, EP 9
RI.2.30	EP 1–EP 5, EP 11–EP 13
RI.2.40	EP 2
RI.2.50	EP 1–EP 4, EP 7
RI.2.70	EP 4
RI.2.80	EP 2, EP 4, EP 6–EP 7, EP 9, EP 20–EP 21
RI.2.90	EP 1–EP 3
RI.2.100	EP 3–EP 4
RI.2.110	EP 2, EP 4–EP 7
RI.2.120	EP 1–EP 5, EP 7, EP 9
RI.2.130	EP 1–EP 6
RI.2.150	EP 2

RI.2.170	EP 1, EP 3
RI.2.180	EP 1–EP 8
RI.2.190	EP 2–EP 5
RI.2.200	EP 1
RI.2.210	EP 2–EP 3
RI.2.220	EP 1–EP 2
RI.2.240	EP 1
RI.2.250	EP 1–EP 2
RI.2.260	EP 3–EP 5
RI.2.270	EP 1–EP 3
RI.2.280	EP 1–EP 5
RI.2.290	EP 1–EP 5
RI.3.10	EP 3–EP 4
	Provision of Care, Treatment, and Services (PC)
PC.1.10	EP 2, EP 4, EP 9
PC.2.120	EP 8, EP 17
PC.2.130	EP 1–EP 2, EP 4–EP 5
PC.2.150	EP 1–EP 2
PC.3.230	EP 1–EP 3
PC.4.10	EP 4, EP 8, EP 12–EP 13, EP 16
PC.5.10	EP 1
PC.5.30	EP 1–EP 5
PC.5.40	EP 2–EP 4
PC.5.50	EP 4–EP 5
PC.6.10	EP 2
PC.6.30	EP 5
PC.7.10	EP 2–EP 5, EP 11, EP 17
PC.8.10	EP 1, EP 3, EP 6–EP 7
PC.8.20	EP 1–EP 9
PC.8.30	EP 1
PC.8.40	EP 1, EP 3
PC.8.70	EP 2
PC.9.10	EP 10

(continued)

PC.11.90	EP 1–EP 2, EP 14, EP 17
PC.13.20	EP 7–EP 8
PC.13.30	EP 2
PC.13.40	EP 2, EP 5
PC.15.10	EP 4
PC.15.20	EP 1–4, EP 6–EP 10
PC.15.30	EP 1–EP 2
PC.16.10	EP 2, EP 6
PC.16.50	EP 4–EP 5
PC.16.60	EP 1–EP 2
	Medication Management (MM)
MM.1.10	EP 3
MM.2.20	EP 1–EP 2, EP 4, EP 11, EP 15
MM.2.30	EP 4, EP 6
MM.3.10	EP 1
MM.3.20	EP 13
MM.4.10	EP 1
MM.4.20	EP 4–EP 6
MM.4.40	EP 3–EP 4
MM.4.80	EP 4
MM.5.10	EP 2–EP 7
MM.5.20	EP 2–EP 3
MM.6.10	EP 1–EP 2, EP 5–EP 6
MM.6.20	EP 2–EP 3
MM.7.10	EP 3
	Surveillance, Prevention, and Control of Infection (IC)
IC.4.10	EP 5–EP 7
	Leadership (LD)
LD.01.07.01	EP 2
LD.04.02.03	EP 15
	Management of the Environment of Care (EC)
EC.1.10	EP 5–EP 6
EC.1.20	EP 2–EP 3

EC.1.30	EP 4–EP 5
EC.2.10	EP 4, EP 6
EC.3.10	EP 3, EP 6, EP 11–EP 12
EC.5.30	EP 1, EP 4
EC.5.40	EP 1–EP 2, EP 4–EP 8, EP 11–EP 14, EP 16
EC.6.20	EP 1, EP 4, EP 6
EC.7.10	EP 14
EC.7.20	EP 2, EP 4
EC.7.30	EP 1, EP 5
EC.7.40	EP 1–EP 4
EC.8.10	EP 4
EC.8.20	EP 1–EP 2, EP 6–EP 7
EC.9.20	EP 2
	Life Safety (LS)
LS.01.02.01	EP 4, EP 8–EP 9, EP 12, EP 14
	Management of Human Resources (HR)
HR.1.20	EP 2, EP 4–EP 7, EP 11–EP 12
HR.2.10	EP 2–EP 5, EP 7–EP 9
HR.2.20	EP 1–EP 4
HR.2.30	EP 2–EP 8
HR.3.10	EP 8–EP 9
HR.3.20	EP 1–EP 2, EP 4
HR.4.10	EP 24
HR.4.20	EP 4, EP 6
HR.4.50	EP 2
	Management of Information (IM)
IM.2.10	EP 6, EP 8
IM.6.10	EP 4–EP 6
IM.6.20	EP 1–EP 3
IM.6.50	EP 2
IM.6.70	EP 1–EP 2
IM.6.80	EP 1–EP 2
IM.6.90	EP 1–EP 2

(continued)

IM.6.100	EP 1–EP 7
IM.6.110	EP 1–EP 4
IM.6.120	EP 1–EP 2
IM.6.130	EP 1
IM.6.140	EP 1
IM.6.150	EP 1
IM.6.160	EP 1
IM.6.170	EP 1–EP 2

Appendix 2
Worksheets to Facilitate Survey Logistics Planning

- ☑ **Worksheet 1. Joint Commission Survey Planning Master List**
- ☑ **Worksheet 2. Documents for Preliminary Planning Session**
- ☑ **Worksheet 3. Opening Conference and Orientation to the Organization**
- ☑ **Worksheet 4. Environment of Care**
- ☑ **Worksheet 5. Individual-Based System Tracer: Medication Management**
- ☑ **Worksheet 6. Individual-Based System Tracer: Infection Control**
- ☑ **Worksheet 7. Individual-Based System Tracer: Data Use**
- ☑ **Worksheet 8. Leadership**

To help organizations logistically prepare for the unannounced survey, worksheets pertaining to several different survey activities (such as the Opening Conference and Orientation to the Organization, the competency assessment process, and the individual-based system tracers) have been included. These worksheets should be filled out prior to the unannounced survey and should help keep important information at the forefront of staff members' minds during each survey activity.

☑ Worksheet 1. Joint Commission Survey Planning Master List

Key Contact Staff for Surveyors:

1.______________________________ Dept:__________ Phone:__________

2.______________________________ Dept:__________ Phone:__________

3.______________________________ Dept:__________ Phone:__________

Survey Activity	Primary Lead (phone #)	Secondary Lead (phone #)	Survey Day & Time	Meeting Room	Approx. # Participants
Surveyor Arrival ■ Information or Security Desk ■ Internal calling tree, e-mails ❑ 10 minutes to bring key documents to surveyor meeting room for review or surveyors begin tracers ■ Waiting location for surveyor(s) ■ Check *The Joint Commission Connect*™ for letter, surveyor bios, PFP & ORYX® Reports Login ID: ________ Password: ________			Day 1 7:00 A.M. eastern time		Number of Surveyor(s)
1st Hour Surveyor Planning Session			Day 1 7:00–8:00 A.M.		Number of Surveyor(s)
Opening Conference and Orientation to the Organization			Day 1 8:00–9:00 A.M.		
2nd Hour Surveyor Planning Session			Day 1 9:00–10:00 A.M.		Number of Surveyor(s)
Individual Tracers					
Life Safety Code®* Building Assessment†					

* *Life Safety Code*® is a registered trademark of the National Fire Protection Association, Quincy, MA.

† Not applicable to Medicare/Medicaid certification–based accreditation.

Survey Activity	Primary Lead (phone #)	Secondary Lead (phone #)	Survey Day & Time	Meeting Room	Approx. # Participants
Environment of Care Session					
Daily Briefing			Beginning of most days		
Special Issue Resolution			End of each day		Number of Surveyor(s)
Surveyor Team Meeting, if applicable			End of each day		Number of Surveyor(s)
Competence Assessment Process					
Individual-Based System Tracer: Data Use					
Individual-Based System Tracer: Medication Management					
Individual-Based System Tracer: Infection Control					
Leadership Session			Morning last day		
Surveyor Report Preparation			Afternoon last day		Number of Surveyor(s)
Exit Briefing & Exit Conference			Afternoon last day		Number of Surveyor(s)

Note: *Please refer to your survey agenda on* The Joint Commission Connect *extranet site.*

☑ Worksheet 2. Documents for Preliminary Planning Session

This time is set aside for the surveyor(s) to review and discuss pertinent data and plan the survey agenda. The surveyor(s) reviews the following:

✓	Document	Location	Staff Assignment - Bring to Surveyor Meeting Room
	Performance improvement data from the last 12 months		1. 2.
	Infection control surveillance data from last 12 months		1. 2.
	Environment of Care management plans and annual reviews		1. 2.
	Environment of Care multidisciplinary team meeting minutes for the 12 months prior to survey if available		1. 2.
	Electronic Statement of Conditions (e-SOC) and Plans For Improvement (PFIs)		1. 2.
	Organizational chart		1. 2.
	Map of the organization, if available		1. 2.
	List of departments/units/areas/programs within the organization		1. 2.
	Staffing effectiveness data (last 12 months) including annual report to the board		1. 2.
	Any reports or lists of residents (resident census roster including room numbers and quality indicators) that help identify residents to trace		1. 2.
	Name of key contact person who can assist surveyors in planning tracer selection		1. 2.
	Priority Focus Process (PFP) data	*The Joint Commission Connect* extranet site (morning of the survey)	1. 2.
	Measures of Success (MOS) data for any standard or element of performance that required a Plan of Action and MOS during completion of the Periodic Performance Review (PPR)		

✓	Document	Location	Staff Assignment - Bring to Surveyor Meeting Room
	ORYX data (last 12 months) ❑ Core Measure data ❑ MDS data ❑ ORYX/QI/QM data		1. 2.
	Organization's MDS Quality Measure Reports*		1. 2.
	Most recent CMS state certification report (that is, CMS form 2567)*		1. 2.

Notes:

1. If staff members are not able to bring documents within 10 minutes to the surveyor meeting room you have assigned, the surveyor(s) will begin individual tracers, giving your staff some additional time to obtain the needed documents.
2. Assign a backup person to bring the documents in case the first person is absent that day.

* These documents are required only for organizations accredited by the Medicare/Medicaid certification–based option.

☑ Worksheet 3. Opening Conference and Orientation to the Organization

- First 15 minutes – Introductions, surveyor describes on-site survey process
- Next 45 minutes –Interactive discussion session on the topics below. Consider assigning two people to each discussion point to get each conversation topic started. Others should join into the discussion as appropriate.

Topics	Discussion Points	
Include *all* accreditation programs (if applicable)	❑ Hospital ❑ Home Care ❑ Behavioral Health ❑ Long Term Care ❑ ______________	
Mission, vision, goals, and strategic directions		
Organization structure		
Oversight and responsibilities: ❑ Governance ❑ Senior leadership		
Planning, allocating resources, and decision making (including oversight by Board or Trustees), and staffing effectiveness		
Operational management		
Contract management		
Health care errors reduction and resident safety (including root cause analysis)		
National Patient Safety Goals		
Community involvement		
Leaders role in emergency management planning		
Other:		
Identify "your" priority focus areas (PFAs)	Strengths:	Weaknesses:
Identify "your" baseline assessment of systems/processes from a leadership/ management perspective with other leadership responsibilities		
Leaders' approach to Periodic Performance Review (PPR) and methods used to address improvements needed		

Topics	Discussion Points	
Leaders' role in performance improvement (PI)	**Specific Examples:**	**Achieved & Sustained?**
	1. ______	❑ Yes ❑ No
Ongoing initiatives to improve health care and resident safety and future project prioritization	2. ______	❑ Yes ❑ No
❑ PPR review methods in context of PI	3. ______	❑ Yes ❑ No
❑ Prioritization of future projects	4. ______	❑ Yes ❑ No
❑ How do you set expectations, plan, assess, and measure for PI?	5. ______	❑ Yes ❑ No
❑ What are your proactive risk assessment topic areas and resulting improvements?	6. ______	❑ Yes ❑ No
❑ Is the board involved in safety issues?	7. ______	❑ Yes ❑ No
❑ Is there provision of staff time, training, information technology (IT), and data management/analysis?	8. ______	❑ Yes ❑ No
❑ What are the residents' perceptions of care?	9. ______	❑ Yes ❑ No
Are there any potential issues for system or individual tracers?		

Participants: At least one member of the governing body or organization trustee (can be available by conference call) should attend if at all possible; senior organization leaders from all accreditation programs should attend; participation of department directors is not required.

☑ Worksheet 4. Environment of Care

Discuss the organization's approach to managing risks in the environment of care.

Participants: Individuals responsible for issues related to the management of the environment of care in all major areas (including safety management coordinator, security management, facility management, building utilities management, medical/laboratory equipment management, leader of the environment of care team or safety committee, and organizational leaders)

SAFETY

Topics	Discussion Points
❑ Plan - What specific risks have been identified?	
❑ Teach - How have roles/responsibilities for staff and volunteers been communicated? (The human resources department may be involved in this step.)	
❑ Implement - What procedures and controls (human and physical components) have been implemented to minimize risk to residents, visitors, and staff?	
❑ Respond - What procedures have been implemented to respond to an EC incident/failure? - How, when, and to whom are EC problems, incidents, or failures reported within the organization?	
❑ Monitor - How is EC performance (both human activities and physical components) monitored by the organization? - What monitoring activities have taken place within the last 12 months?	
❑ Improve - What EC issues are currently being analyzed? - What actions have been taken as a result of EC monitoring activities?	

SECURITY*

Topics	Discussion Points
❑ Plan - What specific risks have been identified?	
❑ Teach - How have roles/responsibilities for staff and volunteers been communicated? (The human resources department may be involved in this step.)	
❑ Implement - What procedures and controls (human and physical components) have been implemented to minimize risk to residents, visitors, and staff?	
❑ Respond - What procedures have been implemented to respond to an EC incident/failure? - How, when, and to whom are EC problems, incidents, or failures reported within the organization?	
❑ Monitor - How is EC performance (both human activities and physical components) monitored by the organization? - What monitoring activities have taken place within the last 12 months?	
❑ Improve - What EC issues are currently being analyzed? - What actions have been taken as a result of EC monitoring activities?	

HAZARDOUS MATERIAL

Topics	Discussion Points
❑ Plan - What specific risks have been identified?	
❑ Teach - How have roles/responsibilities for staff and volunteers been communicated? (The human resources department may be involved in this step.)	
❑ Implement - What procedures and controls (human and physical components) have been implemented to minimize risk to residents, visitors, and staff?	

(continued)

* Not applicable to organizations seeking accreditation under the Medicare/Medicaid certification–based long term care option.

HAZARDOUS MATERIAL *(continued)*

Topics	Discussion Points
❑ Respond - What procedures have been implemented to respond to an EC incident/failure?	
- How, when, and to whom are EC problems, incidents, or failures reported within the organization?	
❑ Monitor - How is EC performance (both human activities and physical components) monitored by the organization? - What monitoring activities have taken place within the last 12 months?	
❑ Improve - What EC issues are currently being analyzed? - What actions have been taken as a result of EC monitoring activities?	

FIRE*

Topics	Discussion Points
❑ Plan - What specific risks have been identified?	
❑ Teach - How have roles/responsibilities for staff and volunteers been communicated? (The human resources department may be involved in this step.)	
❑ Implement - What procedures and controls (human and physical components) have been implemented to minimize risk to residents, visitors, and staff?	
❑ Respond - What procedures have been implemented to respond to an EC incident/failure? - How, when, and to whom are EC problems, incidents, or failures reported within the organization?	
❑ Monitor - How is EC performance (both human activities and physical components) monitored by the organization? - What monitoring activities have taken place within the last 12 months?	
❑ Improve - What EC issues are currently being analyzed? - What actions have been taken as a result of EC monitoring activities?	

* Not applicable to organizations seeking accreditation under the Medicare/Medicaid certification–based long term care option.

MEDICAL/LABORATORY EQUIPMENT

Topics	Discussion Points
❑ Plan - What specific risks have been identified?	
❑ Teach - How have roles/responsibilities for staff and volunteers been communicated? (The human resources department may be involved in this step.)	
❑ Implement - What procedures and controls (human and physical components) have been implemented to minimize risk to residents, visitors, and staff?	
❑ Respond - What procedures have been implemented to respond to an EC incident/failure? - How, when, and to whom are EC problems, incidents, or failures reported within the organization?	
❑ Monitor - How is EC performance (both human activities and physical components) monitored by the organization? - What monitoring activities have taken place within the last 12 months?	
❑ Improve - What EC issues are currently being analyzed? - What actions have been taken as a result of EC monitoring activities?	

UTILITIES

Topics	Discussion Points
❑ Plan - What specific risks have been identified?	
❑ Teach - How have roles/responsibilities for staff and volunteers been communicated? (The human resources department may be involved in this step.)	
❑ Implement - What procedures and controls (human and physical components) have been implemented to minimize risk to residents, visitors, and staff?	
❑ Respond - What procedures have been implemented to respond to an EC incident/failure?	

(continued)

UTILITIES *(continued)*

Topics	Discussion Points
- How, when, and to whom are EC problems, incidents, or failures reported within the organization?	
❑ Monitor - How is EC performance (both human activities and physical components) monitored by the organization? - What monitoring activities have taken place within the last 12 months?	
❑ Improve - What EC issues are currently being analyzed? - What actions have been taken as a result of EC monitoring activities?	

CONSTRUCTION

Topics	Discussion Points
❑ Plan - What specific risks have been identified?	
❑ Teach - How have roles/responsibilities for staff and volunteers been communicated? (The human resources department may be involved in this step.)	
❑ Implement - What procedures and controls (human and physical components) have been implemented to minimize risk to residents, visitors, and staff?	
❑ Respond - What procedures have been implemented to respond to an EC incident/failure? - How, when, and to whom are EC problems, incidents, or failures reported within the organization?	
❑ Monitor - How is EC performance (both human activities and physical components) monitored by the organization? - What monitoring activities have taken place within the last 12 months?	
❑ Improve - What EC issues are currently being analyzed? - What actions have been taken as a result of EC monitoring activities?	

☑ Worksheet 5. Individual-Based System Tracer: Medication Management

➤ **Select a high-risk medication a resident is receiving such as:**
❑ Antibiotic ❑ Anticoagulant ❑ Insulin
❑ Pain Medication ❑ ______________

➤ **Trace the medication:**
- ❑ Nursing unit or department
- ❑ Pharmacy
- ❑ Lab
- ❑ Dietary
- ❑ Warehouse/Materials Management

❑ Conference Room (10 minutes) to summarize, clarify, and share insights

❑ Other issues:
- Implementation of USP-797 standard
- Error reporting process
- Data collection, analysis, use
- Meds brought in to the facility by physicians, family members or residents
- Education (staff and resident)
- Information management systems
- Resident involvement in safe medication management

Processes	Discussion Points
Selection and procurement	
Storage	
Prescribing, ordering, transcribing	
Preparation and dispensing	
Administration	
Monitoring effects on residents	

Participants: Pharmacist (if nursing home operates a pharmacy; also consider pharmacy staff members involved in delivery of medications to units and a clinical educator). Focus will be on staff involved in the medication processes and any physicians encountered while tracing the selected high-risk medication.

☑ Worksheet 6. Individual-Based System Tracer: Infection Control

Part 1 – (20 minutes) Discussion of the infection control processes

Processes	Discussion Points
Infection Control Program ❑ Planning ❑ Implementation ❑ Evaluation	
Processes to reduce infection (will also be observed during tracer)	
Infection Control Plan ❑ Plan development: 1. Risk prioritization 2. Goal setting 3. Strategies to meet goals 4. Measurement and evaluation ❑ Outcome of annual evaluation process ❑ Oversight of opportunities for improvement	

Part 2 – (40 minutes) Tracing the IC processes for a selected resident

- ❑ Individuals seen with fever of unknown origin
- ❑ Postoperative infection, if applicable
- ❑ Readmitted surgical resident
- ❑ Resident on new (formulary) antibiotic
- ❑ Isolation
- ❑ Emergency management and infection control
- ❑ Immunocompromised resident
- ❑ Construction effect on infection control

Topics of Discussion

- ❑ How individuals with infections are identified by the organization
- ❑ What process exists for laboratory confirmation (for example, physician's request for testing, physician order, communication to the lab, collection of specimen, transportation to the lab, turn-around time of results, communication of results from lab to physician)
- ❑ How individuals with infections are considered within the context of the infection control program
- ❑ Current and past surveillance activity—taking place in the last 24 months
- ❑ Type of analysis conducted on infection control data, including comparisons
- ❑ Reporting of infection control data—frequency and audience

- ❑ Prevention and control activities (for example, staff training, housekeeping procedures, organizationwide hand hygiene, food sanitation, the appropriate storage, cleaning, disinfection, sterilization and/or other disposal of supplies and equipment)
- ❑ Interventions for licensed independent practitioners, staff, students/trainees, independent practitioners, and volunteers that include screening for exposure and/or immunity to infectious diseases they come in contact with, and the referral for assessment, potential testing, immunization and/or prophylaxis treatment and counseling of those who have potentially been identified with an infectious disease
- ❑ Physical facility changes, either completed or in progress, that have an impact on infection control
- ❑ Actions taken as a result of surveillance and the outcomes of those actions

Participants: Clinical staff (physicians, nurses, pharmacists, laboratorians) as applicable, infection control staff, facility manager, and leaders.

☑ Worksheet 7. Individual-Based System Tracer: Data Use

Surveyor will select one subprocess based on prior review of data:

Processes	Strengths	Weaknesses
Planning - Selection of Measures: Understand your organization's planning process for data use including how your organization identifies and prioritizes measures.		
Data Collection: Understand your organization's methodology for ensuring that all data are collected as planned.		
Data Aggregation and Analysis: Understand your organization's processes for turning data into useful information.		
Data Use: Understand how your organization uses the information obtained from data analysis.		

Additional data-related topics may be discussed:

ORYX	❑ MDS data ❑ ORYX/QI/QM data
Infection Control Data Use Issues	❑ Types of data collected - Whether infection-related data are collected per the Centers for Disease Control's (CDC) National Nosocomial Infection Surveillance (NNIS) system guidelines - Whether the organization has developed and implemented a system for measuring improvements in adherence to the CDC's Hand Hygiene and World Health Organization's (WHO) Hand Hygiene Guidelines ❑ Use of standardized definitions ❑ Control methods (includes data dissemination to physicians, staff, leaders, external entities) ❑ The organization's plans to collect data are relevant to the infection control plan

Staffing Effectiveness (HR.1.30)	Which inpatient nursing units were selected and why? (minimum of 2) What indicators were selected? 1. HR:______________ 2. HR:______________ 3. C/S:______________ 4. C/S:______________ ❑ What were the findings? ❑ Improvements? ❑ Annual report to leaders? **Revisions to Staffing Effectiveness Standard** (HR.1.30 for Long Term Care) ❑ Detailed introduction to standard added to clarify intent and provide guidance ❑ Focus narrowed to a minimum of two units/divisions in long term care organizations ❑ Input from clinical staff required in selection of areas of focus and indicators ❑ Focus on nurse staffing, with option to include other care providers - Effective as soon as published in *The Joint Commission Perspectives®* ❑ Revised list of indicators to include National Quality Forum staffing measures at http://www.qualityforum.org/
Performance Improvement (PI.1.10, PI.2.10, PI.3.20)	❑ Staff opinions and needs ❑ Staff perceptions of risks to individuals and suggestions for improving resident safety ❑ Staff willingness to report unanticipated adverse events ❑ Resident-specific needs and expectations ❑ How well the organization meets these needs and expectations ❑ How the organization can improve resident safety ❑ The effectiveness of pain management ❑ High-risk process: medication management - All serious adverse drug events (ADEs), if applicable and as defined by the organization - All significant medication errors, if applicable and as defined by the organization ❑ High-risk process: blood and blood product use - All confirmed transfusion reactions, if applicable to the organization ❑ High-risk process: restraint use; seclusion use; behavior management and treatment ❑ High-risk process: resuscitation and its outcomes ❑ Incorporate risk management ❑ Utilization management ❑ Infection control surveillance and reporting ❑ Quality control ❑ Research, when applicable ❑ Autopsy findings, when applicable ❑ Annual proactive risk assessment prevention activity:____________

(continued)

Medication Management Data Use Issues	Medication management data collection issues are addressed here in shorter surveys where only one system tracer (data use) is scheduled. Discussion explores the following:
	❑ Data collected on the performance of the organization's medication management system and processes, including trends or issues that have been identified, and changes made as a result of that review
	❑ Medication data the organization is collecting. Medication management data collection should be relevant to the services provided by the organization and residents served. The organization should be collecting data related to the "risk points" it has identified in its medication management system. Examples of such data based on an assessed risk point might include but are not limited to:
	  ❑ Turn-around times from order to administration
	  ❑ ADEs
	  ❑ Use of high-risk medications

National Patient Safety Goal Monitoring	
Data Related to Timeliness of Critical Values	❑ Critical tests (time from order to result known) ❑ Critical values (time from value available to physician notification)
Enhancing Hand Hygiene	❑ How are you measuring? ❑ What improvements have you seen?
Fall Reduction Program	❑ How are you measuring? ❑ What improvements have you seen?
New Goals for 2009	❑ How are you monitoring implementation successes and weaknesses for improvements?

Participants: The surveyor will inform the organization about who should attend as active participants. (Whenever possible and based on the focus, physician involvement is desired.)

☑ Worksheet 8. Leadership

Discussion will be guided by observations made throughout the survey within the context of Priority Focus Areas (PFAs) and organizationwide processes and functions. Organization leaders should provide the surveyor(s) with their views and perspectives about an area or topic being discussed.

The following may be relevant to the discussion points:

- Planning (Leadership Structure)
- Communication (Leadership Relationships)
- People (Leadership Relationships)
- Changing Performance (Organization Culture and System Performance)
- Data Use (Organization Culture and System Performance)

Topics	**Discussion Points**
Discuss leaders' role related to PFA: ________________ Safety and quality? Performance evaluated?	
Discuss leaders' role related to PFA: ________________ Safety and quality? Performance evaluated?	
Discuss leaders' role related to PFA: ________________ Safety and quality? Performance evaluated?	
Discuss leaders' role related to PFA: ________________ Safety and quality? Performance evaluated?	
Performance improvement in organizationwide functions	
Support and direction, including planning and resource allocation	
Design and implementation of supporting processes and structures?	
Comprehensive implementation throughout the organization	

Participants: At least one member from governing body, senior organization leaders (CEO, COO, CNO, CFO, CIO), elected and appointed leaders of the medical staff (if applicable).